Case Files™: Psychiatry

NOTICE

Medicine is an ever-changing science. As new research and clinical experience broaden our knowledge, changes in treatment and drug therapy are required. The authors and the publisher of this work have checked with sources believed to be reliable in their efforts to provide information that is complete and generally in accord with the standard accepted at the time of publication. However, in view of the possibility of human error or changes in medical sciences, neither the editors nor the publisher nor any other party who has been involved in the preparation or publication of this work warrants that the information contained herein is in every respect accurate or complete, and they disclaim all responsibility for any errors or omissions or for the results obtained from use of the information contained in this work. Readers are encouraged to confirm the information contained herein with other sources. For example and in particular, readers are advised to check the product information sheet included in the package of each drug they plan to administer to be certain that the information contained in this work is accurate and that changes have not been made in the recommended dose or in the contraindications for administration. This recommendation is of particular importance in connection with new or infrequently used drugs.

Case Files™: Psychiatry

Second Edition

EUGENE C. TOY, MD
THE JOHN S. DUNN SENIOR ACADEMIC CHAIR AND PROGRAM DIRECTOR
THE METHODIST HOSPITAL, OBSTETRICS AND GYNECOLOGY RESIDENCY PROGRAM
HOUSTON, TEXAS
CLERKSHIP DIRECTOR, ASSISTANT CLINICAL PROFESSOR
DEPARTMENT OF OBSTETRICS AND GYNECOLOGY
UNIVERSITY OF TEXAS—HOUSTON MEDICAL SCHOOL
HOUSTON, TEXAS

DEBRA KLAMEN, MD, MPHE
ASSOCIATE DEAN OF EDUCATION AND CURRICULUM
CHAIR, DEPARTMENT OF MEDICAL EDUCATION
PROFESSOR, DEPARTMENT OF PSYCHIATRY
SOUTHERN ILLINOIS UNIVERSITY SCHOOL OF MEDICINE
SPRINGFIELD, ILLINOIS

Lange Medical Books/McGraw-Hill

MEDICAL PUBLISHING DIVISION

New York Chicago San Francisco
Lisbon London Madrid Mexico City
Milan New Delhi San Juan Seoul
Singapore Sydney Toronto

The McGraw-Hill Companies

Case Files™: Psychiatry, Second Edition

1 2 3 4 5 6 7 8 9 0 DOC/DOC 0 9 8 7 6

ISBN 13: 978-0-07-146282-2
ISBN 10: 0-07-146282-1

This book was set in Times Roman by International Typesetting and Composition.
The editors were Catherine A. Johnson and Penny Linskey.
The production supervisor was Catherine Saggese.
The cover designer was Aimee Nordin.
The index was prepared by Susan Hunter.
RR Donnelley was printer and binder.

This book is printed on acid-free paper.

Library of Congress Cataloging-in-Publication Data

Case files™: Psychiatry / [edited by] Eugene C. Toy, Debra Klamen. —2nd ed.
p. ; cm.
Includes index.
ISBN 0-07-146282-1
1. Psychiatry—Case studies. I. Toy, Eugene C. II. Klamen, Debra L. III. Title: Phychiatry
[DNLM: 1. Mental Disorders—therapy—Case Report. 2. Phychology, Clinical—Case Report. WM 40 C3364 2006]
RC465.C285 2006
616.89'09—dc22

2006042047

International Edition ISBN 13: 978-0-07-110465-4; ISBN 10: 0-07-110465-8

DEDICATION

To my grandmother, Lew Yook Toy, who at the age of 96 is still vibrant and active, and in loving memory of my grandfather, Manway Toy, who courageously pioneered our family's legacy in this great country.

—ECT

To my wonderful husband, Phil,
who loves me and supports me in all things.
To my mother, Bonnie Klamen, and to my late father,
Sam Klamen, who were and are, always there.

—DLK

CONTENTS

❖ CONTRIBUTORS

Joan Anzia, MD
Associate Professor and
Medical Director of Outpatient Services
Department of Psychiatry
Northwestern University
Chicago, Illinois
Acute Stress Disorder
Bipolar Disorder (Manic)
Conversion Disorder
Dissociative Fugue
Factitious Disorder
Histrionic Personality Disorder
Neurosis
Panic Disorder
Posttraumatic Stress Disorder
Psychosis Secondary to a General Medical Condition
Schizoid Personality Disorder
Social Phobia

Sean Blitzstein, MD
Director, Third Year Clerkship
University of Illinois at Chicago
Clinical Assistant Professor of Psychiatry
University of Illinois at Chicago
Staff Psychiatrist, Veterans Administration
Chicago Healthcare System
Chicago Illinois
Alcohol Dependence
Cocaine Intoxication
Dependent Personality Disorder
Dysthymic Disorder
Generalized Anxiety Disorder
Hypochondriasis
Major Depression in the Elderly
Major Depression, Recurrent
Mood Disorder Secondary to a General Medical Condition
Narcissistic Personality Disorder
Obsessive-Compulsive Disorder (Child)
Obsessive-Compulsive Personality Disorder
Pain Disorder
Primary Insomnia

Neeta V. Gautam, MD
Faculty, The Methodist Hospital Family Medicine Residency
Houston, Texas
Attention-Deficit/Hyperactivity Disorder
Psychosis Secondary to General Medical Conditions
Schizophrenia

Philip Pan, MD
Director, Outpatient Services
Assistant Professor of Psychiatry
Southern Illinois University
Springfield, Illinois
Alcohol Withdrawal
Antisocial Personality Disorder
Benzodiazepine Withdrawal
Delirium
Dementia
Fetishism
Malingering
Opioid Withdrawal
Paranoid Personality Disorder
Paranoid Schizophrenia
Phencyclidine Intoxication
Somatization Disorder

Kimberly Rutter, MD
Faculty in Obstetrics and Gynecology
University of Texas Galveston Medical Branch at Brackenridge Hospital
Austin, Texas
Generalized Anxiety Disorder

Amber D. Shamburger, MD
Resident in Obstetrics and Gynecology
The Methodist Hospital Obstetrics and Gynecology Residency
Houston, Texas
Bipolar Disorder (Child)
Bipolar Disorder (Adult)

Steve Soltys, MD
Professor and Chair, Department of Psychiatry
Southern Illinois University
Springfield, Illinois
Anorexia
Attention-Deficit/Hyperactivity Disorder
Avoidant Personality Disorder
Bipolar Disorder (Child)
Bulimia
Hallucinogen Persisting Perception Disorder
Major Depression with Psychosis
Mental Retardation
Psychosis Not Otherwise Specific (Postpartum Depression)
Schizotypal Personality Disorder
Sleep Terror Disorder
Substance-Induced Mood Disorder

Tom Wright, MD
Medical Director and Interim
Executive Director
Community Partnerships, Inc.
Madison, Wisconsin
Adjustment Disorder
Amphetamine Intoxication
Anxiety Secondary to a General Medical Condition
Autism
Borderline Personality Disorder
Conduct Disorder
Gender Identity Disorder
Obsessive-Compulsive Disorder (Child)
Obsessive-Compulsive Personality Disorder
Schizoaffective Disorder (Child)
Separation Anxiety Disorder
Tourette Disorder

❖ PREFACE

We appreciate all the kind remarks and suggestions from the many medical students over the past 2 years. Your positive reception has been an incredible encouragement, especially in light of the short life of the Case Files series. In this second edition of *Case Files: Psychiatry,* the basic format of the book has been retained. Improvements were made in streamlining many of the chapters. Also, numerous clinical cases were rewritten to be representative of more typical patient presentations rather than the "flamboyant" presentation. We debated about whether to group the cases together so that students could compare related disorders such as cases 1–10 would be "personality disorders" to allow for side-by-side comparison. We decided not to use this systematic grouping approach, since patients do not present to their doctors in the real world in this manner. Rather, patients present with symptoms and signs, and it is the "job" of the student and clinician to sort out whether there is a psychiatric issue, and which one is likely. Nevertheless, the case listing in the back of the book and the index will allow a student to quickly reference similar cases for the sake of comparison. The multiple choice questions have been carefully reviewed and rewritten to ensure that they comply with the National Board and USMLE Step 2 format. Some new psychiatric medications have been introduced as well. By using this second edition, we hope that the reader will continue to enjoy learning psychiatry through the simulated clinical cases. It is certainly a privilege to be a teacher for so many students, and it is with humility that we present this edition.

The Authers

ACKNOWLEDGMENTS

The curriculum from which the ideas for this series evolved was inspired by two talented, forthright students, Philbert Yau and Chuck Rosipal, who have since graduated from medical school. It has been a great joy to work with Debra Klamen, a brilliant psychiatrist, educator, and lover of horses, and with all the excellent contributors. I am greatly indebted to my editor, Catherine Johnson, whose exuberance, experience, and vision helped to shape this series. I appreciate McGraw-Hill's belief in the concept of teaching through clinical cases, and I would especially like to acknowledge Penny Linskey for her editing expertise. At Southern Illinois University, I thank Dr. Kevin Dorsey for his help and support in completing this project. At the Methodist Hospital, I applaud the finest administrators I have encountered: Dr. Marc Boom, Dr. Judy Paukert, Dr. H. Dirk Sostman and Michael Brown, for their commitment to medical education, and Jo McMains and Dorothy Mersinger for their sage advice and support. I am indebted to John N. Lyle VII, a brilliant administrator, and Amy Reddell, the most talented attorney I have encountered. Without my esteemed colleagues, Drs. Saul Soffar, Earl Lord, and Jeane Simmons, this book could not have been written. Most of all, I appreciate my loving wife, Terri, and my four wonderful children, Andy, Michael, Allison, and Christina, for their patience and understanding.

Eugene C. Toy

❖ INTRODUCTION

Mastering the cognitive knowledge within a field such as psychiatry is a formidable task. It is even more difficult to draw on that knowledge, procure and filter through the clinical and mental status data, develop a differential diagnosis, and finally form a rational treatment plan. To gain these skills, the student often learns best by directly interviewing patients, guided and instructed by experienced teachers and inspired toward self-directed, diligent reading. Clearly, there is no replacement for education at the patient's side. Unfortunately, clinical situations usually do not encompass the breadth of the specialty. Perhaps the best alternative is to prepare carefully crafted cases designed to simulate the clinical approach and decision making. In an attempt to achieve this goal, we have constructed a collection of clinical vignettes to teach diagnostic or therapeutic approaches relevant to psychiatry. Most importantly, the explanations for the cases emphasize mechanisms and underlying principles rather than merely rote questions and answers.

This book is organized for versatility: to allow the student "in a rush" to read the scenarios quickly and check the corresponding answers, as well as to provide more detailed information for the student who wants thought-provoking explanations. The answers are arranged from simple to complex: a summary of the pertinent points, the bare answers, an analysis of the case, an approach to the topic, a comprehension test at the end for reinforcement and emphasis, and a list of resources for further reading. The clinical vignettes are purposely presented in random order to simulate the way that real patients present to a practitioner. A listing of cases is included in Section IV to aid students who desire to test their knowledge of a certain area or to review a topic, including the basic definitions. Finally, we intentionally did not primarily use a multiple-choice question (MCQ) format because clues (or distractors) are not available in the real world. Nevertheless, several MCQs are included at the end of each scenario to reinforce concepts or introduce related topics.

HOW TO GET THE MOST OUT OF THIS BOOK

Each case is designed to simulate a patient encounter by using open-ended questions. At times, the patient's complaint differs from the issue of greatest concern, and sometimes extraneous information is given. The answers are organized into four different parts.

PART I

1. A **Summary:** The salient aspects of the case are identified, filtering out extraneous information. The student should formulate a summary of the case before looking at the answers. A comparison with the summation appearing in the answer will help improve the student's ability to focus on the important data while appropriately discarding irrelevant information, a fundamental skill required in clinical problem solving.
2. A **Straightforward Answer** to each open-ended question.
3. An **Analysis of the Case** consisting of two parts:
   a. **Objectives:** A listing of the two or three main principles that are crucial for a practitioner in treating the patient. Again, the student is challenged to make "educated guesses" about the objectives of the case on initial review of the case scenario, which helps to sharpen his or her clinical and analytical skills.
   b. **Considerations:** A discussion of the relevant points and a brief approach to the specific patient.

PART II

An Approach to the Disease Process consisting of two distinct parts:

   a. **Definitions:** Terminology pertinent to the disease process.
   b. **Clinical Approach:** A discussion of the approach to the clinical problem in general, including tables and figures.

PART III

Comprehension Questions: Each case contains several MCQs that reinforce the material presented or introduce new and related concepts. Questions about material not found in the text are explained in the answers.

PART IV

Clinical Pearls: A listing of several clinically important points that are reiterated as a summation of the text and allow for easy review, such as before an examination.

SECTION I

How to Approach Clinical Problems

PART 1. APPROACH TO THE PATIENT

It is a difficult transition from reading about patients with psychiatric disorders, and reading the diagnostic criteria from the *Diagnostic and Statistical Manual of Mental Disorders, 4th edition (DSM-IV),* to actually developing a psychiatric diagnosis for a patient. It requires the physician to understand the criteria and be able to sensitively elicit symptoms and signs from patients, many of whom have difficulty providing a clear history. The clinician must then put together the pieces of a puzzle in order to find the single best diagnosis for the patient. This process can require further information from the patient's family, additions to the medical and psychiatric history, careful observation of the patient, a physical examination, selected laboratory tests, and other diagnostic studies. Establishing rapport and a good therapeutic alliance with patients is critical to both their diagnosis and their treatment.

CLINICAL PEARL

❖ A patient's history is the single most important tool in establishing a diagnosis. Developing good rapport with patients is key to effective interviewing and thorough data gathering. Both the content (what the patient says and does not say) and the manner in which it is expressed (body language, topic shifting) are important.

History

1. **Basic information:**
   a. Identifying information includes name, age, marital status, gender, occupation, and language spoken other than English. Ethnic background and religion can also be included if they are pertinent.
   b. It is helpful to include the circumstances of the interview because they provide information about potentially important patient characteristics that can be relevant to the diagnosis, the prognosis, or compliance. Circumstances include where the interview was conducted (emergency setting, outpatient office, in leather restraints) and whether the episode reported was the first occurrence for the patient.
   c. Sources of the information obtained and their reliability should be mentioned at the beginning of the psychiatric history.

2. **Chief complaint:** The chief complaint should be written exactly as the patient states it, no matter how bizarre. For example, "The space aliens

are attacking outside my garage so I came in for help." Other individuals accompanying the patient can then add their versions of why the patient is presenting currently, but the chief complaint stated in the patient's words helps with the initial formulation of a differential diagnosis. For example, if a patient comes in with a chief complaint about aliens, as just noted, one would immediately begin to consider diagnoses that have psychosis as a component and conduct the interview accordingly.

CLINICAL PEARLS

❖ When recording a chief complaint in the patient's own words, put quotation marks around the patient's statements to indicate that they are indeed the patient's words, not the writer's.

❖ A 45-year-old woman comes to the emergency department with the chief complaint, "I know everyone is going to try to hurt me."

3. **History of present illness (HPI):** This information is **probably the most useful part of the history** in terms of **making a psychiatric diagnosis.** It should contain a **comprehensive, chronological picture** of the circumstances leading up to the encounter with the physician. It is important to include details such as when symptoms first appeared, in what order, and at what level of severity, as this information is critical in making the correct diagnosis. Relationships between psychological stressors and the appearance of psychiatric and/or physical symptoms should be carefully outlined. In addition, details of the history such as the use of drugs or alcohol, which are normally listed in the social history, should be put in the HPI if they are thought to make a significant contribution to the presenting symptoms.

4. **Psychiatric history:** The patient's previous encounters with psychiatrists and other mental health therapists should be listed in chronological order. Past psychiatric hospitalizations, the treatment received, and the length of stay should be recorded. Whether or not the patient has received psychotherapy, what kind, and for how long, are also important. Any pharmacotherapy received by the patient should be recorded, and details such as dosage, response, length of time on the drug, and compliance with the medication should be included. Any treatments with electroconvulsive therapy (ECT) should be noted as well, including the number of sessions and the associated effects.

5. **Medical history:** Any medical illnesses should be listed in this category along with the date of diagnosis. Hospitalizations and surgeries should also be included with their dates. Episodes of **head trauma, seizures, neurologic illnesses** or tumors, and positive assays for **human immunodeficiency virus (HIV)** are all pertinent to the psychiatric history. If it is felt that some aspect of the medical history is directly pertinent to the current chief complaint, it should be mentioned in the HPI.

6. **Medications:** A list of medications including their doses and their duration of use should be obtained. All medications, including over-the-counter, herbal, and prescribed, are relevant and should be delineated.

7. **Allergies:** A list of agents causing allergic reactions, including medications and environmental agents (dust, henna, etc.) should be obtained. For each, it is important to describe what reaction actually occurred, such as a skin rash or difficulty breathing. Many patients who have a dystonic reaction to a medication consider it an allergy, although it is actually a side effect of the medication.

8. **Family history:** A brief statement about the patient's family history of psychiatric as well as medical disorders should be included. Listing each family member, his or her age, and medical or psychiatric disorders is generally the easiest, clearest way to do this.

9. **Social history:**
   a. The **prenatal and perinatal history** of the patient is probably relevant for all young children brought to a psychiatrist. It can also be relevant in older children and/or adults if it involves birth defects or injuries.
   b. A **childhood history** is important when evaluating a child and can be important in evaluating an adult if it involves episodes of trauma, long-standing personal patterns, or problems with education. For a child, issues such as age of and/or difficulty in toilet training, behavioral problems, social relationships, cognitive and motor development, and emotional and physical problems should all be included.
   c. Occupational history, including military history.
   d. Marital and relationship history.
   e. Education history.
   f. Religion.
   g. Social history, including the nature of friendships and interests.
   h. Drug and alcohol history.
   i. Current living situation.

10. **Review of systems:** A systematic review should be performed with emphasis on common side effects of medications and common

symptoms that might be associated with the chief complaint. For example, patients taking typical antipsychotic agents (such as haloperidol) might be asked about dry mouth, dry eyes, constipation, and urinary hesitancy. Patients with presumed panic disorder might be questioned about cardiac symptoms such as palpitations and chest pain or neurologic symptoms such as numbness and tingling.

Mental Status Examination

The **mental status examination** comprises the **sum total** of the **physician's observations** of the patient at the time of the interview. Of note is that this examination can change from hour to hour, whereas the patient's history remains stable. The mental status examination includes impressions of the patient's **general appearance, mood, speech, actions, and thoughts.** Even a mute or uncooperative patient reveals a large amount of clinical information during the mental status examination.

CLINICAL PEARL

❖ The mental status examination provides a snapshot of the patient's symptoms at the time of the interview. It can differ from the patient's history, which is what has happened to the patient **up until the time** of the interview. If a patient has thought about suicide for the past 3 weeks but during the interview says that he is not feeling suicidal while speaking with the psychiatrist, his **history** is considered **positive for suicidal ideation** although the **thought content** section of the **mental status examination** is said to be **negative** for (current) **suicidal ideation.**

1. **General description**
   a. **Appearance:** A description of the patient's overall appearance should be recorded, including posture, poise, grooming, and clothing. Signs of anxiety and other mood states should also be noted, such as wringing of hands, tense posture, clenched fists, or a wrinkled forehead.
   b. **Behavior and psychomotor activity:** Any bizarre posturing, abnormal movements, agitation, rigidity, or other physical characteristics should be described.
   c. **Attitude toward examiner:** The patient's attitude should be noted using terms such as "friendly," " hostile," "evasive," "guarded," or any of a host of descriptive adjectives.

2. **Mood and affect**
   a. **Mood:** The emotion (anger, depression, emptiness, guilt, etc.) that underlies a person's perception of the world. Although mood can often be inferred throughout the course of an interview, it is best to ask the patient directly, "How has your mood been?" Mood should be **quantified wherever possible**—a **scale from 1 to 10** is often used. For example, a person rates his depression as 3 on a scale of 1 to 10 where 10 is the happiest he has ever felt.
   b. **Affect:** The person's emotional responsiveness during the examination as inferred from his/her expressions and behavior. In addition to the affect noted, the **range (variation) of the affect** during the interview, as well as its **congruency** with (consistency with) the stated mood, should be noted. A **blunted** or **constricted** affect means that there is little variation in facial expression or use of hands; a **flat affect** is even further reduced in range.

3. **Speech:** The physical characteristics of the patient's speech should be described. Notations as to the **rate, tone, volume, and rhythm** should be made. Impairments of speech, such as stuttering, should also be noted.

4. **Perception:** Hallucinations and illusions reported by the patient should be listed. The sensory system involved (tactile, gustatory, auditory, visual, or olfactory) should be indicated, as well as the content of the hallucination (e.g., "It smells like burning rubber," "I hear two voices calling me bad names.") Of note is that whereas some clinicians use perception as a separate category, others combine this section with the thought content portion of the write-up/presentation.

5. **Thought process:** Thought process refers to the *form* of thinking or *how* a patient thinks. It does not refer specifically to *what* a person thinks, which is more appropriate to the thought content. In order of most logical to least logical, thought process can be described as **logical/coherent, circumstantial, tangential, flight of ideas, loose associations, and word salad/incoherence.** Neologisms, punning, or thought blocking also should be mentioned here.

6. **Thought content:** The actual thought content section should include **delusions (fixed, false beliefs), paranoia, preoccupations, obsessions and compulsions, phobias, ideas of reference, poverty of content, and suicidal and homicidal ideation.** Patients with suicidal or homicidal ideation should be asked whether, in addition to the presence of the ideation, they have a *plan* for carrying out the suicidal or homicidal act as well as about their *intent* to do so.

7. **Sensorium and cognition:** This portion of the mental status examination assesses **organic brain function, intelligence, capacity for abstract thought**, and **levels of insight and judgment.** The basic tests of sensorium and cognition are performed on every patient. Those whom the clinician suspects are suffering from an organic brain disorder can be tested with further cognitive tests beyond the scope of the basic mental status examination.
   a. **Consciousness:** Common descriptors of levels of consciousness include "alert," "somnolent," "stuporous," and "clouded consciousness."
   b. **Orientation and memory:** The classic test of orientation is to discern the patient's ability to locate himself or herself in relation to person, place, and/or time. Any impairment usually occurs in this order as well (i.e., a sense of time is usually impaired before a sense of place or person). Memory is divided into four areas: immediate, recent, recent past, and remote. **Immediate memory** is tested by asking a patient to **repeat numbers** after the examiner, in both forward and backward order. **Recent memory** is tested by asking a patient **what she ate for dinner the previous night** and asking if she remembers the examiner's name from the beginning of the interview. **Recent past memory** is tested by asking about news items publicized in the past several months, and **remote memory** is assessed by asking patients about their childhood. Note that information must be verified to be sure of its accuracy because confabulation (making up false answers when memory is impaired) can occur.
   c. **Concentration and attention: Subtracting serial 7s from 100** is a common way of testing concentration. Patients who are unable to do this because of educational deficiencies can be asked to subtract serial 3s from 100. Attention is tested by asking a patient to spell the word "world" forward and backward. The patient can also be asked to name five words that begin with a given letter.
   d. **Reading and writing:** The patient should be instructed to read a given sentence and then do what the sentence asks, for example, "Turn this paper over when you have finished reading." The patient should also be asked to write a sentence. Examiners should be aware that illiteracy might impact a patient's ability to follow instructions during this part of the examination.
   e. **Visuospatial ability:** The patient is typically asked to **copy the face of a clock** and fill in the numbers and hands so that the clock shows the correct time. Images with **interlocking shapes or angles** can also be used—the patient is asked to copy them.
   f. **Abstract thought:** Abstract thinking is the ability to deal with concepts. Can patients distinguish the similarities and differences

between two given objects? Can patients understand and articulate the meaning of simple proverbs? (Be aware that patients who are immigrants and have learned English as a second language can have problems with proverbs for this reason rather than because of a mental status disturbance.)

g. **Information and intelligence:** Answers to questions related to a general fund of knowledge (presidents of the United States, mayors of the city in which the mental status examination is conducted), vocabulary, and the ability to solve problems are all factored in together to come up with an estimate of intelligence. A patient's educational status should of course be taken into account as well.
h. **Judgment:** During the course of the interview, the examiner should be able to get a good idea of the patient's ability to understand the likely outcomes of his or her behavior and whether or not this behavior can be influenced by knowledge of these outcomes. Having the patient predict what he or she would do in an imaginary scenario can sometimes help with this assessment. For example, what would the patient do if he or she found a stamped envelope lying on the ground?
i. **Insight:** Insight is the degree to which a patient understands the nature and extent of his or her own illness. Patients can express a complete denial of their illnesses or progressive levels of insight into knowing that there is something wrong within them that needs to be addressed.

CLINICAL PEARL

❖ Almost all of the mental status examination can be made by careful observation of the patient while obtaining a detailed, complete history. Only a few additional questions need to be addressed to the patient directly, for example, those regarding the presence of suicidal ideation and specific cognitive examination questions.

Physical Examination

The physical examination can be an important component of the assessment of a patient with a presumed psychiatric illness. Many physical illnesses masquerade as psychiatric disorders, and vice versa. For example, a patient with **pancreatic cancer** can first present to a psychiatrist with symptoms of **major depression.** Thus an examiner should be alert to all of a patient's signs and symptoms, physical and mental, and be prepared to perform a physical examination, especially in an emergency department setting. Some patients can be too agitated or paranoid to undergo parts of the physical examination, but when possible, all elements should be completed.

1. **General appearance:** Cachetic versus well-nourished, anxious versus calm, alert versus obtunded.
2. **Vital signs:** Temperature, blood pressure, heart rate, respiratory rate, and weight.
3. **Head and neck examination:** Evidence of trauma, tumors, facial edema, goiter (indicating hyper- or hypothyroidism), and carotid bruits should be sought. Cervical and supraclavicular nodes should be palpated.
4. **Breast examination:** Inspection for symmetry, skin or nipple retraction with the patient's hands on hips (to accentuate the pectoral muscles), and with arms raised. With the patient supine, the breasts should then be palpated systematically to assess for masses. The nipple should be examined for discharge, and the axillary and supraclavicular regions for adenopathy.
5. **Cardiac examination:** The point of maximal impulse should be ascertained, and the heart auscultated at the apex of the heart as well as at the base. Heart sounds, murmurs, and clicks should be characterized.
6. **Pulmonary examination:** The lung fields should be examined systematically and thoroughly. Wheezes, rales, rhonchi, and bronchial breath sounds should be recorded.
7. **Abdominal examination:** The abdomen should be inspected for scars, distension, masses or organomegaly (i.e., spleen or liver), and discoloration. Auscultation of bowel sounds should be accomplished to identify normal versus high-pitched and hyperactive versus hypoactive sounds. The abdomen should be percussed for the presence of shifting dullness (indicating ascites).
8. **Back and spine examination:** The back should be assessed for symmetry, tenderness, or masses.
9. **Pelvic examination:** Although this examination is not often done in the emergent setting of psychiatric illness, it is important to realize that many patients with a psychiatric illness do not see their physicians regularly and that this important preventive maintenance procedure is often neglected. Patients should be reminded of the need for this examination.
10. **Extremities and skin:** The presence of tenderness, skin edema, and cyanosis should be recorded.
11. **Neurologic examination:** Patients require a thorough assessment including evaluation of the cranial nerves, strength, sensation, and reflexes.

Laboratory Tests

Compared to other medical practitioners, psychiatrists depend more on the patient's signs and symptoms and the clinician's examination than on laboratory tests. There are no definitive tests for bipolar disorder, schizophrenia, or major depression. However, tests can be used to identify potential medical problems appearing as psychiatric disturbances, as well as to look for substances such as lysergic acid diethylamide (LSD) or cocaine in a patient's system. Laboratory tests are also useful in long-term monitoring of medications such as lithium and valproic acid.

I. Screening tests
   - A. A complete blood count (CBC) to assess for anemia and thrombocytopenia
   - B. Renal function tests
   - C. Liver function tests
   - D. Thyroid function tests
   - E. Laboratory studies including determinations of chloride, sodium, potassium, bicarbonate, serum urea nitrogen, creatinine, and blood sugar levels
   - F. Urine toxicology or serum toxicology tests when drug use is suspected by the interviewer

II. Tests related to psychotropic drugs
   - A. **Lithium:** A CBC, a serum electrolyte determination, **kidney function tests,** a fasting blood glucose determination, **a pregnancy test,** and an **electrocardiogram (ECG)** are recommended before treatment and yearly thereafter. **Lithium levels** should also be monitored.
   - B. **Clozapine:** Because of the risk of developing **agranulocytosis,** patients taking this medication should have their white blood cell (WBC) and differential count measured at the onset of treatment, weekly during treatment, and weekly for 4 weeks after discontinuation of treatment.
   - C. **Tricyclic and tetracyclic antidepressants:** An **ECG** should be obtained before a patient begins treatment with these medications.
   - D. **Carbamazepine:** A pretreatment CBC including a platelet count should be obtained to assess for **agranulocytosis.** Reticulocyte and serum iron levels should also be determined and all these tests performed monthly thereafter. Liver function tests should be performed every 3 to 6 months, and carbamazepine levels should be monitored this often as well.
   - E. **Valproate:** Valproate levels should be monitored every 6 to 12 months, along with liver function tests.

III. Psychometric testing

A. **Structured clinical diagnostic assessments**

1. Tests based on structured or semistructured interviews designed to produce numerical scores
2. Scales useful in determining the severity of an illness and in monitoring the patient's recovery
3. Examples: **Beck Rating Scale for Depression, Hamilton Anxiety Rating Scale, Brief Psychiatric Rating Scale,** and Structured Clinical Interview for DSM-IV Dissociative Disorders (SCID-IV)

B. **Psychological testing of intelligence and personality**

1. Tests designed to measure aspects of the patient's intelligence, ability to process information, and personality.
2. Tests generally **administered by psychologists** trained to administer and interpret them.
3. Such tests play a relatively small role in the diagnosis of psychiatric illness: The psychiatric interview and other observable signs and symptoms play a much larger role. These tests are therefore reserved for special situations.
4. Objective tests generally consisting of pencil-and-paper examinations based on specific questions. They yield numerical scores and are statistically analyzed.
   a. **Minnesota Multiphasic Personality Inventory:** This self-report inventory is widely used and has been thoroughly researched. It assesses personality using an objective approach.
   b. **Projective tests:** These tests present stimuli that are not immediately obvious. The **ambiguity of the situation forces patients to project their own needs into the test situation.** Therefore, there are no right or wrong answers.
      i. **Rorschach test:** This projective test is used to assess personality. A series of 10 inkblots are presented to the patient, and the psychologist keeps a verbatim record of the patient's responses to each one. The test brings the patient's thinking and association patterns into focus. In skilled hands, it is helpful in bringing out defense mechanisms, subtle thought disorders, and pertinent patient psychodynamics.
      ii. **Thematic Apperception Test (TAT).** This test also assesses personality but does so by presenting patients with selections from 30 pictures and 1 blank card. The patient is required to create a story about each picture presented. Generally, the TAT is most useful for investigating personal motivation (e.g., why a patient does what he or she does) than it is in making a diagnosis.

iii. **Sentence completion test:** A projective test in which the patient is given part of a sentence and asked to complete it. It taps the unconscious associations of the patient to locate areas of functioning in which the interviewer is interested, for example, "My greatest fear is. . . ."

c. **Intelligence tests:** These tests are used to establish the degree of mental retardation in situations where this is the question. The Wechsler Adult Intelligence Scale is the test most widely used in clinical practice today.

d. **Neuropsychologic tests:** The aim of these tests is to compare the patient being tested with "normal" people of similar background and age. They are used to identify cognitive deficits, assess the toxic effects of substances, evaluate the effects of treatment, and identify learning disorders.

i. **Wisconsin Card Sorting Test:** This test assesses abstract reasoning and flexibility in problem solving by asking the patient to sort a variety of cards according to principles established by the rater but not known to the sorter. Abnormal responses are seen in patients with damaged frontal lobes and in some patients with schizophrenia.

ii. **Wechsler Memory Scale:** This is the most widely used battery of tests for adults. It tests rote memory, visual memory, orientation, and counting backward, among other dimensions. It is sensitive to amnestic conditions such as Korsakoff syndrome.

iii. **Bender Visual Motor Gestalt Test:** A test of visuomotor coordination. Patients are asked to copy nine separate designs onto unlined paper. They are then asked to reproduce the designs from memory. This test is used as a screening device for signs of organic dysfunction.

IV. Further diagnostic tests

A. Additional psychiatric diagnostic interviews (e.g., the Diagnostic Interview Schedule for Children)

B. Interviews conducted by a social worker with family members, friends, or neighbors

C. Electroencephalogram to rule in or rule out a seizure disorder

D. Computed tomography scan to assess intracranial masses

E. Magnetic resonance imaging to assess intracranial masses or any other neurologic abnormality

F. Tests to confirm other medical conditions.

PART 2. APPROACH TO CLINICAL PROBLEM SOLVING

A clinician typically undertakes four distinct steps to solve most clinical problems systematically:

1. Making a diagnosis
2. Assessing the severity of the disease
3. Rendering treatment based on the disease
4. Following the patient's response to the treatment

Making a Diagnosis

A diagnosis is made by careful evaluation of the database, analysis of the information, assessment of the risk factors, and development of a list of possibilities (the differential diagnosis). The process involves knowing which pieces of information are meaningful and which can be discarded. Experience and knowledge help the physician to "key in" on the most important possibilities. A good clinician also knows how to ask the same question in several different ways and to use different terminology. For example, patients at times can deny having been treated for bipolar disorder but answer affirmatively when asked if they have been hospitalized for mania. A diagnosis can be reached by systematically reading about each possible disease. The patient's presentation is then matched up against each of the possibilities, and each disorder is moved higher up or lower down on the list as a potential etiology based on the prevalence of the disease, the patient's presentation, and other clues. The patient's risk factors can also influence the probability of a diagnosis.

Usually, a long list of possible diagnoses can be pared down to the two or three most likely ones based on a careful delineation of the signs and symptoms displayed by the patient, as well as on the time course of the illness. For example, a patient with a history of depressive symptoms, including problems with concentration, sleep, appetite, *and* symptoms of psychosis that started *after* the mood disturbances can have major depression with psychotic features, whereas a patient with a psychosis that started *before* the mood symptoms can have schizoaffective disorder.

CLINICAL PEARL

❖ The first step in clinical problem solving is **making a diagnosis.**

Assessing the Severity of the Disease

After ascertaining the diagnosis, the next step is to characterize the severity of the disease process; in other words, describe "how bad" it is. With a malignancy, this is done formally by staging the cancer. With some infections, such as syphilis, staging depends on the duration and extent of the infection and follows its natural history (i.e., primary syphilis, secondary syphilis, latent period, and tertiary/neurosyphilis). Some major mental illnesses, such as schizophrenia, can be characterized as acute, chronic, or residual, whereas the same clinical picture, occurring with less than a 6-month duration, is termed schizophreniform disorder. Other notations frequently used in describing psychiatric illnesses include "mild," "moderate," "severe," "in partial remission," and "in full remission."

CLINICAL PEARL

The second step is to establish the severity or subcategory of the disease. This categorization usually has prognostic or treatment significance.

Treating Based on Stage

Many illnesses are stratified according to severity because prognosis and treatment often vary based on these factors. If neither the prognosis nor the treatment is influenced by the stage of the disease process, there is no reason to subcategorize a disease as mild or severe. For example, some patients with **suicidal ideation but no intent or plan** can be **treated as outpatients,** but other patients who report **intent and a specific plan, must be immediately hospitalized** and even committed if necessary.

CLINICAL PEARL

❖ The third step requires that, for most conditions, **the treatment be tailored** to the extent or severity of the disease.

Following the Response to Treatment

The final step in the approach to disease is to follow the patient's response to the therapy. The measure of response should be recorded and monitored. Some responses are clinical, such as improvement (or lack of improvement) in the level of depression, anxiety, or paranoia. Obviously, the student must work on becoming skilled in eliciting the relevant data in an unbiased, standardized manner. Other responses can be followed by laboratory tests, such as a urine toxicology screening for a cocaine abuser or a determination of lithium level for a bipolar patient. The student must be prepared to know what to do if the measured marker does not respond according to what is expected. Is the next step to reconsider the diagnosis, to repeat the test, or to confront the patient about the findings?

CLINICAL PEARL

❖ The fourth step is to monitor treatment response or efficacy, which can be measured in different ways. It can be based on symptoms (the patient feels better) or on a laboratory or some other test (a urine toxicology screening).

PART 3. APPROACH TO THE *DIAGNOSTIC AND STATISTICAL MANUAL OF MENTAL DISORDERS*

The *Diagnostic and Statistical Manual of Mental Disorders*, currently in its fourth edition, text revision *(DSM-IV-TR),* is published by the American Psychiatric Association. It is the official psychiatric coding system used in the United States. The *DSM-IV-TR* describes mental disorders and only rarely attempts to account for how these disturbances come about. Specified diagnostic criteria are presented for each disorder and include a list of features that must be present for the diagnosis to be made. The *DSM-IV-TR* also systematically describes each disorder in terms of its associated descriptors such as age, gender, prevalence, incidence, and risk; course; complications; predisposing factors; familial pattern; and differential diagnosis.

The *DSM-IV-TR* uses a five-axis system that evaluates patients along several dimensions. Axes I and II make up the entire classification of mental disorders. **Each patient should receive a five-axis diagnosis,** which usually appears at the end of a write-up in the assessment section.

Axis I: Clinical disorders and other disorders that can be the focus of clinical attention.

Axis II: Personality disorders and mental retardation only.

Axis III: Physical disorders and other general medical conditions. The physical condition can be causing the psychiatric one (e.g., delirium, coded on axis I, caused by renal failure, coded on axis III), be the result of a mental disorder (e.g., alcoholic cirrhosis, coded on axis III, secondary to alcohol dependence, coded on axis I), or be unrelated to the mental disorder (e.g., chronic diabetes mellitus).

Axis IV: This axis is used to code the psychosocial problems contributing to the patient's psychiatric problem. Information about these stressors can be helpful when it is time to develop treatment plans for the patient. Problems can include those involving the primary support group, educational problems, job problems, housing problems, economic problems, problems with access to health care, or problems related to the legal system/crime.

Axis V: This axis is used to provide a global assessment of functioning (GAF). The scale is based on a continuum of health and illness, using a 100-point scale on which 100 is the highest level of functioning. People who had high GAF values before an episode of illness often have a better prognosis than those whose functioning was at a lower level.

PART 4. APPROACH TO READING

The clinical problem-oriented approach to reading is different from the classic "systematic" researching of a disease. Patients rarely present with symptoms that permit a clear diagnosis; hence, the student must become skilled in applying textbook information in the clinical setting. Furthermore, a reader retains more information when reading with a purpose. In other words, the student should read with the goal of answering specific questions. There are several fundamental questions that facilitate **clinical thinking:**

1. What is the most likely diagnosis?
2. What should the next step be?
3. What is the most likely mechanism for this process?
4. What are the risk factors for this condition?
5. What complications are associated with this disease process?
6. What is the best therapy?
7. How can you confirm the diagnosis?

Note that questions 3 through 5 are probably used less in the field of psychiatry than in other specialties, such as medicine, where the pathophysiology and risk factors of a particular disease process are known. Likewise,

CLINICAL PEARL

❖ Reading with the purpose of answering the seven fundamental clinical questions improves retention of information and facilitates the application of book knowledge to clinical knowledge.

confirmation of a diagnosis (question 7) is less often made by further laboratory tests or other diagnostic studies but can be achieved by carefully obtaining additional history from family, colleagues, and so on. The preceding questions should, however, be kept in mind for all patients.

What Is the Most Likely Diagnosis?

The method of establishing a diagnosis was covered in the previous section. One way to attack this problem is to develop standard "approaches" to common clinical situations. It is helpful to understand the most common presentation of a variety of illnesses, for example, a common presentation of major depression. (Clinical pearls appear at the end of each case.)

The clinical scenario might be the following:

A 36-year-old woman presents to her physician with the chief complaint of a depressed mood and difficulty sleeping. What is the most likely diagnosis?

With no other information to go on, the student notes the depressed mood and the vegetative symptom of insomnia. Using the "common presentation" information, the student might make an educated guess that the patient has **major depression.**

However, what if the scenario also includes the following?

She states that she has been depressed and has had trouble sleeping since she was raped 2 weeks ago.

Then the student would use the clinical pearl: A diagnosis of acute stress disorder should be considered in a patient with a depressed mood, insomnia, and a history of recent trauma.

CLINICAL PEARLS

❖ A common presentation of major depression is depressed mood and the vegetative symptom of insomnia. These symptoms, however, are common in instances of trauma and bereavement as well, and so these details must be investigated in reference to the patient.

❖ If mood changes and insomnia are secondary to an emotional and/or physical trauma, the clinician should consider a diagnosis of acute stress disorder.

What Should the Next Step Be?

This question is difficult because *the next step* has many possibilities: The answer can be to obtain more diagnostic information, rate the severity of the illness, or introduce therapy. It is often a more challenging question than what is the most likely diagnosis because there can be insufficient information to make a diagnosis and the next step can be to pursue more diagnostic information. Another possibility is that there is enough information for a probable diagnosis and that the next step is to assess the severity of the disease. Finally, the most appropriate answer can be to start treatment. Hence, based on clinical data, a judgment needs to be rendered regarding how far along one is in the following process:

(1) Make a diagnosis → (2) Stage the severity of the disease → (3) Treat based on the severity of the disease → (4) Follow the response

Frequently, students are taught to "regurgitate" information that someone has written about a particular disease but are not skilled in describing the next step. This ability is learned optimally at the bedside, in a supportive environment, with freedom to make educated guesses and with constructive feedback. A sample scenario describes a student's thought process as follows:

1. **Make a diagnosis:** "Based on the information I have, I believe that Ms. Smith has major depression because she has a depressed mood, problems with concentration, anhedonia, insomnia, loss of appetite, anergia, and a weight loss of 10 lb in 3 weeks."
2. **Stage the severity of the disease:** "I don't believe that this is severe disease because the patient does not have suicidal ideation or any psychotic symptoms."
3. **Treat based on the severity of the disease:** "Therefore, my next step is to treat her with a selective serotonin reuptake inhibitor (SSRI) such as paroxetine."
4. **Follow the response:** "I want to follow the treatment by assessing her depressed mood (I will ask her to rate her mood on a scale of 1 to 10 weekly), her insomnia (I will ask her to keep a sleep log), and her appetite (I will weigh her weekly)."

In a similar case, when the clinical presentation is unclear, perhaps the best next step should be diagnostic in nature, such as a thyroid function test to rule out hypothyroidism.

CLINICAL PEARL

❖ Usually, the vague query, "what is the next step?" is the most difficult question because the answer can be diagnostic, involve staging, or be therapeutic.

What Is the Likely Mechanism for this Process?

This question goes further than making the diagnosis and also requires the student to understand the underlying mechanism of the process. For example, a clinical scenario can describe a 26-year-old man who develops a sudden onset of blindness 3 days after being told of his mother's death. The student must first diagnose a conversion disorder, which can occur after an emotionally traumatic event, once physical explanations for blindness have been ruled out. Then the student must understand that there is a psychodynamic explanation for the particular nature of the symptoms as they have arisen. The mechanism for the conversion disorder, blindness in this scenario, is the patient's fear (and guilt) about never "seeing" his mother again. Although many mechanisms of disease are not well understood in psychiatry at the present time, it is anticipated that they will be further elucidated as the fields of neuropsychiatry and neuroimaging continue to grow.

What Are the Risk Factors for this Process?

Understanding the risk factors helps a practitioner to establish a diagnosis and to determine how to interpret tests. For example, understanding the risk factor analysis can help in treating a 56-year-old man who presents to a physician with a chief complaint of loss of memory. If the man does not have a family history of (and thus a risk for) Huntington's chorea, an autosomally transmitted disease, the workup for memory loss would not likely include an examination of his genotype. Thus, the presence of risk factors helps to categorize the likelihood of a disease process.

CLINICAL PEARL

❖ When patients are at high risk for a disease based on risk factors, more testing can be indicated.

What Are the Complications of this Process?

Clinicians must be cognizant of the complications of a disease so that they understand how to follow and monitor the patient. Sometimes the student has to make a diagnosis from clinical clues and then apply the knowledge of the consequences of the pathologic process. For example, a woman who presents with a depressed mood, anhedonia, anergia, loss of concentration, insomnia, and weight loss is first diagnosed as having major depression. A complication of this process includes psychosis or suicidal ideation. Therefore, understanding the types of consequences helps the clinician to become aware of the dangers to the patient. Not recognizing these possibilities might lead the clinician to miss asking about psychotic symptoms (and treating them) or to overlook a potentially fatal suicidal ideation.

What Is the Best Therapy?

To answer this question, the clinician needs to make the correct diagnosis, assess the severity of the condition, and weigh the situation to determine the appropriate intervention. For the student, knowing exact doses is not as important as understanding the best medication, route of delivery, mechanism of action, and possible complications. It is important for the student to be able to verbalize the diagnosis and the rationale for the therapy. A common error is for a student to "*jump*" *to a treatment* by making a random guess; as a result, he or she receives *correct or incorrect* feedback. In fact, the student's guess can be correct, but for the wrong reason; conversely, the answer can be a reasonable one with only one small error in thinking but can simply be labeled "wrong." Instead, the student should verbalize the steps so that feedback can be given at every reasoning point.

For example, if the question is what is the best therapy for a 24-year-old woman with an elated mood, lack of a need for sleep, excessive buying behavior, hypersexuality, and psychomotor agitation, the incorrect manner of responding is for the student to blurt out "a mood stabilizer." Rather, the student's reasoning should resemble the following: "The most common cause of these kinds of symptoms is mania, which would make the diagnosis bipolar disorder. There was no mention of a general medical condition (such as hyperthyroidism) or a substance abuse problem (such as cocaine use) that would account for these symptoms. Therefore, the best treatment for this patient with probable bipolar disorder would be lithium or valproic acid (after the final diagnosis is made)."

CLINICAL PEARL

Therapy should be logically based on the severity of disease. There is no need to hospitalize all patients with major depression, but it can be lifesaving to do so if suicidal ideation with intent and plan are present.

How Can You Confirm the Diagnosis?

In the previous scenario, the 24-year-old woman is likely to have bipolar disorder, manic phase. Confirmation can be achieved by obtaining an additional history of manic or depressive episodes from the patient and/or from family members and friends who have observed her behavior over a period of time. Further information about the presence of other symptoms common in mania can also be helpful, as is ruling out any general medical conditions or substance abuse problems. The student should strive to know the limitations of various diagnostic tests and the manifestations of disease.

SUMMARY

1. There is no replacement for a meticulously constructed history and physical examination.
2. There are four steps in the clinical approach to a patient: making a diagnosis, assessing the severity of the disease, treating based on the severity of the disease, and following the response to treatment.
3. There are seven questions that help to bridge the gap between the textbook and the clinical arena.
4. The *DSM-IV* describes five axes:
   - Axis I: Clinical disorders other than those listed in axis II
   - Axis II: Personality disorders, mental retardation
   - Axis III: Physical disorders
   - Axis IV: Psychosocial problems
   - Axis V: Global assessment of functioning

REFERENCES

Ebert M, Loosen P, Nurcombe B, eds. Current diagnosis and treatment in psychiatry. New York: McGraw-Hill, 2000:115–121.

Goldman HH, ed. Review of general psychiatry, 5th ed. New York: McGraw-Hill, 2000:171–189.

Kaplan H, Sadock B. Synopsis of psychiatry, 9th ed. Baltimore: Lippincott Williams & Wilkins, 2004:185–254.

SECTION II

Psychiatric Therapeutics

PART 1. PSYCHOTHERAPY

Psychological, or "talking therapy" treatments fall into four broad categories: (1) individual psychotherapy, (2) behavior modification, (3) cognitive therapies, and (4) social therapies.

I. **Individual psychotherapy:** Varies according to the time frame used (psychotherapy can be either brief or protracted). It can be *supportive, directive, and reality-oriented* versus *expressive, exploratory, and oriented toward a discussion of unconscious material.*

   A. **Supportive psychotherapy**

      1. Goals: Form a **close alliance with the patient,** help the patient **define current problems,** consider and implement possible problem solutions, and "shore up" the patient's current ego defenses.
      2. Indicated in the treatment of **adjustment disorders, acute emotional crises,** and when a long-lasting "cure" is not expected but **improved functioning** is hoped for (as in the case of chronic schizophrenia).

   B. **Insight-oriented psychotherapy**

      1. Goals: Form an alliance with the patient, recognize **transference/countertransference feelings** as they occur, and **uncover unconscious wishes and defenses** that have caused the patient to become maladaptive.
      2. Indicated in the treatment of **anxiety, depression in all of its forms, somatoform and dissociative disorders, personality disorders, neuroses, and trauma.** It should be noted that although psychotherapy can be indicated for all these disorders, the degree of patient insight and motivation for undergoing treatment are critical to its success.

II. **Behavior modification/therapy:** Includes a group of loosely related therapies that work according to the principles of learning. A short list of examples of these therapies follows.

   A. **Systematic desensitization:** Exposing the patient to increasingly anxiety-provoking stimuli and at the same time teaching him or her to relax. This therapy is used in the treatment of phobias and in preventing compulsions.

   B. **Substitution:** Replacing an undesirable behavior (smoking) with a desirable one (chewing gum).

   C. **Hypnosis:** Induction of an advanced state of relaxation or a "trance" during which suggestions can be made. Hypnosis works in selected patients in the management of pain, the resolution of conversion disorders, and relaxation training.

III. **Cognitive therapy**
   A. Focuses on the cognitive responses that are the primary targets for intervention.
   B. Used in changing maladaptive behavior occurring as a result of cognitive responses.
   C. The most common use for this form of therapy is in the **treatment of major depression,** where the **self-defeating attitudes** that are so common are identified, challenged, and **replaced with more realistic thoughts.**

IV. **Social therapies:** These therapies use the principles of supportive and individual or **marital therapy,** but occur in groups of similar patients, a family, or a couple.

PART 2. PSYCHOPHARMACOTHERAPY

Medications can be subdivided into **antidepressants,** including miscellaneous and mood-stabilizing agents, **antipsychotic** medications, and **anxiolytic/hypnotic** medications. Tables II-1 through II-9 summarize the characteristics of these agents. Many of these medications affect neurotransmitters (Figure II-1). The main neurotransmitters are monoamines (norepinephrine, dopamine, serotonin, acetylcholine, histamine), amino acids (gamma-aminobutyric acid), and glutamic acid.

I. Antidepressants: Antidepressants can be placed in three main categories.
   1. **Tricyclics and heterocyclics** once represented the first line of treatment. These drugs work by **increasing the level of monoamines in the synapse by reducing the reuptake of norepinephrine and serotonin.** Although they are quite effective, they are dangerous in overdose, **causing fatal cardiac arrhythmias (Table II-1).**
   2. **Selective serotonin reuptake inhibitors (SSRIs) are the most commonly used antidepressants today. Major side effects include gastrointestinal and sexual dysfunction (Table II-2).**
   3. **Monoamine oxidase inhibitors (MAOIs) are not commonly used** because **a tyramine-free diet (no wine or cheese) must be followed or a hypertensive crisis can result.** These agents can be more helpful in depression with atypical features (overeating, oversleeping, irritability) (Table II-3).
   4. Miscellaneous medications (Table II-4).
   5. **Mood stabilizers:** These medications are used to treat mania and include agents such as lithium, valproic acid, and carbamazepine. **Lithium** has many adverse effects including **tremor, polyuria/diabetes insipidus, acne, hypothyroidism, cardiac dysrhythmias, weight gain, edema, and**

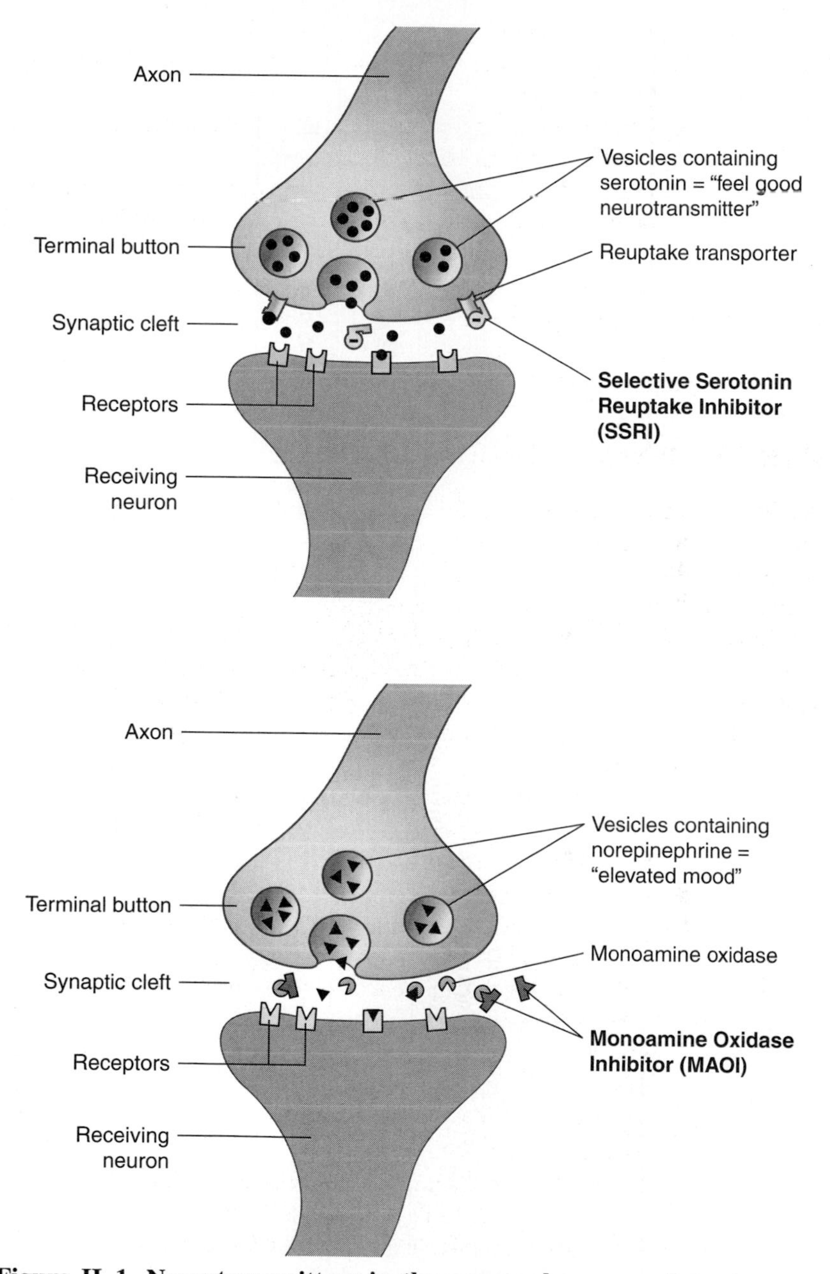

Figure II–1. Neurotransmitters in the neuronal synapse. Selective serotonin reuptake inhibitors block the reuptake of serotonin by the presynaptic neuron (top), allowing more serotonin to be available at the postsynaptic receptor. Monoamine oxidase inhibitors block the ability of this enzyme to inactivate monoamines such as norepinephrine in the synaptic cleft (bottom), allowing more neurotransmitter to bind to the postsynaptic receptor.

Table II–1

TRICYCLIC/TETRACYCLIC MEDICATIONS

NAME*	CLASS OF COMPOUND	SIDE EFFECTS	COMMENTS	HALF-LIFE (H)
All tricyclics and tetracyclics		**Anticholinergic: dry mouth, blurry vision, urinary retention, constipation,** **Sedation** **Orthostatic hypotension (alpha-adrenergic blockade)** **Tachycardia, prolongation of QT interval** **Weight gain (antihistamine-1 effect)**	Concern about a risk of falling in elderly patients	16
Amitriptyline (Elavil)	Tertiary amine		Highly anticholinergic, very sedating	20
Doxepin	Tertiary amine		Highly anticholinergic, very sedating	16
Imipramine (Tofranil)	Tertiary amine		Highly anticholinergic	20
Trimipramine (Surmontil)	Tertiary amine		Highly anticholinergic, very sedating	22
Desipramine (Norpramin)	Secondary amine		Least anticholinergic, not sedating	24

Nortriptyline (Pamelor)	Secondary amine		Less anticholinergic	12
Protriptyline (Vivactil)	Secondary amine	Psychomotor stimulation	Less anticholinergic, not sedating	6
Amoxapine (Asendin, Asendas)	Tetracyclic	**May cause extrapyramidal syndrome (metabolite of loxapine)**	Less anticholinergic	30

*Proprietary names are given in parentheses.
†Secondary amines and tetracyclic compounds tend to have fewer anticholinergic and sedating effects.

Table II–2

SELECTIVE SEROTONIN REUPTAKE INHIBITORS

NAME*	HALF-LIFE	SIDE EFFECTS	COMMENTS
Nearly all selective serotonin reuptake inhibitors (SSRIs)		Agitation, akathisia, anxiety, panic, insomnia, diarrhea, gastrointestinal distress, headache, Sexual dysfunction: delayed ejaculation or impotence (male); anorgasmia (female)	**To avoid fatal serotonin syndrome[†] no SSRI should be combined with a monoamine oxidase inhibitor (MAOI), and an SSRI should be discontinued at least 5 weeks before starting an MAOI**
Fluoxetine (Prozac)	1–3 d		
Sertraline (Zoloft)	25 h		Cause **diarrhea** more commonly than others
Paroxetine (Paxil)	24 h		Mildly **anticholinergic**
Fluvoxamine (Luvox)	15 h		**Nausea and vomiting more common**
Citalopram (Celexa)	35 h		**Possibly fewer sexual side effects**
Escitalopram (Lexapro)	27–30 h		

*Proprietary names are given in parentheses.

†**Serotonin syndrome is similar to neuroleptic malignant syndrome. It is characterized by confusion, muscle rigidity, high temperature, muscle twitching, shivering, and loss of consciousness, and it may be fatal.**

leukocytosis. Lithium is cleared through the **kidneys** and must be used carefully in older patients and in those with renal insufficiency. **Lithium and valproic acid are both teratogenic** and must be used with caution in women of childbearing age (Table II-5).

II. Antipsychotic agents

A. **First-generation antipsychotics (typical antipsychotics)**

1. These medications work by **blocking central dopamine receptors.** They are most effective in reducing the positive symptoms of schizophrenia, including hallucinations and delusions.

Table II–3
MONOAMINE OXIDASE INHIBITORS

NAME*	HALF-LIFE (H)	SIDE EFFECTS	COMMENTS
Phenelzine (Nardil)	4–5	Orthostatic hypotension, somnolence, weight gain	**All cheese, fermented or aged foods, wine, and liver should be avoided** **Should not be coadministered with SSRIs** Should never be coadministered with drugs that increase intrasynaptic levels of amine neurotransmitters
Tranylcypromine (Parnate)	2–3	Orthostatic hypotension, somnolence, weight gain	**All cheese, fermented or aged foods, wine, and liver should be avoided** **Should never be coadministered with SSRIs** Should never be coadministered with drugs that increase intrasynaptic levels of amine neurotransmitters

*Proprietary names are given in parentheses.

2. Side effects (Table II-6) include the following:
   a. **Central nervous system effects:**
      i. **Extrapyramidal symptoms (EPS):** Parkinsonian syndrome, acute dystonias, akathisia.
      ii. **Tardive dyskinesias: Late onset** of choreiform and athetoid movements of the trunk, extremities, or mouth.
      iii. **Sedation.**
      iv. **Neuroleptic malignant syndrome (NMS):** Can occur at any time with an antipsychotic agent; typically movement disorder (muscle rigidity, dystonia, agitation) and autonomic symptoms (high fever, sweating, tachycardia, hypertension). Treatment is mostly supportive but can include medication with dantrolene and/or bromocriptine.

Table II–4

MISCELLANEOUS ANTIDEPRESSANT MEDICATION

NAME*	MECHANISM OF ACTION	HALF-LIFE (H)	SIDE EFFECTS	COMMENTS
Venlafaxine (Effexor)	Serotonin and norepinephrine reuptake inhibitor	5	Anxiety; may increase blood pressure at higher doses, headache, insomnia, sweating	
Nefazodone (Serzone)	Serotonin-2 antagonist and serotonin reuptake inhibitor	2–4	Sedation, hepatotoxicity	Decreased sexual dysfunction occurs with this drug
Trazodone (Desyrel)	Serotonin-2 antagonist and serotonin reuptake inhibitor	10–15	**Priapism: prolonged erection may lead to impotence,** orthostatic hypotension, sedation	Can be used in lower doses to manage sleep problems Should be avoided with monoamine oxidase inhibitors
Mirtazapine (Remeron)	Noradrenergic and specific serotonin antagonist	20–40	Weight gain, sedation	No interference with sexual function, no nausea or diarrhea
Bupropion (Wellbutrin)	Norepinephrine reuptake inhibitor and dopamine reuptake inhibitor	14	Gastrointestinal: nausea, anorexia Risk of seizures at higher doses, less sexual dysfunction	Used for smoking cessation Contraindicated in patients with an eating disorder or a seizure disorder

*Proprietary names are given in parentheses.

Table II–5
MOOD STABILIZERS

NAME*	MECHANISM OF ACTION	HALF-LIFE (H)	SIDE EFFECTS	TESTING	COMMENTS
Lithium	Inhibits adenylate cyclase enzyme	24	Nausea, tremor, hypothyroidism, cardiac dysrhythmias, diarrhea **Diabetes insipidus:** thirst, urination, weight gain, acne At toxic levels, significant alterations in consciousness, seizures, coma, and death may occur	**Serum levels** every 5–7 days with each dose change; every 6–12 months when stable **Renal function tests** (creatinine clearance, serum urea nitrogen, and serum creatinine) every 6–12 months **Thyroid function tests** every 6–12 months, serum human chorionic gonadotropin (hCG) level in women of childbearing age, electrocardiogram	Propranolol may help with tremor; benign increase in white blood cell (WBC) count seen
Valproic acid, valproate (Depakene)	Opens chloride channels, unknown	8	Thrombocytopenia, pancreatitis, weight gain, hair loss, gastrointestinal distress, cognitive dulling, **neural tube defects in pregnancy**	Complete blood count (CBC), liver function tests, pancreatic enzyme levels, serum hCG level in childbearing women	

(Continued)

Table II–5

MOOD STABILIZERS *(Continued)*

NAME*	MECHANISM OF ACTION	HALF-LIFE (H)	SIDE EFFECTS	TESTING	COMMENTS
Carbamazepine (Tegretol)	Inhibits kindling, inhibits repetitive firing of action potentials by inactivating sodium channels	18–55	Nausea, vomiting, slurred speech, dizziness, drowsiness, low WBC count, high liver function tests, cognitive slowing, may cause craniofacial defects in newborn	CBC, liver function tests, pancreatic enzyme levels, serum hCG level in child-bearing women	Potent inducer of P450 system
Lamotrigine (Lamictal)		15	Leukopenia, rash, hepatic failure, nausea, vomiting, diarrhea, somnolence, dizziness	CBC with platelet count every 6–12 months	Alternative choice, may have acute antidepressant effect; dose must be increased slowly to avoid rash
Gabapentin (Neurontin)		5–9	Somnolence, dizziness, ataxia, fatigue, leukopenia, weight gain	Rash can be fatal	No drug interactions

*Proprietary names are given in parentheses.

Table II–6
FIRST-GENERATION ANTIPSYCHOTIC AGENTS

NAME*	HALF-LIFE (H)	POTENCY	COMMENTS
Chlorpromazine (Thorazine)	24	Low	Sedation and orthostatic hypotension are very common
Haloperidol (Haldol)	24	High	**Extrapyramidal syndrome very common;** available in a long-acting intramuscular depot
Thioridazine (Mellaril)	24	Low	Higher incidence of cardiac disturbances, **retinitis pigmentosa**
Mesoridazine (Serentil)	30	Low	Cardiac arrhythmias (torsade de pointe)
Molindone (Lidone, Moban)	12	Medium	
Fluphenazine (Prolixin)	18	High	Available in a long-acting intramuscular depot
Trifluoperazine (Stelazine)	18	High	
Thiothixene (Navane)	34	High	
Perphenazine (Etrafon, Trilafon)	12	High	
Loxapine (Loxitane)	8	Medium	
Pimozide (Orap)	55	High	

*Proprietary names are given in parentheses.

b. **Anticholinergic effects**
c. **Cardiovascular effects**
   i. **Alpha-adrenergic blockade,** which causes **orthostatic hypotension.**

ii. **Cardiac rhythm disturbances,** especially prolongation of the **QT interval.**

d. **Endocrine effects:** Decreasing the amount of dopamine in the pituitary gland leads to increased **prolactin levels,** which can cause gynecomastia and **galactorrhea** as well as sexual dysfunction.

e. **Weight gain.**

B. **Second-generation antipsychotics (atypical antipsychotics):** These medications are more commonly used than first-generation antipsychotics because they are **less likely to produce EPS, tardive dyskinesia, and NMS.** However, many have significant side effects (Table II-7) of their own that limit their use (e.g., **clozapine can cause fatal agranulocytosis).** There is also new concern that the atypical antipsychotics can increase the risk of Type 2 diabetes. The two of most concern are Zyprexa (olanzapine) and Clozaril (clozapine).

III. Anxiolytics and sedative/hypnotics

A. **Benzodiazepines:** These drugs work by binding to sites on gamma-aminobutyric acid (GABA) receptors. They are effective in anxiety and sleep disorders and in anxiety and agitation in other disorders such as acute psychosis. They are generally safe in overdose if used alone. They are metabolized mainly in the liver. Their side effects include sedation, behavioral disinhibition (especially in the young or the elderly), psychomotor impairment, cognitive impairment, confusion, and ataxia. They are **addictive,** and after prolonged use, **withdrawal can cause seizures and death.** Shorter-acting benzodiazepines carry a higher risk for dependency, although they carry less risk of a "hangover" after use. Table II-8 lists commonly used benzodiazepines. Table II-9 lists other anxiolytics.

IV. Drugs used to treat the **side effects** of other psychotropic medications

1. **Anticholinergic agents** used to **treat dystonias** (caused by the use of antipsychotic medication) include benztropine, biperiden, diphenhydramine, and trihexyphenidyl.
2. Medications used to treat **akathisias** (restlessness caused by the use of antipsychotic medication) include **propranolol and benzodiazepines.**
3. Medications used to treat parkinsonian side effects (caused by the use of antipsychotic medication) include **amantadine and levodopa.**

Table II–7
SECOND-GENERATION ANTIPSYCHOTIC AGENTS

NAME*	SITE OF ACTION	HALF-LIFE (H)	SIDE EFFECTS	COMMENTS
Clozapine (Clozaril)	Serotonin-dopamine antagonist	5–15	**Agranulocytosis,** anticholinergic side effects, weight gain, sedation, neuroleptic malignant syndrome	Complete blood count and differential counts required weekly for the first 6 months and biweekly thereafter
Risperidone (Risperdal)	Serotonin-dopamine antagonist	3 in fast metabolizers, 120 in poor metabolizers	Extrapyramidal syndrome with high doses, postural hypotension, increased prolactin; weight gain, sedation, decreased concentration	Present in breast milk
Olanzapine (Zyprexa)	Serotonin-dopamine antagonist	31	Increased prolactin, orthostatic hypotension, anticholinergic side effects, weight gain, **somnolence**	Alanine aminotransferase levels as drug affects the liver
Quetiapine (Seroquel)	Serotonin-dopamine antagonist	7	Orthostatic hypotension, somnolence, transient increase in weight	Slitlamp eye examination at baseline and every 6 months for those at risk for developing cataracts
Ziprasidone (Geodon, Zeldox)	Serotonin-dopamine antagonist	7	Dose-related **QT interval prolongation,** postural hypotension, sedation	Present in breast milk; baseline potassium and magnesium measurements
Aripiprazole	Partial agonist at dopamine and serotonin-1A receptors and antagonist at postsynaptic serotonin-2A receptors	75	Headache, nausea, anxiety, insomnia, somnolence	

*Proprietary names are given in parentheses.

Table II–8
BENZODIAZEPINES

NAME	PROPRIETARY NAME	HALF-LIFE (INCLUDING METABOLITES) (H)
Diazepam	Valium	20–70
Lorazepam	Ativan	10–70
Clonazepam	Klonopin	19–50
Alprazolam	Xanax	8–15
Oxazepam	Serax	5–15
Temazepam	Restoril	8–12
Midazolam	Versed	1.5–3.5
Triazolam	Halcion	1.5–5

Table II-9
OTHER ANXIOLYTICS/SEDATIVE-HYPNOTICS

NAME*	INDICATION	HALF-LIFE (H)	SIDE EFFECTS	COMMENTS
Buspirone (BuSpar)	Generalized anxiety	5–11	Headache, gastrointestinal distress, dizziness	Less useful in patients who have used benzodiazepines; should not be used with monoamine oxidase inhibitors
Zolpidem (Ambien)	For insomnia disorder	2–4	Headache, drowsiness, dizziness, nausea, diarrhea	Increased effect with alcohol or selective serotonin reuptake inhibitors
Zaleplon (Sonata)	For insomnia	1	Headache, peripheral edema, amnesia, dizziness, rash, nausea, tremor	

*Proprietary names are given in parentheses.

Comprehension Questions

[2.1] A 43-year-old woman with a long history of schizophrenia complains of a loss of night vision. Which of the following medications is most likely responsible?

A. Haloperidol
B. Thioridazine
C. Risperidone
D. Chlorpromazine
E. Clozapine

[2.2] A 28-year-old man with a history of a psychiatric admission 6 months previously is seen in the emergency department with a painful erection, which he says has persisted for 18 hours. Which of the following is the best next step?

A. Epinephrine injection into the penis
B. Follow-up in 12 hours
C. Oral benzodiazepines and careful observation
D. Magnetic resonance imaging of the lumbosacral spine
E. IM injection of benztropine

[2.3] A 57-year-old woman complains of feeling dizzy when she gets up in the morning and when standing. She takes imipramine each evening for depression. Which of the following is the most likely cause of her symptoms?

A. Hypovolemia from decreased appetite
B. Hypoglycemia
C. Diabetes insipidus
D. Alpha-adrenergic blockade
E. Dehydration

[2.4] A 34-year-old man is seen in the emergency department with a headache, dizziness, and blood pressure of 210/150 mm Hg. He has no medical problems, states that he feels fine, and says that last night he even had a nice meal with wine. Which of the following medications is he most likely taking?

A. Bupropion
B. Lithium
C. Amitriptyline
D. Phenelzine
E. Fluoxetine

[2.5] A 22-year-old college student with a history of depression is being treated with sertraline. He enjoys drinking beer on the weekends. Which of the following side effects is most likely to occur?

A. Alcohol potentiation
B. Alcohol withdrawal
C. Sexual dysfunction
D. Diabetes insipidus
E. Serotonin syndrome

[2.6] Because of the side effects of his original antidepressant, the college student in question [2.5] is switched to another agent. He comes to the emergency department several days later with muscle spasms, confusion, fever, tachycardia, and hypertension. Which of the following is the most likely cause?

A. Serotonin syndrome
B. Cocaine intoxication
C. Meningitis
D. Alcohol withdrawal (delirium tremens)
E. Neuroleptic malignant syndrome (NMS)

[2.7] A 17-year-old adolescent suffers from bulimia nervosa and is very depressed. She is also suffering from insomnia and apathy. Which of the following medications should be avoided?

A. Fluoxetine
B. Trazodone
C. Imipramine
D. Bupropion
E. Amitriptyline

[2.8] A 32-year-old woman has been taking medication (the name of which she does not remember) for her psychiatric condition. She complains of excessive thirst and urinating "all the time." Which of the following is the most likely diagnosis?

A. Bipolar disorder
B. Major depression
C. Panic disorder
D. Schizophrenia
E. Social phobia

[2.9] A 29-year-old man who "hears voices" at times, complains of a fever and chills. His temperature is 102°F (38.9°C) with no findings of infection. His white blood cell count is 800 cells/mm^3. Which of the following medications is most likely responsible?

A. Haloperidol
B. Risperidone
C. Clozapine
D. Thioridazine
E. Fluphenazine

[2.10] A 38-year-old woman is admitted to the hospital for an elective hysterectomy. On hospital day 3, she experiences auditory and visual hallucinations, has tremors, and is agitated. Which of the following would be the best therapy?

A. Selective serotonin reuptake inhibitor (SSRI)
B. Propranolol
C. Imipramine
D. Benzodiazepine
E. An atypical antipsychotic

[2.11] A 35-year-old African American woman with bipolar disorder delivers a male newborn who has spina bifida. Which of the following is the most likely etiology?

A. Advanced maternal age
B. Mood-stabilizing medication
C. Folate excess
D. Ethnicity
E. Maternal malnutrition

[2.12] A 39-year-old man tries to commit suicide by taking an overdose of amitriptyline tablets. He is rushed to the emergency room where resuscitation is attempted but fails. Which of the following is most likely to be noted during the attempted resuscitation or the autopsy?

A. Massive coronary artery occlusion
B. Aortic valve stenosis
C. Electrocardiographic conduction abnormalities
D. Cardiac tamponade
E. Massive pulmonary embolism

Match the following therapies (A through F) to the clinical scenarios listed (questions [2.13] through [2.16]).

A. Benztropine
B. Propranolol
C. Amantadine
D. Dantrolene
E. Dialysis
F. Flumazenil

[2.13] A 25-year-old man with bipolar disorder took too many pills, had two seizures, and is now in a coma.

[2.14] A 38-year-old schizophrenic woman feels restless and cannot sit still; her physician states that this behavior is caused by her medication.

[2.15] A 32-year-old woman with panic disorder and anxiety took an overdose of diazepam and is taken to the emergency department with somnolence and hypoventilation.

[2.16] A 30-year-old man being treated for schizophrenia complains of tremor and a slow gait.

Answers

[2.1] **B.** High doses of thioridazine are associated with irreversible pigmentation of the retina, leading initially to symptoms of night vision difficulty and ultimately to blindness.

[2.2] **A.** This priapism is most likely caused by trazodone. One treatment is epinephrine injected into the corpus of the penis.

[2.3] **D.** The mechanism for orthostatic hypotension caused by tricyclic/heterocyclic antidepressants is alpha-adrenergic blockade.

[2.4] **D.** This patient probably experienced a hypertensive crisis induced by an interaction between the wine and phenelzine, a MAOI.

[2.5] **C.** Sexual dysfunction is a very common side effect of SSRI medications.

[2.6] **A.** This patient was likely switched from a SSRI, sertraline, to a MAOI, such as phenelzine. Because both agents increase serotonin levels, 5 weeks should elapse between discontinuation of one medication and initiation of the other. The danger is very serious serotonin syndrome, which has features similar to those of NMS.

[2.7] **D.** Seizure disorders and eating disorders are contraindications for bupropion because of its possible lowering of the seizure threshold and its anorectic effects.

[2.8] **A.** This patient has symptoms of diabetes insipidus, a side effect of lithium used in the treatment of bipolar disease.

[2.9] **C.** This individual has neutropenic fever as a result of agranulocytosis, a side effect of the atypical antipsychotic agent clozapine.

[2.10] **D.** This woman is probably experiencing either alcohol or benzodiazepine withdrawal; in either case, benzodiazepines would be the treatment.

[2.11] **B.** This woman was likely taking valproic acid, a mood stabilizer used in treating bipolar disorder, which increases the risk for teratogenicity (e.g., a neural tube defect).

[2.12] **C.** A tricyclic antidepressant overdose can lead to increased QT intervals and ultimately to cardiac dysrhythmias.

[2.13] **E.** Dialysis is used to treat lithium toxicity when it is severe and life-threatening, such as causing seizures or coma.

[2.14] **B.** Akathisia (restlessness) can be treated with propranolol.

[2.15] **F.** A benzodiazepine overdose can be treated with flumazenil, which is a benzodiazepine antagonist.

[2.16] **C.** The parkinsonian-like symptoms of neuroleptic agents are treated with amantadine or levodopa.

CLINICAL PEARLS

- In general, the side effects of tricyclic/heterocyclic antidepressant agents are anticholinergic effects, sedation, orthostatic hypotension, cardiac rhythm disturbances, and weight gain.
- Usually, tricyclic/heterocyclic antidepressants do not cause EPS. An exception to this rule is amoxapine.
- Selective serotonin reuptake inhibitors are the most commonly used medications for depression but should *not* be used in conjunction with MAOIs. One medication should be discontinued for at least 5 weeks before the other is initiated to avoid serotonin syndrome.
- Serotonin syndrome is similar to NMS and is characterized by confusion, muscle rigidity, high temperature, muscle twitching, shivering, and loss of consciousness. It can be fatal.
- The most common side effects of SSRIs are gastrointestinal and sexual dysfunction.
- Individuals taking MAOIs should avoid cheese, wine, liver, and aged foods (tyramine) or an acute hypertensive crisis can ensue.

- Trazodone can lead to priapism; thus, a prolonged painful erection that is trazodone-induced is considered an emergency and is treated with an intracorporeal injection of epinephrine or drainage of blood from the penis.
- Bupropion is used for smoking cessation but must be avoided in patients with eating disorders or seizures.
- Lithium has numerous side effects, including tremor, polyuria/diabetes insipidus, acne, hypothyroidism, cardiac dysrhythmias, weight gain, edema, and leukocytosis.
- Lithium is cleared through the kidneys and must be used with caution in older patients and in those with renal insufficiency.
- Lithium and valproic acid can be teratogenic and must be used with caution in women of childbearing age.
- Antipsychotic agents produce many adverse effects, including EPS, sedation, and orthostatic hypotension.
- Neuroleptic malignant syndrome can be caused at any time by an antipsychotic agent. It typically includes a movement disorder (muscle rigidity, dystonia, agitation) and autonomic symptoms (high fever, sweating, tachycardia, hypertension). White blood cell (WBC) and creatine kinase (CPK) levels are both typically high.
- Clozapine can cause fatal agranulocytosis, and thus leukocyte-count monitoring is mandatory.
- Benzodiazepine withdrawal resembles alcohol withdrawal and can be fatal.

SECTION III

Clinical Cases

❖ CASE 1

A 42-year-old man comes to his outpatient psychiatrist with complaints of a depressed mood, which he states is identical to depressions he has experienced previously. He was diagnosed with major depression for the first time 20 years ago. At that time, he was treated with imipramine, up to 150 mg/day, with good results. During a second episode, which occurred 15 years ago, he was treated with imipramine, and once again his symptoms remitted after 4 to 6 weeks. He denies illicit drug use or any recent traumatic events. The man states that although he is sure he is experiencing another major depression, he would like to avoid imipramine this time because it produced unacceptable side effects such as dry mouth, dry eyes, and constipation.

◆ **What is the best therapy?**

◆ **What are the side effects of the proposed therapy?**

ANSWERS TO CASE 1: Major Depression, Recurrent

Summary: A 42-year-old man complains of symptoms of major depression identical to two prior episodes he experienced in the past. Previously, he was successfully treated with a tricyclic antidepressant (TCA), although this class of medication often produces anticholinergic side effects such as dry mouth, dry eyes, and constipation, which this patient complains about. The question becomes what medication should be used to treat recurrent major depression when tricyclics are not an option.

- **Best therapy:** A selective serotonin reuptake inhibitor (SSRI) such as sertraline, paroxetine, citalopram, or fluoxetine is one of the first-line choices of medication for this patient.

- **Common side effects: Gastrointestinal symptoms**—stomach pain, nausea, and diarrhea—occur in early stages of the treatment. Minor sleep disturbances—either sedation or insomnia—can occur. Other common side effects include tremor, dizziness, increased perspiration, and **male and female sexual dysfunction** (most commonly delayed ejaculation in men and decreased libido in women).

Analysis

Objectives

1. Understand the treatment of uncomplicated major depression without psychotic features.
2. Be able to counsel a patient in regard to the common side effects of SSRIs.

Considerations

Although the patient has been successfully treated with a **TCA** (imipramine) two times in the past, these medications are no longer considered first-line treatments because of their **common side effects and their potential lethality in overdose** (cardiac arrhythmias). For a patient such as this one, one might consider using imipramine again. However, the patient specifically requests another type of medication because of his previous discomfort with the side effects. One of the current first-line treatments for patients with major depression, SSRIs are thus the logical choice; they have fewer side effects and are safer.

Table 1–1 lists the criteria for major depression, recurrent.

Table 1–1
DIAGNOSTIC CRITERIA FOR MAJOR DEPRESSIVE DISORDER, RECURRENT

- Two or more episodes of major depression diagnosed by the following:
  Five or more of the following symptoms have been present most of the time for at least 2 weeks:
  1. Depressed mood
  2. Anhedonia
  3. Significant weight change or change in appetite
  4. Insomnia or hypersomnia
  5. Psychomotor agitation or retardation
  6. Fatigue or loss of energy
  7. Feelings of worthlessness or excessive guilt
  8. Decreased ability to concentrate or indecisiveness
  9. Thoughts of death or suicidal ideation
- There has never been a manic, hypomanic, or mixed episode.
- Symptoms cause significant distress or impairment in functioning.
- Symptoms are not caused by a substance of abuse, medication, or a medical condition.
- Symptoms are not better accounted for by schizophrenia, schizoaffective disorder, delusional disorder, or a psychotic disorder not otherwise specified.
- Symptoms are not better accounted for by bereavement (i.e., symptoms last longer than 2 months; marked functional impairment, suicidal ideation, and/or psychotic symptoms are noted)

APPROACH TO MAJOR DEPRESSIVE DISORDER, RECURRENT

Definitions

Anhedonia: Loss of interest or pleasure in activities that were previously pleasurable.

Selective serotonin reuptake inhibitor: An agent that blocks the reuptake of serotonin from presynaptic neurons without affecting norepinephrine or dopamine reuptake. These agents are used as antidepressants and in treating eating disorders, panic, obsessive-compulsive disorder, and borderline personality disorder.

Clinical Approach

Major depression is a common problem. In the United States, approximately one in seven individuals will suffer from this disorder at some time in their lives. Women are affected twice as often as men, with a mean age of occurrence at 40 years. A common hypothesis concerning the etiology of major depressive disorder involves the alteration of biogenic amines, particularly norepinephrine and serotonin. Genetics plays a role, as evidenced by family studies.

Given the frequency with which depression is a presenting complaint in the primary care setting, a mnemonic is helpful in remembering the criteria for an episode of major depression. As lack of energy is common to most of these episodes, the mnemonic relates to "treating" this symptom by "prescribing energy capsules" and is written on a prescription as **SIG: E**(nergy) **CAPS.** Each letter stands for a criteria (except for depressed mood) used in diagnosing an episode of major depression:

S—sleep changes

I—(decreased) interest

G—(excessive) guilt

E—(decreased) energy

C—(decreased) concentration

A—appetite changes

P—psychomotor agitation or retardation

S—suicidal ideation

Differential Diagnosis

It is important to rule out other disorders that could be causing a depressed state, including medical diseases (e.g., hypothyroidism or multiple sclerosis), medications (e.g., antihypertensives), or substances (e.g., alcohol use or cocaine withdrawal). Obtaining a thorough history, performing a physical examination, and ordering appropriate laboratory studies are crucial in the assessment of any new onset of depression.

Many psychiatric illnesses are characterized by depressive symptoms, including psychotic disorders, anxiety disorders, and personality disorders. A critical distinction to make, especially in recurrent episodes of depression, is between major depressive disorder, recurrent, and bipolar disorder, depressed. This distinction is essential not only for making the correct diagnosis but also for proper treatment. **Standard therapies for major depression can be less effective and actually worsen bipolar** illnesses. It is necessary to obtain any current or past history of episodes of mania, as well as any family history of bipolar disorder.

Assessment of Suicide Risk

One of the most important determinations a clinician must make in the case of a depressed individual is the risk of suicide. The best approach is to ask the patient directly using questions such as, Are you or have you ever been suicidal? Do you want to die? A patient with a specific suicide plan is of special concern. Also, the psychiatrist should be alert to warning signs such as an individual becoming uncustomarily quiet and less agitated after a previous expression of suicidal intent or making a will and giving away personal property. Risk factors for suicide include older age, alcohol or drug dependence, prior suicide attempts, male gender, and a family history of suicide.

The results of a careful mental status examination, risk factors, prior suicidal attempts, and suicidal thoughts and intent must be all considered.

Postpartum Depression

As many as 20% to 40% of U.S. women report some emotional disturbance or problem with cognitive functioning during the postpartum period. Many experience what is known as **postpartum blues,** in which there **is sadness, strong feelings of dependency, frequent crying spells, and dysphoria.** These feelings, which do not constitute major depression and therefore should not be treated as such, seem to be attributable to a combination of the rapid hormonal shifts occurring during the postpartum period, the stress of childbearing, and the sudden responsibility of caring for another human being. Postpartum blues **usually lasts for only several days to a week.** In rare cases, postpartum **depression** exceeds in both severity and length that observed in postpartum blues and is **characterized by suicidality and severely depressed feelings.** Women with postpartum depression need to be treated as one would treat a patient with major depression, taking care to educate them as to the risks of breast-feeding an infant when the antidepressant appears in the milk. Left untreated, postpartum depression can worsen to a point where the patient becomes **psychotic,** in which case antipsychotic medication and hospitalization can be necessary as well.

Treatment

In individuals who suffer from one episode of major depression, there is a **50% to 85% chance of having another episode.** The risk of recurrence increases not only with each subsequent episode but also with the occurrence of residual symptoms of depression between episodes, comorbid psychiatric disorders, and chronic medical conditions. Therefore, adequate treatment resulting in full remission is the goal. The treatment options for recurrent episodes of major depression are not significantly different from those for a first episode: pharmacotherapy, psychotherapy (for mild or moderate symptomatology), a combination of the two, or **electroconvulsive therapy** (ECT) in **major depression with psychotic features or where a rapid response is required.**

Common first-line pharmacotherapy for episodes of major depression includes SSRIs (such as fluoxetine, sertraline, paroxetine, and citalopram), venlafaxine, bupropion, mirtazapine, and duloxetine. Side effects vary among the specific medications and include sedation or activation, weight gain, headache, gastrointestinal symptoms, tremor, elevated blood pressure (for venlafaxine at higher doses), and **sexual dysfunction,** particularly with **SSRIs and venlafaxine.** Although efficacy is essentially equivalent among all classes of antidepressants, **TCAs** such as desipramine and nortriptyline are usually **not considered first-line agents** because their **side effects are less well tolerated,** including **anticholinergic effects, orthostasis, and cardiac effects** leading to lethality in overdose. **Monoamine oxidase inhibitors (MAOIs)** are used less frequently because of their significant **drug–drug interactions** and because **dietary restrictions** are necessary.

A rule of thumb in managing recurrent episodes of major depression is that the particular medication that achieved remission in past episodes is likely to achieve remission in subsequent episodes, often at the same dose. Additional factors to consider when choosing a medication are prior side effects, drug–drug interactions, cost, and patient preference.

Comprehension Questions

[1.1] A 70-year-old woman presents to her primary care provider complaining of fatigue for the past 7 weeks. She admits to difficulty falling asleep, a poor appetite with a 10-lb weight loss, and thoughts of wanting to die. She admits to having had symptoms similar to these on several occasions in the past, but "never this bad." Her medical problems include asthma and a high cholesterol level. She uses an albuterol inhaler only as needed. Which of the following symptoms is necessary in order to make a diagnosis of major depressive disorder?

A. Depressed mood
B. Decreased appetite
C. Fatigue
D. Suicidal ideation
E. Excessive guilt

[1.2] A 44-year-old woman comes to your office for a follow-up visit. She recently received a diagnosis of major depressive disorder and began treatment with citalopram (an SSRI) 6 weeks ago. She claims to feel "happy again," without further depression, crying spells, or insomnia. Her appetite has improved, and she has been able to focus at work and enjoy time with her family. Although she experienced occasional headaches and loose stools at the beginning of her treatment, she no longer complains of any side effects. Which of the following is the most appropriate next step in her treatment?

A. Lower the dose of citalopram
B. Maintain the current dose of citalopram
C. Increase the dose of citalopram
D. Discontinue the citalopram

[1.3] Which of the following side effects common to SSRIs is the woman in question [1.2] most likely to complain of in the future?

A. Anorgasmia
B. Insomnia
C. Nausea
D. Tremor

[1.4] The woman in questions [1.2] and [1.3] is seen one year later for a return visit. She has remained on the citalopram at the same dose, and she is tolerating it well, but she worries about "always having to take medication." What is her risk of recurrence if she is not maintained on antidepressant medication?

A. 0%–20%
B. 20%–50%
C. 50%–85%
D. 85%–100%

Answers

[1.1] **A.** Although a change in appetite, decreased energy, fatigue, and suicidal ideation are all criteria used in diagnosing major depressive disorder, one of the symptoms must be either a depressed mood or anhedonia.

[1.2] **B.** The proper strategy in the management of an episode of major depression that has recently remitted is to continue treatment at the same dose if it can be tolerated. Early discontinuation of medication can lead to an early relapse. A general rule of thumb is, "The dose that got you better will keep you well." A reasonable duration for continuing the medication is 6 to 9 months.

[1.3] **A.** Although activation (causing insomnia), gastrointestinal symptoms (including nausea), and tremor are common side effects of SSRIs, only sexual dysfunction generally occurs later in the treatment course (after weeks to months).

[1.4] **C.** The recommendations for maintenance therapy in major depressive disorder should be made on a case by case basis. However, the illness tends to run a chronic course, especially if treatment is discontinued. Indeed, 50% to 85% of individuals will suffer from at least one further episode, most likely within 2 to 3 years.

CLINICAL PEARLS

- It is important to rule out an underlying substance, medication, or medical condition causing depression, especially if the patient does not have a prior history of depression.
- More than 50% of patients who have had one episode of major depression will have recurrent episodes.
- The risk of further episodes of major depression increases with the number of prior episodes, the occurrence of residual symptoms of depression between episodes, and any comorbid psychiatric or chronic medical illnesses.
- The treatment that was successful for prior episodes of major depression has a higher likelihood of achieving remission in future episodes.
- Selective serotonin reuptake inhibitors, as well as bupropion, venlafaxine, mirtazapine, and duloxetine, are all first-line treatment options for major depressive disorder.

REFERENCES

American Psychiatric Association. Practice guidelines for the treatment of major depressive disorder. Available at: http://www.psych.org/clin_res/depression2e.book.cfm. Accessed July 14, 2005.

Stoudemire A. Clinical psychiatry for medical students, 3rd ed. Philadelphia: Lippincott Williams & Wilkins, 1998:243–245; 257–260.

❖ CASE 2

A 21-year-old man is brought to the emergency department by the police after he was found sitting in the middle of a busy street. By way of explanation, the patient states, "The voices told me to do it." The patient says that for the past year he has felt that "people are not who they say they are." He began to isolate himself in his room and dropped out of school. He claims that he hears voices telling him to do "bad things." There are often two or three voices talking, and they often comment to each other on his behavior. He denies that he currently uses drugs or alcohol, although he reports that he occasionally smoked marijuana in the past. He says that he has discontinued this practice over the past 6 months because "it makes the voices louder." He denies any medical problems and is taking no medication.

On a mental status examination, the patient is noted to be dirty and disheveled, with poor hygiene. He appears somewhat nervous in his surroundings and paces around the examination room, always with his back to a wall. He states that his mood is "Okay." His affect is congruent, although flat. His speech is of normal rate, rhythm, and tone. His thought processes are tangential, and loose associations are occasionally noted. His thought content is positive for delusions and auditory hallucinations. He denies any suicidal or homicidal ideation.

◆ **What is the most likely diagnosis for this patient?**

◆ **What conditions are important to rule out before a diagnosis can be made?**

◆ **Should this patient be hospitalized?**

ANSWERS TO CASE 2: Schizophrenia, Paranoid

Summary: A 21-year-old man is brought to the emergency department after exhibiting bizarre and dangerous behavior. For at least 1 year, he experienced delusions and auditory hallucinations. The hallucinations consist of several voices commenting on the patient's behavior and giving him commands. He became socially isolated and dysfunctional as a result of these symptoms. He denies current drug use or medical problems. A mental status examination shows several abnormalities. Disturbances in grooming, hygiene, and behavior (paranoia) are noted, and he has a flat affect. His thought processes are occasionally loose, and he reports auditory hallucinations and delusions.

- **Most likely diagnosis:** Schizophrenia, probably paranoid type.
- **Important conditions to rule out:** To make a diagnosis of schizophrenia, psychosis secondary to substance abuse and general medical conditions must be ruled out. In addition, schizoaffective disorder and mood disorders must also be excluded.
- **Should this patient be hospitalized:** Yes. He clearly poses a danger to himself (and potentially to others based on the nature of "bad things" he is being commanded to perform) because he listens to the voices and acts on their instructions so as to put himself at risk for serious physical harm (i.e., sitting in the middle of a busy street).

Analysis

Objectives

1. Understand diagnostic criteria of schizophrenia.
2. Understand that other conditions must be ruled out before such a diagnosis can be made.
3. Understand involuntary admission criteria and know when a patient should be admitted.

Considerations

This patient demonstrates the two main diagnostic criteria for schizophrenia: **delusions** (thinks people are not who they say they are) and **auditory hallucinations.** (See Table 2–1 for diagnostic requirements.) The hallucinations are characteristic of those seen in schizophrenia, as there are several voices speaking to each other, and there is both a commentary and command nature to the hallucinations. On a mental status examination, the patient shows loosening of associations as well. He meets the criterion for **social and/or occupational dysfunction,** as he has dropped out of school and socially isolated himself. He has had the disorder for at least 1 year. He denies mood symptoms, drug abuse, and medical problems, although of course these issues would need to be further

Table 2–1
DIAGNOSTIC CRITERIA FOR SCHIZOPHRENIA

- At least two of the following symptoms of psychosis have been present for 1 month:
  1. Delusions
  2. Hallucinations
  3. Disorganized speech
  4. Disorganized or catatonic behavior
  5. Negative symptoms.

Only one of the proceding is needed if the delusions are bizarre, the auditory hallucinations involve comments on the patient, or there are two or more voices talking to each other

- There has to be significant social and/or occupational dysfunction
- Some symptoms are required to be present for at least 6 months; they can include only negative symptoms or less intense positive symptoms
- Both schizoaffective disorder and mood disorder with psychotic features need to be ruled out
- A substance (either of abuse or medication) or general medical condition cannot cause the symptoms

investigated by obtaining a more complete history, performing a physical examination, and ordering the appropriate laboratory tests.

APPROACH TO SCHIZOPHRENIA

Definitions

Bizarre delusions: Delusions that are totally implausible (e.g., having been captured by aliens).

Delusions: Fixed, false beliefs that remain despite clear evidence to the contrary, that are not culturally sanctioned.

Flat affect: The absence of a noticeable emotional state (e.g., no facial expression).

Ideas of reference: False beliefs that, for example, a television or radio performer, a song, or a newspaper article refers to oneself.

Loose associations: Thoughts that are not connected to one another or illogical answers to questions.

Tangentiality: Thoughts can be connected to each other although the patient does not come back to the original point or answer the question.

Negative symptoms of schizophrenia: Affective flattening, alogia (diminished flow and spontaneity of speech), and avolition (lack of initiative or goals).

Positive symptoms of schizophrenia: Ideas of reference, grossly disorganized speech or behavior, delusions (such as paranoia), and hallucinations.

Clinical Approach

Schizophrenia is defined as a disturbance that lasts at least 6 months and includes at least 1 month of active-phase symptoms (two or more of the following: delusions, hallucinations, disorganized speech, grossly disorganized or catatonic behavior, loose associations). There is a 1% lifetime prevalence in the general population, but only about half of those affected ever obtain treatment. The average age of onset is 18 to 25 years in men and 25 to 35 years in women. Women tend to have better outcomes than men. Between 20% and 40% of schizophrenics attempt suicide. Specific risk factors include depressive symptoms—especially hopelessness, under 45 years of age, male gender, unemployment, and recent discharge from the hospital. Ten percent of schizophrenics will successfully complete suicide. The course of schizophrenia is variable. Some individuals demonstrate exacerbations and remissions, whereas others remain chronically ill. Complete remission is unlikely. Significant lifelong impairment is experienced by 40% to 60% of patients.

There are five subtypes of schizophrenia:

1. **Paranoid:** Characterized by preoccupation with one or more delusions or frequent auditory hallucinations.
2. **Disorganized:** Usually characterized by disorganized speech and behavior, with flat or inappropriate affect.
3. **Catatonic:** Characterized by two or more of the following: (a) motor immobility (catalepsy/stupor), (b) excessive purposeless motor activity, (c) extreme negativism (maintenance of rigid posture) or mutism, (d) peculiar voluntary movements such as posturing, stereotyped movements, prominent mannerisms or grimacing, and (e) echolalia/echopraxia.
4. **Undifferentiated:** Two or more of the following are present: delusions, hallucinations, disorganized speech, grossly disorganized behavior, and negative symptoms, but the patient does not meet the criteria for the other subtypes of this disorder.
5. **Residual:** Characterized by the absence of prominent delusions, hallucinations, disorganized speech, or grossly disorganized/catatonic behavior. Continuing evidence of disturbance is indicated by the presence of negative symptoms or two or more criteria in an attenuated form.

Differential Diagnosis

Most important and immediate in the differential diagnosis are **medical conditions characterized by psychotic symptoms** such as **deliria, dementias,**

severe hypothyroidism, and hypercalcemia. Clues are usually provided by the patient's history or the presentation (e.g., no prior psychiatric history, a late age of onset, a positive review of systems). The physical examination, and/or results from laboratory studies (e.g., thyroid function tests, determination of electrolyte levels, rapid plasma reagin [RPR] assist in clarifying the diagnosis.

Alcohol and illicit drugs, either during intoxication (hallucinogens, cocaine, phencyclidine, methamphetamine) or withdrawal (alcohol, benzodiazepines), can produce psychotic symptoms. In particular, phencyclidine intoxication can appear identical to those of schizophrenia. A thorough substance use history, a physical examination including the measurement of vital signs, a determination of blood alcohol level, and a urine toxicology screening reveal substance use as a causal factor in most cases.

A careful examination of the medications a patient is taking, including over-the-counter and herbal supplements, is also important, as **many medications (e.g., steroids and anticholinergics) can cause psychotic states.** Distinguishing schizophrenia from both schizoaffective disorder and mood disorders with psychotic features (such as major depression or bipolar disorder) can be difficult. Patients are frequently poor historians given their psychotic symptoms, and so gathering information from other sources such as prior records, family members, or significant others is imperative because a complete history is needed to clarify the issue. Table 2–2 highlights these differences. The previous distinctions are important not only for the diagnosis but also in determining the treatment and the prognosis. In general, a mood disorder with psychotic features has a better prognosis than schizoaffective disorder, which has a better prognosis than schizophrenia.

Table 2–2
CHARACTERISTICS OF SCHIZOPHRENIA AND MOOD DISORDERS

DIAGNOSIS	PSYCHOTIC SYMPTOMS	MOOD DISORDER
Schizophrenia	Present	Brief duration of mood symptoms
Schizoaffective disorder	Present along with *and* in the absence of mood disorder	Present only with psychotic symptoms
Mood disorder with psychotic features (e.g., major depression with psychosis)	Present only during mood disorder	Present in the absence of psychotic symptoms

Treatment

The cornerstone in the treatment of schizophrenia is the use of newer, **atypical antipsychotic** medications, including risperidone, olanzapine, quetiapine, ziprasidone, and aripiprazole. Although **clozapine** is beneficial, especially in treatment-resistant schizophrenia, the possibility of **agranulocytosis** prevents it from being a first-line drug. Atypical antipsychotics have several advantages over older "typical" antipsychotics such as chlorpromazine and haloperidol. Although typical medications adequately treat the positive symptoms of schizophrenia, they can worsen or actually cause negative symptoms. Atypical medications appear to treat the positive symptoms (at least as well as the older medications) and also treat the negative symptoms. Metabolic syndrome, consisting of obesity, glucose intolerance, hypertension, and dyslipidemia has been identified as a significant issue in treatment with atypical antipsychotics. Clozapine and olanzapine tend to be the worst, whereas ziprasidone and aripiprazole have the least associated problems with metabolic syndrome.

Older antipsychotics also have a higher likelihood of causing unwanted side effects, namely, **extrapyramidal symptoms** (dystonias, parkinsonian symptoms, and akathisia), hyperprolactinemia (leading to impotence, amenorrhea, or gynecomastia), and tardive dyskinesia. Acute symptoms such as **dystonic reactions and parkinsonian symptoms can be managed** by **reducing the dose or adding an anticholinergic drug such as benztropine.** In addition, **akathisia can respond to benzodiazepines or a beta-blocker such as propranolol.** Unfortunately, **tardive dyskinesia is usually a permanent condition** and can be both disfiguring and disabling. **Neuroleptic malignant syndrome (NMS) is the most severe potential side effect and can occur with any antipsychotic at any time during treatment.** Treatment of NMS is largely supportive; dantrolene and bromocriptine are commonly used therapeutic agents.

Comprehension Questions

[2.1] Which of the following symptoms is most specific to a diagnosis of schizophrenia?

A. Auditory hallucinations
B. Belief that one has the power of an alien species
C. Catatonic symptoms
D. Depression
E. Inappropriate affect

Match the most likely diagnosis (A through D) with the following case scenarios (questions [2.2] through [2.4]):

A. Major depression with psychotic features
B. Schizoaffective disorder
C. Schizophrenia
D. Psychosis secondary to a general medical condition

[2.2] A 46-year-old man presents with a long-standing belief that his thoughts are being taken from his head and used to create a blockbuster movie. He is certain that the government is involved because they often communicate with him through a microchip they have implanted in his brain. Although he feels frustrated at being taken advantage of, he denies any significant depressive symptoms and is often able to enjoy playing cards with his peers at the group home.

[2.3] A 58-year-old man presents with 4 weeks of significant depression following the sudden, premature death of his wife of 35 years. He reports difficulty sleeping, a 10-lb weight loss, frequent crying spells, and profound guilt over surviving her. For the last several days, he has been convinced that his body is literally decaying. He admits to seeing his wife's face during the day, as well as hearing her voice telling him to kill himself and join her.

[2.4] A 27-year-old woman states that for approximately 6 months she has believed that Michael Jackson is in love with her. She insists that he has professed his intentions to marry her through messages in his song lyrics. She has written numerous letters to him and loitered around his home, resulting in several arrests. She is irritated because, although he won't meet with her in person, he often calls her name outside her window when no one else is around. For the past several weeks, she has slept approximately only 2 hours a night but still has enough energy to continuously redecorate her apartment in preparation for her wedding to Mr. Jackson. She admits to feeling "on top of the world" because Michael Jackson has chosen her and that she "can't stop talking about it."

Answers

[2.1] **B.** Although all these symptoms can be seen in various psychotic disorders, the presence of a bizarre delusion is the most specific to schizophrenia. Only one psychotic symptom is needed to diagnose schizophrenia if there are bizarre delusions, auditory hallucinations commenting on the patient, or two or more voices speaking to each other.

[2.2] **C.** The most likely diagnosis for this man is schizophrenia. He has been suffering from psychotic symptoms including delusions and auditory hallucinations for more than 6 months. Although he can have brief periods of depressed mood, he does not have a history of major mood disorder.

[2.3] **A.** The most likely diagnosis for this man is major depression with psychotic features. Significant depression and neurovegetative symptoms are present, as well as delusions and auditory and visual hallucinations. Although he has mood symptoms and psychotic symptoms, his history is consistent with major depression because his mood symptoms preceded his psychotic symptoms.

[2.4] **B.** The most likely diagnosis for this woman is schizoaffective disorder. She describes a 6-month history of ideas of reference, delusions, and auditory hallucinations. In addition, she has had clear manic symptoms for the past month, including an elevated mood, a decreased need for sleep, increased energy, increased goal-directed activities, and talkativeness. Although she has symptoms consistent with schizophrenia, she has had a significant episode of mood disorder during her psychotic illness. Her psychotic symptoms, which preceded and occurred in the absence of mood symptoms, make primary mood disorder (mania) with psychotic features less likely.

CLINICAL PEARLS

- ❖ Before diagnosing schizophrenia, remember to rule out any substance abuse, medications, or medical conditions that could be causing the psychotic symptoms.
- ❖ Schizophrenia is a chronic illness, as the diagnosis requires more than 6 months of psychotic symptoms.
- ❖ Positive symptoms of schizophrenia include hallucinations, delusions, ideas of reference, paranoia, grossly disorganized speech or behavior, and loose associations.
- ❖ Negative symptoms of schizophrenia include affective flattening, alogia (diminished flow and spontaneity of speech), and avolition (lack of initiative or goals).
- ❖ Overall, major depression with psychotic features has a better prognosis than schizoaffective disorder, which has a better prognosis than schizophrenia.
- ❖ Clozapine is beneficial, especially in treatment-resistant schizophrenia, but has a significant adverse effect in that it can cause agranulocytosis.
- ❖ Neuroleptic malignant syndrome can occur with any antipsychotic at any time during treatment. Treatment is largely supportive, often including dantrolene or bromocriptine.

REFERENCES

American Psychiatric Association. Practice guidelines for treatment of schizophrenia. Available at: http://www.psych.org/clin_res/pg_schizo.cfm.

Ebert M, Loosen P, Nurcombe B, eds. Current diagnosis and treatment in psychiatry. New York: McGraw-Hill, 2000:260–277.

Kaplan H, Sadock B. Synopsis of psychiatry, 8th ed. Philadelphia: Lippincott Williams & Wilkins, 1998:456–491.

❖ CASE 3

A 36-year-old woman comes to the emergency department with a chief complaint of "I think that I am going crazy." She states that for the past 2 months, she has been experiencing sudden episodes of palpitations, sweating, trembling, shortness of breath, chest pain, dizziness, and feeling as if she is going to die. She has been to the emergency department twice in the past 2 weeks, convinced that she is having a heart attack. However, the results of all her physical and laboratory examinations have been within normal limits. She states that the first episode occurred when she was walking down the street, not thinking about "anything in particular." The episode lasted approximately 15 minutes, although the patient says that it felt like it lasted much longer. Since that time she has had similar episodes once or twice a day, every day. As a result she finds herself worrying almost constantly about when she is going to have another attack. She denies having any other symptoms. She denies drug use and uses alcohol only "occasionally." Her alcohol intake has decreased since the episodes began. Her only medical problem is a 1-year history of hypothyroidism for which she takes Synthroid (levothyroxine).

◆ **What is the differential diagnosis?**

 **What is the next diagnostic step?**

ANSWERS TO CASE 3: Panic Disorder versus Thyroid Medication Overuse

Summary: A 36-year-old woman comes to the emergency department with a chief complaint and symptoms consonant with panic disorder (feeling as if she is going crazy or going to die, chest pain, shortness of breath, palpitations, sweating, trembling, and dizziness). She has been to the emergency department several times with the same symptoms, and no physical problems were found. The episodes have occurred once or twice a day for several months, and nothing in particular seems to precipitate them. The patient spends a lot of time between attacks worrying about when she is going to have another attack. The episodes last approximately 15 minutes. The patient denies alcohol or drug abuse, and her only medical problem is hypothyroidism.

- **Top two diagnoses in the differential:** Panic disorder versus medication (Synthroid)-induced anxiety disorder.

- **Next diagnostic step:** Obtain a thyroid profile and look for elevated levels of thyroid hormone, which if present could explain her symptoms.

Analysis

Objectives

1. Correctly diagnose panic disorder in a patient.
2. Be aware that medical illnesses (or some substances) can cause panic attacks.
3. Understand how to rule out a medical illness or substance use issue by requesting the appropriate laboratory studies.

Considerations

This woman presents with classic symptoms of a panic attack. The **attacks first appeared "out of the blue"** and have occurred **once or twice a day, every day, for the past several months.** They are short-lived in duration, lasting about 15 minutes per episode. The patient spends a lot of time in between the attacks worrying about having another attack, a classic feature of the disease. The patient does not seem to have any symptoms of any other psychiatric disorder. She denies drug or alcohol use other than the occasional use of alcohol (which should be carefully quantified). She has hypothyroidism that is being treated with Synthroid (levothyroxine), which has been known to cause panic attacks when the dose is too high; thyroid studies should be used to rule out this possibility. If the thyroxine level is too high, the diagnosis will be substance-induced anxiety disorder and not anxiety disorder secondary to hyperthyroidism, as might be considered. If the patient has panic disorder, she should be treated with a combination of a selective serotonin reuptake inhibitor (SSRI) and a course of cognitive-behavioral therapy; a short-acting benzodiazepine (alprazolam) can be added for immediate control of her symptoms. The use of benzodiazepine should be discontinued after the first several weeks. If the patient has an anxiety disorder because of a substance (thyroid medication), the dose should be decreased, and the panic symptoms should remit.

APPROACH TO PANIC DISORDER

Definitions

Agoraphobia: Anxiety about being in places or situations from which escape might be difficult (or embarrassing) or in which help can not be available in the event of experiencing a panic attack. These situations include being outside the home alone, being in a crowd, being on a bridge, or traveling on a bus, train, or automobile.

Panic attack: A period of intense fear lasting for a discrete period of time, associated with at least four of the symptoms listed in Table 3–1. The criteria for panic disorder are denoted in Table 3–2.

Clinical Approach

Attacks can vary from several a day to only a few during the course of an entire year. Prior to publication of the *Diagnostic and Statistical Manual of Mental Disorders, 4th edition (DSM-IV),* panic disorders were defined by

Table 3–1
DEFINITION OF PANIC ATTACK

Panic attack consists of discrete episodes of at least four of the following:

1. Palpitations
2. Sweating
3. Trembling
4. Shortness of breath
5. Feeling of choking
6. Chest pain
7. Nausea
8. Dizziness
9. Derealization or depersonalization
10. Fear of losing control or going crazy
11. Fear of dying
12. Numbness or tingling
13. Chills or hot flashes

Table 3–2
DIAGNOSTIC CRITERIA FOR PANIC DISORDER

1. Recurrent, unexpected panic attacks.
2. Attacks followed by 1 month of one of the following: concerns about having additional attacks, worry about the consequences of attacks, or a change in behavior as a result of attacks.
3. Attacks are not caused by substance abuse, by medication, or by a general medical condition.
4. Attacks are not better accounted for by another mental illness.
5. Can occur with or without agoraphobia.

placing boundaries on the quantity and/or minimal time frame necessary between attacks. The *DSM-IV* does not specify the number of attacks necessary nor does it give a time frame. It requires that at least one panic attack be followed by **concern about another attack, fear of the implications of the attack, or a change in behavior related to the attack.** The *DSM-IV* has established two diagnostic criteria for this disorder: **panic disorders with agoraphobia** (anxiety about being in places or situations from which escape would be difficult) and **without agoraphobia.** It is theorized that agoraphobia stems from the fear of having a panic attack in a place from which escape would prove difficult.

Typically, the first panic attack an individual experiences is spontaneous; however, it can also follow excitement, exertion, or an emotional event. The attack begins within a 10-minute period of rapidly intensifying symptoms (extreme fear or a sense of impending doom) and can last up to 20 to 30 minutes. Patients with agoraphobia avoid being in situations where obtaining help from friends or loved ones would be difficult. These individuals typically need to be accompanied when traveling on busy streets or in enclosed areas (tunnels, elevators). Severely affected individuals do not even leave their own homes.

In the general population, the lifetime prevalence rates of panic disorder ranges from 1.5% to 5%. The mean age of presentation is about 25 years of age, with women being two or three times more likely to be affected than men. Approximately one third of patients with panic disorder also have agoraphobia.

Differential Diagnosis

At the top of the differential diagnosis list for panic disorder are the numerous medical conditions that can cause panic attacks. Table 3–3 lists some of them. Intoxication caused by amphetamines, cocaine, or hallucinogens and by withdrawal from alcohol or other sedative-hypnotic agents can mimic panic disorder. Medications such as steroids, anticholinergics, and theophylline are also well known to produce anxiety. Obtaining a thorough history (including details of alcohol and substance use) and performing a physical examination can usually clarify the issue. Except for the elevated blood pressure and pulse rate found in anxious states, no abnormalities are seen on examination. Any significant abnormal findings discovered should prompt a further workup for a nonpsychiatric cause. Treating the underlying conditions, adjusting medications, and/or initiating a detoxification process are also likely to resolve the anxiety symptoms.

Table 3–3
MEDICAL CONDITIONS CAUSING PANIC ATTACKS

Cardiovascular diseases
- Anemia
- Angina
- Congestive heart failure
- Myocardial infarction

Endocrine diseases
- Addison disease
- Carcinoid syndrome
- Hyperthyroidism
- Hypoglycemia
- Hypoparathyroidism
- Pheochromocytoma

Neurologic diseases
- Epilepsy
- Huntington's chorea
- Migraine
- Multiple sclerosis
- Transient ischemic attacks
- Wilson disease

Pulmonary diseases
- Asthma
- Hyperventilation
- Pulmonary embolus

Other diseases
- Anaphylaxis
- Electrolyte disturbances
- Heavy-metal poisoning
- Systemic lupus erythematosus
- Uremia
- Vitamin B_{12} deficiency

Reproduced, with permission, from Kaplan H, Sadock B. Synopsis of psychiatry, 8th ed. Baltimore: Lippincott Williams & Wilkins, 1998:586.

Distinguishing panic disorder from other anxiety disorders can often be confusing. Panic attacks can be seen in many other anxiety states, as well as in depression. In fact, major depressive disorder has a high rate of comorbidity with panic disorder. The **hallmark of panic disorder is *unexpected* panic attacks not provoked by any particular stimulus.** This condition is distinct from other anxiety disorders, where panic attacks are the result of exposure to a certain cue. For example, a car backfiring might provoke a panic attack in a patient with posttraumatic stress disorder, or being near a dog might provoke a panic attack in someone with a specific phobia to dogs. The other important aspect to remember is that in panic disorder, the *fear is actually of having an attack,* not of a specific situation (contamination in the case of obsessive-compulsive disorder or performance in the case of social phobia) or of a number of activities (as in generalized anxiety disorder).

Treatment

Antidepressants such as SSRIs, tricyclic antidepressants, and monoamine oxidase inhibitors are highly effective in treating panic disorder. Best results are obtained when medication is used in combination with a course of cognitive behavioral therapy (CBT). As in depression, a significant therapeutic effect can not be seen for several weeks. Treatment with a **benzodiazepine may be needed on a short-term basis to provide more immediate relief.** Given the addictive potential of benzodiazepines, as well as the significant comorbidity of alcohol abuse in panic disorder, the goal should be to use as small a dose for as short a period of time as possible, with the intention of discontinuing this medication once the antidepressant reaches full effect. Cognitive behavioral therapy teaches the patient about the disorder, helps reduce or eliminate core fears, and specifically addresses the restrictions on lifestyle present in individuals with this condition.

Comprehension Questions

[3.1] A 28-year-old man describes a persistent fear of speaking in public. Although he does not have difficulty with one-on-one situations, when giving a lecture he becomes extremely anxious, worrying that he will be humiliated. He relates one episode in which he was forced to speak at the last minute, which resulted in his experiencing panic, shaking, abdominal cramps, and a fear that he would defecate on himself. Because of this problem, he has been held back from promotion at his place of business. Which of the following is the most likely diagnosis?

A. Generalized anxiety disorder
B. Panic disorder
C. Social phobia
D. Specific phobia

[3.2] A 40-year-old woman presents with complaints of not being able to leave her house. For the past 5 years, she has had increasing difficulty traveling far from home. She constantly worries that she will not be able to get help if she "freaks out." In fact, she has had numerous unprovoked episodes of intense fear, associated with shortness of breath, chest pain, diaphoresis, and dizziness, that lasted for 20 minutes. She is convinced that if she drives too far from home, she will have an attack and not be able to obtain help. Which of the following is the most likely diagnosis?

A. Generalized anxiety disorder
B. Panic disorder
C. Social phobia
D. Specific phobia

[3.3] A 25-year-old woman describes a lifelong history of being "scared of heights." She becomes uncomfortable when higher than three stories and whenever traveling or shopping becomes preoccupied with knowing the heights of buildings. On finding herself at a significant elevation, she has severe anxiety symptoms such as trembling, lightheadedness, numbness and tingling, and a fear of dying. Which of the following is the most likely diagnosis?

A. Generalized anxiety disorder
B. Panic disorder
C. Social phobia
D. Specific phobia

[3.4] The chief complaint of a 33-year-old man is, "I'm going to have a heart attack like my father." He explains that his father died of a myocardial infarction at 45 years of age. He is convinced that he is experiencing angina attacks consisting of nervousness, sweating, palpitations, flushing, and numbness in his hands and lasting approximately 5 minutes. He is anxious about having these symptoms and, despite negative results from a cardiology workup, remains certain that he will suffer a heart attack. His behavior and lifestyle have not been otherwise affected. Which of the following is the most likely diagnosis?

A. Generalized anxiety disorder
B. Panic disorder
C. Social phobia
D. Specific phobia

Answers

[3.1] **C.** The most likely diagnosis for this man is social phobia. Although he suffers from panic attacks, they are not unprovoked as in panic disorder because they occur in response to public speaking. His fear is not of having further attacks but rather of being embarrassed or humiliated.

[3.2] **B.** This woman most likely has panic disorder with agoraphobia. She experiences recurrent spontaneous panic attacks and between attacks worries about having further attacks. She avoids driving away from her home for fear of being unable to obtain help in the event of an attack.

[3.3] **D.** Specific phobia is the most likely diagnosis for this woman. Although she has panic attacks, they are not unexpected and result from being in a high place. Her fears are actually of a situation (heights) rather than of having further panic attacks.

[3.4] **B.** The most likely diagnosis for this man is panic disorder without agoraphobia. He displays characteristic features of panic attacks, such as recurrent episodes of anxiety associated with physical symptoms. These episodes are spontaneous, and he worries about the consequences of having an additional attack, namely, a myocardial infarction.

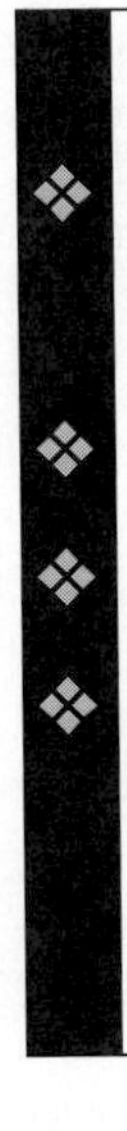

CLINICAL PEARLS

- Panic disorder is characterized by recurrent, unexpected panic attacks associated with worry about having additional attacks, the consequences of attacks, or a change in behavior as a result of attacks.
- Any medical conditions, medications, or substance abuse that can cause panic attacks should be ruled out.
- Major depressive disorder is commonly seen in patients with panic disorder.
- Selective serotonin reuptake inhibitors or other antidepressants, in combination with cognitive behavioral therapy, are used in the pharmacologic treatment of panic disorder. If benzodiazepines are also administered, they should be used in as low a dose and for as short a time as possible.

REFERENCES

American Psychiatric Association. Treatment guidelines for panic disorder. Available at: http://www.psych.org/clin_res/panic_disorder_qrg9402.pdf.

Ebert M, Loosen P, Nurcombe B, eds. Current diagnosis and treatment in psychiatry. New York: McGraw-Hill, 2000:330–334.

Foa EB, Franklin MF, Moser J. Context in the clinic: How well do cognitive-behavioral therapies and medications work in combination? Biol Psychiatry 2002;52(10):987–997.

Kaplan H, Sadock B. Synopsis of psychiatry, 8th ed. Baltimore: Lippincott Williams & Wilkins, 1998:586,596–597.

Roy-Byrne PP, Craske MG, Stein MB, et al. A randomized effectiveness trial of cognitive-behavioral therapy and medication for primary care panic disorder. Arch Gen Psychiatry 2005;62(3):290–298.

❖ CASE 4

A 55-year-old woman comes to a psychiatrist complaining of experiencing a depressed mood over the past 3 months. She notes that her mood has been consistently low, and she describes her condition as "just not me." She has also noticed a decrease in energy and a weight gain of 6 to 7 lb occurring over the same period of time, although her appetite has not increased. She has never visited a psychiatrist before and does not remember ever feeling this depressed for this long before. She states that she has no medical problems that she is aware of and that she takes no medication. Her family history is positive for a history of schizophrenia in one maternal aunt.

On a mental status examination the patient appears depressed and tired, although she has a normal range of affect. Her thought processes are linear and logical. She is not suicidal or homicidal and does not report hallucinations or delusions. Her physical examination reveals a blood pressure of 110/70 mm Hg and a temperature of 98°F (36.7°C). Her thyroid gland is diffusely enlarged but not painful. Her heart has a regular rate and rhythm. She has coarse, brittle hair but no rashes.

- **What is the most likely diagnosis?**

- **What is the next diagnostic step?**

ANSWERS TO CASE 4: Hypothyroidism with Depression

Summary: A 55-year-old woman presents to a psychiatrist with a depressed mood, decreased energy, and a weight gain. She has never had these symptoms before. The results of the rest of her mental status examination are normal. Her physical examination is notable for a diffusely enlarged thyroid gland.

 **Most likely diagnosis:** Mood disorder secondary to a general medical condition.

◆ **Next diagnostic step:** Obtain thyroid studies for this patient, including determinations of thyroid stimulating hormone (TSH), triiodothyronine, and thyroxine levels.

Analysis

Objectives

1. Recognize mood disorder occurring secondary to a general medical condition.
2. Use the most likely diagnosis for this patient to guide the laboratory examination required for a patient with suspected hypothyroidism.

Considerations

Although this patient's history is consistent with that of major depression, two elements are atypical, and one very much so. A weight gain is observed in patients with atypical major depression, but this condition is usually accompanied by an increase in appetite. A weight gain in the absence of an increase in appetite is a clue to the metabolic changes caused by this patient's hypothyroidism. At times the clinical features of hypothyroidism are evident. An enlarged thyroid is not seen in patients with major depression but is a clue that guides the specific laboratory examinations chosen in this case.

APPROACH TO MOOD DISORDER BECAUSE OF A GENERAL MEDICAL CONDITION

Clinical Approach

Diagnosis of this disorder requires a disturbance in mood that causes significant distress or an impairment in functioning. It can resemble either an episode of depression (depressed mood or decreased pleasure) or an episode of mania (elevated or irritable mood). The history, the physical examination, or the laboratory findings must demonstrate a causal physiologic relationship between the medical illness and the change in mood. In other words, the depression or mania cannot result only from the *stress* of having a medical condition. The mood episode also should not occur only during a delirium.

Differential Diagnosis

The differential diagnosis for mood disorder because of a general medical condition is large given the numerous medical and neurologic conditions that can cause depression or another mood state. Table 4–1 lists many of them. Also

Table 4–1
MEDICAL CONDITIONS CAUSING MOOD DISORDER

MEDICAL CONDITION	MOOD DISORDER
Parkinson disease	Depression
Huntington disease	Depression or mania
Wilson disease	Mania
Cerebrovascular accident	Depression or mania
Cerebral neoplasm	Depression or mania
Cerebral trauma	Depression or mania
Encephalitis	Depression or mania
Multiple sclerosis	Depression or mania
Temporal lobe epilepsy	Mania
Hyperthyroidism	Depression or mania
Hypothyroidism	Depression
Hyperparathyroidism	Depression
Hypoparathyroidism	Depression
Uremia	Depression or mania
Cushing syndrome	Depression
Addison disease	Depression
Systemic lupus erythematosus	Depression
Rheumatoid arthritis	Depression
Folate deficiency	Depression
Vitamin B_{12} deficiency	Depression or mania
Human immunodeficiency virus disease	Depression

Table 4–2
MEDICATIONS CAUSING DEPRESSIVE SYMPTOMS

Cardiac and antihypertensive drugs	Analgesics and anti-inflammatory medications
Clonidine	Ibuprofen
Hydralazine	Indomethacin
Propranolol	Opiates
Reserpine	**Antimicrobials**
Digitalis	Ampicillin
Procainamide	Clotrimazole
Lidocaine	Griseofulvin
Methyldopa	Metronidazole
Sedatives and hypnotics	Nitrofurantoin
Barbiturates	Streptomycin
Chloral hydrate	Sulfamethoxazole
Benzodiazepines	Sulfonamides
Steroids and hormones	Tetracycline
Corticosteroids	**Antineoplastic medications**
Oral contraceptives	Azathioprine
Prednisone	Vincristine
Triamcinolone	Bleomycin
Neurologic agents	Trimethoprim
Amantadine	
Baclofen	
Bromocriptine	
Carbamazepine	
Levodopa	
Phenytoin	

Reproduced, with permission, from Stoudemire A. Clinical psychiatry for medical students, 3rd ed. Philadelphia, PA: Lippincott Williams & Wilkins. 1998:120–121.

important in this differential diagnosis are substance-induced mood disorders caused not only by alcohol and illicit drugs (in intoxication and in withdrawal) but also by a vast number of medications. See Table 4–2 for a partial list of medications that can cause depressive symptoms. Making a distinction between primary (psychiatric) and secondary (induced) mood disorder can sometimes be difficult, especially because stressors such as medical illnesses themselves can trigger episodes of both major depression and mania.

Treatment

The treatment of mood disorder caused by a general medical condition entails addressing the underlying medical condition first, if possible, and obtaining improvement in the symptoms. For example, in the previously described case, if the woman is found to have hypothyroidism and subsequently treated with thyroid supplementation, she will likely experience an improvement in mood. Mood symptoms caused by medical or neurologic conditions that are recurrent, chronic, or otherwise untreatable (e.g., dementias, strokes, malignancies) often respond to typical psychopharmacologic treatments such as selective serotonin reuptake inhibitors, tricyclic antidepressants, mood stabilizers, and electroconvulsive therapy.

Comprehension Questions

For the following clinical vignettes (questions [4.1] through [4.5]), choose the one most likely diagnosis (A through D):

A. Bipolar disorder, manic
B. Episode of major depression
C. Mood disorder caused by a general medical condition
D. Substance-induced mood disorder

[4.1] An 18-year-old man presents with 3 days of an irritable mood, decreased sleeping, talkativeness, increased energy, and distractibility. He has no personal or family psychiatric history and no current medical problems. His mental status examination is remarkable for psychomotor agitation and an irritable affect. He is paranoid but denies delusions or hallucinations. His physical examination is notable for a slightly elevated pulse rate and blood pressure as well as markedly dilated pupils bilaterally. The results of his urine toxicology screening are positive for cocaine.

[4.2] A 39-year-old woman presents with 1 month of a gradually worsening depressed mood, with increased sleeping, low energy, and difficulty concentrating but no appetite or weight changes. Her medical history is significant for multiple sclerosis, but she is currently not taking any medication. Her mental status examination is notable for psychomotor slowing and depressed facies. Her physical examination demonstrates several different sensory and motor deficits.

[4.3] A 52-year-old male executive presents with an onset of depression, early-morning awakening, decreased energy, distractibility, anhedonia, poor appetite, and weight loss for the past 3 months. His symptoms began shortly after he suffered a myocardial infarction. Although he did not experience significant sequelae, he has felt less motivated and fulfilled in his life and work, believing that he is now "vulnerable." As a result, he does not push himself as he used to, and his output is beginning to decline.

[4.4] An 80-year-old woman without a psychiatric history is examined after a left-sided cerebral vascular accident has left her paralyzed on her right side. Since her stroke, she complains of an absence of pleasure in anything that she formerly enjoyed. She describes frequent crying spells, increased sleeping, a decreased appetite with weight loss, and feelings of hopelessness and helplessness.

[4.5] A 36-year-old man with a past history of a major depressive episode is brought into the emergency room by the police after stopping traffic on the highway proclaiming that he is "the Messiah." His wife is contacted who states that he has been walking throughout the house all night for the last 4 nights, talking "nonstop," and starting many home repair projects that remain unfinished. She believes that he is only taking sertraline for his depression and propranolol for high blood pressure. His blood alcohol level is less than 10, and his urine toxicology screen is negative.

Answers

[4.1] **D.** The most likely diagnosis for this man is substance (cocaine)-induced mood disorder. Although he presents with classic manic symptoms (irritable mood, decreased sleep, etc.), he has no psychiatric or family history of mood disorder. His physical examination reveals several findings not necessarily consistent with mania, namely, elevated vital signs (pulse rate and blood pressure) and dilated pupils. The important factor in this case is his obvious cocaine use, which can produce symptoms mimicking those of acute mania.

[4.2] **C.** The most likely diagnosis in this case is mood disorder caused by a general medical condition, namely, multiple sclerosis. Although this woman displays the characteristic symptoms of an episode of major depression (depressed mood, increased sleeping, low energy), she does not exhibit the appetite or weight changes commonly seen in this illness. Steroids often cause mood symptoms such as depression or mania, but she is currently not taking any medication. The results of her physical examination are also consistent with a flare-up of her multiple sclerosis and demonstrate a temporal relationship to her depression. The central nervous system white matter lesions seen on imaging are known to cause a depressive state.

[4.3] **B.** The most likely diagnosis for this man is major depression. He has symptoms typical of the disorder, both depressed mood and neurovegetative symptoms lasting for more than 2 weeks. Although his condition was preceded by a heart attack, it was not a physiologic cause of his depression. Rather, his medical illness (and subsequent feeling of vulnerability) was the stressor that brought on his episode of depression.

[4.4] **C.** The most likely diagnosis in this case is mood disorder caused by a general medical condition, namely, a cerebral vascular accident. The patient has obvious symptoms of a depressive illness, including anhedonia. These symptoms also have a clear temporal relationship to her stroke, which has left her with significant motor deficits. Cerebral vascular events, especially those affecting the left frontal region (where the stroke occurred), are well known to result in depression.

[4.5] **A.** The most likely diagnosis for this man is bipolar disorder, manic. He has classic symptoms and signs of the illness, such as decreased need for sleep, talkativeness, increased activity, risky behavior, and delusions of grandeur. He also has a history of a major depressive episode and has been taking an antidepressant which can have caused a switch into his current manic episode. Although he is taking a beta-blocker for hypertension, this would be likely to cause a depressive episode rather than a manic episode.

CLINICAL PEARLS

❖ A complete medical history, a physical examination, and routine laboratory tests, including thyroid studies, are essential in the workup for an individual presenting with a first episode of mood disorder.

❖ Atypical symptoms, such as weight gain without an increase in appetite, suggest mood disorder caused by a general medical condition.

❖ The medical condition is required to have a causal physiologic relationship to the mood episode for mood disorder secondary to a medical condition to be diagnosed.

❖ Strokes, especially left frontal strokes, commonly cause subsequent episodes of depression.

REFERENCES

Kaplan H, Sadock B. Synopsis of psychiatry, 9th ed. Baltimore: Lippincott Williams & Wilkins, 2003:738–739.

Stoudemire A. Clinical psychiatry for medical students, 3rd ed. Philadelphia: Lippincott Williams & Wilkins, 1998:120–121.

CASE 5

A 14-year-old boy is brought to the emergency department after being found in the basement of his home by his parents during the middle of a school day. The parents came home after receiving a call from the school reporting that their son had not attended school for 4 days. The boy was furiously working on a project he claimed would solve the fuel crisis. He had started returning home from school after his parents left for work because his science teacher would no longer let him use the school laboratory after school hours. The patient was involved in an altercation with the school janitor after being asked to leave the school because it was so late. The boy claimed that the janitor was a foreign spy trying to stop his progress.

The parents are very proud of their son's interest in science but admit that he has been more difficult to manage lately. He can't stop talking about his project, and others cannot get a word in edgewise. His enthusiasm is now palpable. For the past few weeks, he reads late into the night and gets minimal sleep. Despite this, he seems to have plenty of energy and amazes his parents' friends with detailed plans of how he is going to save the world. His friends have not been able to tolerate his increased interest in his project. His train of thought is difficult to follow. He paces around the examination room, saying "[I am] anxious to get back to my project before it is too late." Although he has no suspects in mind, he is concerned that his life may be in danger because of the importance of his work.

- **What is the most likely diagnosis?**

- **What is the best treatment?**

ANSWERS TO CASE 5: Bipolar Disorder (Child)

Summary: A 14-year-old boy is brought to the emergency department by his parents because he has been skipping school to work feverishly on a project he says will save the world. The problem appears to have escalated over the past few weeks. He does not sleep, yet he has plenty of energy. His thoughts are disordered, and he has no insight into his intrusiveness or how much he annoys people with his excessive, incessant talking. He is irritable and labile. He has paranoid and grandiose thoughts.

Most likely diagnosis: Bipolar I disorder, single manic episode, with psychotic features

Best treatment: Mood stabilizer (such as valproic acid or lithium) and atypical antipsychotic agent. According to American Academy of Child and Adolescent Psychiatry (AACAP) guidelines, monotherapy with the traditional mood stabilizers lithium, divalproex, and carbamazepine or the atypical antipsychotics olanzapine, quetiapine, and risperidone is the first line treatment if no psychosis is present. **The majority of the guideline panel recommended lithium or divalproex as the first medication choice for nonpsychotic mania.** Given that this patient has signs of significant thought disorder and paranoia, he should be started on both a mood stabilizer and an atypical antipsychotic medication.

Analysis

Objectives

1. Understand the diagnostic criteria for bipolar disorder.
2. Understand the criteria for inpatient psychiatric treatment for this disorder.
3. Understand the initial plan for the treatment of bipolar disorder.

Considerations

The patient presents with grandiosity, inflated self-esteem, paranoia, a decreased need for sleep, an increased energy level, pressured speech, and an increased motor activity level. It seems as if the symptoms have been building for several weeks. The boy does not appear distressed and neither were his parents until his behavior became more troublesome, and his school performance was affected. It is unclear whether this is the first such episode for this patient. Although this patient presents with classical euphoric mania, it is important to remember that children with bipolar disorder often present with a mixed or dysphoric picture characterized by short periods of intense mood labiality and irritability. Is there a need for hospitalization? Yes. The patient does not appear to be an acute danger to himself or to others although he has clearly become increasingly difficult to manage. His parents were unaware that he had been leaving school early and are unsure what others activities he engaged in or where he might have been. The patient is at high risk for engaging in impulsive actions that have the potential for painful consequences (sexual indiscretions, buying sprees, or other pleasurable but risky behaviors). An inpatient setting would be ideal for starting treatment with medications rapidly and titrating to efficacy. Because the patient is a minor, his parents can sign him into a hospital voluntarily. After starting a mood stabilizer and atypical antipsychotic medication, the patient would be monitored closely. If there is only a partial response to therapeutic doses of the medications, then addition of another mood stabilizer would be indicated. If no response is seen then a switch to a new mood stabilizer would be the best course of action.

APPROACH TO BIPOLAR DISORDER (CHILD)

Definitions

Bipolar type I disorder: A syndrome with complete manic symptoms occurring during the course of the disorder.

Bipolar type II disorder: Hypomania; characterized by depression and episodes of mania that don't meet the full criteria for manic syndrome. *See* Hypomania.

Hypomania: Symptoms are similar to those of mania, although they do not reach the same level of severity or cause the same degree of social impairment. Although hypomania is often associated with an elated mood and very little insight into it, patients do not usually exhibit psychotic symptoms, racing thoughts, or marked psychomotor agitation.

Rapid-Cycling Bipolar Disorder: Occurrence of at least four episodes—both retarded depression and hypomania/mania—in a year.

Labile: A mood and/or affect that switches rapidly from one extreme to another. For example, a patient can be laughing and euphoric one minute, followed by a display of intense anger and then extreme sadness in the following minutes of an interview.

Clinical Approach

The *Diagnostic and Statistical Manual of Mental Disorders, 4th edition (DSM-IV)* criteria for a diagnosis of bipolar disorder in children (see Table 5–1) are the same as those for adults. **However, current child psychiatric literature suggests that many juveniles with bipolar disorder have a presentation of severe mood dysregulation with multiple intense, prolonged mood swings every day consisting of short periods of euphoria followed by longer periods of irritability.** These children can average between 3 to 4 cycles per day. As a result, the clinician can see youth diagnosed with bipolar disorder

Table 5–1
DIAGNOSTIC CRITERIA FOR BIPOLAR DISORDER IN CHILDREN*

A distinct period of abnormally and persistently elevated, expansive, or irritable mood lasting at least 1 week (or any duration if hospitalization is required). Three or more of the following symptoms during this period: inflated self-esteem or grandiosity; decreased need for sleep; greater talkativeness than usual or pressure to keep talking; flight of ideas or subjective experience that thoughts are racing; distractibility; increase in goal-directed activity or psychomotor agitation; excessive involvement in pleasurable activities with a high potential for painful consequences:

A. Criteria for a mixed episode are not met.
B. Disturbance is severe enough to cause impairment in normal functioning.
C. Symptoms are not caused by the effect of a substance or a medical condition.

*The current *Diagnostic and Statistical Manual of Mental Disorders* diagnosis for bipolar disorder does not have any modifications for the disorder in children.

who do not meet the *DSM-IV* criteria. The incidence of mood disorders increases with increasing age until adulthood. They are rare in pre–school-age children. The rate of occurrence of bipolar I disorder is 0.2% to 0.4% in prepubertal children. Because the symptoms of mania rarely occur before adolescence, it can take years to diagnose a child with bipolar disorder who presents with childhood depressive symptoms. The prevalence of adolescent bipolar disorder in the general population is about 1%.

Mood disorders tend to cluster in families. The rate of mood disorders in the children of adults with these disorders is at least three times the rate seen in the general population with a lifetime risk of 15% to 45%. The finding that identical twins have a concordance rate of 69% for bipolar disorder compared to a 19% rate for dizygotic twins indicates a strong genetic component but also suggests an effect of psychosocial issues on the development of mood disorders.

Bipolar I disorder is rarely diagnosed before puberty because of the absence of episodes of mania. Usually, an episode of major depression precedes an episode of mania in an adolescent with bipolar I. Mania is recognized by a definite change from a preexisting state and is usually accompanied by grandiose and paranoid delusions and hallucinatory phenomena. **In childhood, episodes of mania consist of extreme mood variability, cyclic aggressive behavior, high levels of distractibility, and a poor attention span. In adolescence, episodes of mania are often accompanied by psychotic features,** and hospitalization is frequently necessary. Hypomania must be differentiated from attention-deficit/hyperactivity disorder (ADHD), which is characterized by distractibility, impulsivity, and hyperactivity that is present on a daily basis consistently since before the patient was 7 years old. Children with ADHD will frequently develop oppositional defiant disorder (ODD), where the patient defiantly opposes the wishes of others and breaks minor rules, or conduct disorder (CD), where the youth defiantly breaks major social rules. A youth who has both ADHD and ODD or CD can present with a pattern of distractibility, motor agitation, and impulsive anger outbursts that can be mistaken for bipolar disorder. The history of the behavior in the preschool age then becomes a key piece of information, as bipolar disorder is extremely rare in this age range whereas ADHD and ODD are very common.

Differential Diagnosis

The psychomotor agitation or increase in activity level often associated with bipolar disorder must be carefully differentiated from the symptoms of ADHD, especially if the child also has ODD or CD. If the episode occurring is a depressive one, other mood disorders must be ruled out, including major depression or an adjustment disorder with a depressed mood. Mood disorders related to substance intoxication, anxiety disorders, the side effects of a medication, or a general medical condition must also be excluded.

Working with Children and Their Families

Treatment guidelines of the AACAP note that the family is essential in providing the detailed past history and current observations needed to make an accurate diagnosis. In the process of taking a history, it is critical to consider if the parents or other family members have been diagnosed as having bipolar disorder or if the family members have undiagnosed or untreated bipolar disorder. In such cases, assuring that the family members are receiving adequate treatment for their illness can have major beneficial effects on the child's environment. Finally, it is critical to make sure that the families fully understand what bipolar disorder is, its clinical course, how it can be effectively treated, and the availability of bipolar disorder support groups.

Treatment

Medications play a significant role in the treatment of bipolar disorder, and AACAP treatment algorithms should be consulted when providing care to juveniles with bipolar disorder. Often **mood-stabilizing agents such as lithium carbonate, carbamazepine, and divalproex** can be helpful in preventing and treating manic phases. All must have blood levels monitored to assure dosing in a therapeutic range. Treatment guidelines developed by the AACAP note the lack of good research data in treating depressed bipolar youth but do note that lithium can be recommended as a treatment option in youth with bipolar depression. Selective serotonin reuptake inhibitors and buproprion can also be considered based on the AACAP guidelines, and lamotrigine and divalproex are other treatment options noted. **Many antidepressants are believed to be able to trigger or "unmask" mania,** and so they should be used carefully, and patients should be observed closely for emergent manic symptoms. Patients on lithium need to have thyroid and kidney function monitored on a regular basis, whereas those on carbamazepine need close monitoring for rare aplastic anemia or agranulocytosis. In addition to monitoring for liver function and platelet levels if the patient is on divalproex, a number of studies have suggested a high rate of polycystic ovarian syndrome in women with epilepsy who are treated with divalproex, raising concerns about the long-term used of divalproex in young women with bipolar disorder. Many mood stabilizers have shown evidence of **teratogenic effects.** For this reason, pregnancy tests should be performed on all females of childbearing age before prescribing these drugs. **Atypical antipsychotics such as olanzapine, risperidone, and quetiapine** have **also been used as monotherapy to control episodes of mania.** Patients placed on atypical antipsychotics should be carefully monitored for development of a metabolic syndrome consisting of weight gain, diabetes mellitus, and hypercholesterolemia. **Tardive dyskinesia** is a possible side effect of the atypical antipsychotics, and an assessment of abnormal movements should be done at baseline and regular intervals using the Abnormal Involuntary Movement Scale (AIMS).

The treatment of bipolar disorder in childhood can be very difficult. There are numerous comorbid psychiatric diseases, particularly ADHD. If treatment of the bipolar disorder is adequate, but any comorbid psychiatric disorders are not addressed, the child will continue to have academic and functional impairment. The lack of recognition of the high degree of comorbidity could lead to false assumptions about treatment success and repeated, unnecessary medication trials.

The **treatment of bipolar disorder in children involves both psychotherapy and psychopharmacotherapy.** The school and the family should be included in the treatment, as the ramifications of bipolar disorder in an individual can have far-reaching effects. **Cognitive therapy** is often an important component of treatment and focuses on **reducing negative thoughts and building self-esteem. Family therapy** can be indicated in situations where family dynamics might be a factor contributing to the symptoms.

Comprehension Questions

[5.1] Which of the following medications is used to treat episodes of mania?

A. Accutane (isotretinoin)
B. Beclomethasone
C. Clindamycin
D. Divalproex
E. Erythromycin

[5.2] Which of the following statements is true regarding bipolar disorder in childhood?

A. Current research suggests that many children with bipolar disorder do not present in the same manner as adults.
B. Youth presenting with bipolar mania with psychotic features should initially be treated with either a mood stabilizer or an atypical antipsychotic.
C. The incidence of prepubertal bipolar disorder is the same as in adolescents, both being about 1%.
D. Psychotherapy has little role in the treatment of bipolar disorder.
E. Lithium, divalproex, and carbamazepine can be administered without concern to pregnant women.

[5.3] Which of the following statements is most accurate regarding mood disturbances in childhood and adolescence?

A. Mood-stabilizing agents are relatively safe during pregnancy.
B. Atypical antipsychotic agents can be used to control acute manic symptoms without fear of long-term side effects.
C. The incidence of mood disorders increases with increasing age during childhood and adolescence.
D. Lithium is not always useful for treating the depressive symptoms of bipolar disorder.
E. Hypomania is generally more dangerous than mania.

Answers

[5.1] **D.** Mood stabilizers are used to treat bipolar disorder. Divalproex is the only mood stabilizer listed among these medications.

[5.2] **A.** Current child psychiatric literature suggests that many juveniles with bipolar disorder have a presentation of severe mood dysregulation with multiple intense, prolonged mood swings every day consisting of short periods of euphoria followed by longer periods of irritability that is different from adults.

[5.3] **C.** The incidence of mood disorder increases with increasing age during childhood and adolescence. Mood-stabilizing agents such as lithium and divalproex have significant teratogenic effects. Atypical antipsychotic agents can cause metabolic syndrome or permanent tardive dyskinesia.

CLINICAL PEARLS

- Current child psychiatric literature suggests that many juveniles with bipolar disorder have a presentation of severe mood dysregulation with multiple intense, prolonged mood swings every day consisting of short periods of euphoria followed by longer periods of irritability that is different from adults.
- The majority of the AACAP treatment guideline panel recommended lithium or divalproex as the first medication choice for nonpsychotic mania.
- There is a high degree of psychiatric comorbidity in bipolar disorder in childhood.
- Mood-stabilizing agents have a significant risk for teratogenicity.

REFERENCES

Kowatch RA, Fristad M, Birmaher B, Wagner KD, Findling RL, Hellander M, AACAP Child Psychiatric Workgroup on Bipolar Disorder. Treatment guidelines for children and adolescents with bipolar disorder. J Am Acad Child Adolesc Psychiatry 2005;44(3):213–235.

Pataki CS. Mood disorders and suicide in children and adolescents. In: Sadock, BJ Sadock VA, eds. Kaplan and Sadock's comprehensive textbook of psychiatry, 7th ed. Philadelphia: Lippincott Williams & Wilkins, 2000:2740–2757.

CASE 6

A 36-year-old man visits his primary care physician complaining that he has been "stressed out" since a job change 2 months ago. The patient states that he was doing well in his job as a software developer until he was told that his position was being phased out and that in order to stay with the company, he would need to switch to the sales department. The patient agreed because he did not want to lose his insurance benefits and retirement plan but now states that "he can't stand all those people." He notes that his previous position allowed him to be on his own for most of the work week. However, the new job requires almost constant interaction with colleagues and clients, something he hates. The patient says that he has almost no friends, except for a cousin that he has been close to since childhood. He claims that he has never had a sexual encounter but does not miss not having had this experience or not having friends. He states that he most enjoys spending hours surfing the Internet or playing computer games by himself. He has never seen a psychiatrist and saw no reason to do so before the recent job change occurred.

On a mental status examination, the patient appears notably detached and aloof toward the examiner. His mood is reported as "stressed," but his affect is not congruent with this—he looks emotionally calm, and his range is flat. No other disorders are noted during the mental status examination.

- **What is the most likely diagnosis?**
- **What is the best initial treatment?**

ANSWERS TO CASE 6: Schizoid Personality Disorder

Summary: A 36-year-old man presents to his primary care physician with increased stress after being transferred to a job that requires considerably more interpersonal contact than his previous position. The results of the patient's mental status examination are essentially normal other than showing a restricted emotional range.

- **Most likely diagnosis:** Schizoid personality disorder.
- **Best initial treatment:** Although long-term psychotherapy might help this patient, his condition is ego-syntonic, and thus he will probably not be motivated to undergo such treatment. The best strategy for decreasing this patient's stress is for him to seek another job with a low level of interpersonal interaction.

Analysis

Objectives

1. Recognize schizoid personality disorder in a patient.
2. Know that patients with this disorder tend to do poorly in settings where high amounts of interpersonal interaction are required.

Considerations

This patient likely has schizoid personality disorder. Recent studies indicate that the prevalence of schizoid personality disorder can be as high as 3% in the United States, and there is equal distribution among men and women. Individuals with schizoid personality disorder can be more prone to use alcohol or other substances of abuse. A personality disorder is an inflexible way of thinking about oneself or environment, causing social or occupational difficulties. The patient's life, although very socially isolated, appears adequate for the patient's needs, as he has not sought any kind of psychiatric treatment and is now distressed only because he cannot tolerate the personal interaction the new job requires. The lack of any psychotic symptoms (hallucinations or delusions) as revealed by the patient's mental status examination is also consistent. This patient's visit to the primary care doctor is probably one of the few ways that such patients interact with medical personnel (aside from reporting other physical complaints, as in the general population).

APPROACH TO SCHIZOID PERSONALITY DISORDER

Definitions

Alloplastic defenses: Defenses used by patients with personality disorders. These patients react to stress by attempting to change the external environment, for example, by threatening or manipulating others.

Autoplastic defenses: Defenses used by neurotic patients, who react to stress by changing their internal psychological processes.

Ego-dystonic: Describes a character deficit perceived by a patient as objectionable and alien to the self. Patients blame themselves for their shortcomings.

Ego-syntonic: Describes a character deficit perceived by the patient to be acceptable, unobjectionable, and part of the self. The patient blames others for problems that occur. Personality disorders are ego-syntonic.

Intellectualization: A defense mechanism by which an individual deals with emotional or internal or external stressors by excessive use of abstract thinking or making generalizations to control or minimize disturbing feelings. It is present as a component of brooding in which events are continually rehashed in a distant, abstract, emotionally barren fashion.

Personality disorder: Enduring patterns of perceiving, relating to, and thinking about the environment and oneself that **are inflexible, maladaptive, and cause significant impairment in social or occupational functioning.** They are not caused by the direct physiologic effects of a substance or another general medical condition and are not the consequence of another mental disorder. They are present during the **person's stable functioning** and not only during acute stress.

Personality traits: Enduring patterns of perceiving, relating to, and thinking about the environment and oneself. They are exhibited in a wide range of important social and personal contexts. Everyone has personality traits.

Projection: A defense mechanism by which individuals deal with conflict by falsely attributing to another their own unacceptable feelings, impulses, or thoughts. By blaming others for their sentiments and actions, the focus is removed from the person doing the accusing. For example, a patient who is angry with his therapist suddenly accuses the therapist of being angry with him.

Schizoid fantasy: A defense mechanism whereby fantasy is used as an escape and as a means of gratification so that other people are not required for emotional fulfillment. The retreat into fantasy itself acts as a means of distancing others.

Personality disorder clusters: Three categories into which these disorders are broadly classified: A, B, and C (Table 6–1).

Table 6–1

CLASSIFICATION OF PERSONALITY DISORDERS

Cluster A: "Mad"—odd and eccentric	Schizoid: Loner, detached, flat affect, restricted emotions	Schizotypal: Odd, eccentric, magical thinking, paranoid, not psychotic Defense: projection, regression, fantasy	Paranoid: distrust and suspiciousness; constricted affect Defense: projection	
Cluster B: "Bad"—dramatic and erratic	Histrionic: Excessively emotional, attention-seeking Defense: reaction formation	Narcissistic: Self-important, needs admiration, lacks empathy	Antisocial: Acts out, aggressive, must be older than 18 years of age	Borderline: Impulsive, interpersonal instability, affect instability Defense: splitting, projection
Cluster C: "Sad"—anxious and timid	Obsessive-compulsive: Perfectionism, orderliness Defense: reaction formation	Avoidant: Hypersensitive to criticism, social discomfort	Dependent: Submissive, clinging, needs to be taken care of	

Cluster A: Characterized by odd or eccentric behavior. Schizoid, schizotypal, and paranoid personality disorders fall into cluster A.
Cluster B: Characterized by dramatic or emotional behavior. Histrionic, narcissistic, antisocial, and borderline personality disorders fall into cluster B.
Cluster C: Characterized by anxious or fearful behavior. Obsessive-compulsive, avoidant, and dependent personality disorders fall into cluster C.

CLINICAL PEARL

❖ These clusters can be remembered by the words "mad" (cluster A disorders in which patients display odd or eccentric behavior), "bad" (cluster B disorders in which patients exhibit dramatic or emotional behavior), and "sad" (cluster C disorders in which patients show anxious or fearful behavior).

Clinical Approach

Diagnostic Criteria

Patients with schizoid personality disorders have a pervasive pattern of indifference to social relationships and a restricted range of emotional experience and expression. They have difficulty in expressing hostility and are self-absorbed, detached daydreamers. As a rule, they avoid intimate personal conflict. They can appear quite detached. They are often functional at work as long as it does not require a lot of interpersonal contact. They appear somewhat indifferent to either praise or criticism.

Differential Diagnosis

Patients with schizoid personality disorder do not usually have schizophrenic relatives, and they can have successful work histories, especially if their jobs are performed in an isolated setting. Patients with schizophrenia and schizotypal personality disorder, in contrast, commonly have relatives with schizophrenia and do not have successful work careers. Patients with schizotypal personality disorder often engage in quasi delusional, or magical, thinking. Patients with paranoid personality disorder tend to be more verbally hostile and tend to project their feelings onto others. Although patients with obsessive-compulsive personality disorder and avoidant personality disorder can appear just as emotionally constricted, they experience loneliness as ego-dystonic. They also do not tend to have such a rich fantasy life. Patients with avoidant personality disorder strongly wish for relationships with others but are afraid to reach out. In contrast, patients with schizoid personality disorder do not feel the need for relationships at all.

Tips for Interacting with Schizoid Patients

Patients with schizoid personality disorder need privacy and do not like interpersonal interactions. The needs of such patients should be appreciated. The physician should use a low-key, technical approach (not a "warm and fuzzy" one) when dealing with these patients.

Comprehension Questions

[6.1] To which of the following personality categories is schizoid personality disorder most closely related?

A. Obsessive-compulsive
B. Paranoid
C. Avoidant
D. Histrionic
E. Narcissistic

[6.2] A patient with schizoid personality disorder comes to his primary care physician with a chief complaint of polyuria and polydipsia. He is found to have insulin-dependent diabetes. Which of the following interventions by the physician is likely to be most well received by this patient?

A. Asking the patient to bring in a relative so that he can describe the treatment regimen to the both of them at the same time.
B. Referring the patient to a therapist so that he can talk about the difficult nature of the diagnosis.
C. Giving the patient detailed written information about the disease and telling him the physician will be available to answer any questions.
D. Referring the patient to a group that helps its members learn about diabetes and to better deal with their illness.
E. Scheduling frequent appointments with the patient so that all the treatment details can be explained on a one-to-one basis.

[6.3] A woman with schizoid personality disorder was involved in a motor vehicle accident in which she was rear-ended by another car. The driver of the other car refused to take responsibility for the accident and has hired a lawyer to provide his defense. The woman spends hours every day thinking about the specifics of the accident, including such details as the color of the cars involved and what each party to the accident was wearing. Which of the following defense mechanisms, common to patients with schizoid personality disorder, is the woman using?

A. Sublimation
B. Undoing
C. Projection
D. Intellectualization
E. Introjection

Answers

[6.1] **B.** Cluster A is the "mad" cluster and includes three personality disorders: schizoid, schizotypal, and paranoid.

[6.2] **C.** Patients with schizoid personality disorder generally prefer that social interaction be kept to a minimum. They do well with technical information.

[6.3] **D.** Intellectualization is characterized by rehashing events over and over.

CLINICAL PEARLS

- Patients with schizoid personality disorder show a pervasive, stable pattern of disinterest in interpersonal relationships, coupled with a rich fantasy life. They appear emotionally detached.
- Schizoid personality disorder belongs in cluster A, the "mad" cluster.
- Patients with this disorder can be differentiated from patients with avoidant personality disorder by their lack of interest in interpersonal relationships.
- Patients with schizoid personality disorder can be differentiated from patients with schizotypal personality disorder by the former's lack of a family history of schizophrenia, absence of magical thinking, and their often successful (if isolated) work careers.
- Physicians do well in dealing with such patients when they use a low-key, technical approach.
- Therapy does not tend to work well with these patients, as they are not motivated to undergo treatment. Their disorder is ego-syntonic, as are all personality disorders.

REFERENCES

Ebert M, Loosen P, Nurcombe B, eds. Current diagnosis and treatment in psychiatry. New York: McGraw-Hill, 2000:471–472.

Grant BF, Hasin DS, et al. Prevalence, correlates, and disability of personality disorders in the United States: Results from the national epidemiologic survey on alcohol and related conditions. J Clin Psychiatry 2004;65(1):948–958.

Kaplan H, Sadock B. Synopsis of psychiatry, 9th ed. Baltimore: Lippincott Williams & Wilkins, 2003:1121–1125.

CASE 7

A 79-year old man is brought to the emergency department by his family. Although the patient is essentially mute, his family members report that he has had a long history of episodes of depression, the last occurring 6 years ago. At that time, he was hospitalized and treated with sertraline. He has been hospitalized a total of four times for episodes of depression, but the family denies that he has ever been treated for mania. The patient's only current medication is hydrochlorothiazide, although he has refused to take it for the past 2 days.

The current episode of depression, similar to previous ones, began 3 weeks prior to the emergency department visit. The patient has had frequent crying episodes and has complained of a decrease in energy. He has lost at least 15 lb in the 3 weeks and for the past 2 days has refused to eat anything at all. Three days ago, the patient told his family that he was "sorry for all the pain and suffering I have caused you" and that "it would be better if I were not around any more." Two days ago, he stopped speaking and eating, and for the past 24 hours he has refused to take anything by mouth, even water. After rehydration in the emergency department, the patient was admitted to the psychiatry service. The results of his physical examination were essentially normal, although his blood pressure was 150/92 mm Hg, and he exhibited psychomotor slowing. The patient refused all attempts to feed him by mouth. When asked if he was suicidal, he nodded his assent, as well as assent to the question, "Are you hearing voices?"

- **What is the most likely diagnosis?**

- **What is the best plan of action for this patient?**

ANSWERS TO CASE 7: Major Depression in Elderly Patients

Summary: A 79-year-old man is brought in by his family after refusing to drink fluids for 24 hours. For the past 3 weeks, the patient has shown worsening signs and symptoms of major depression (decreased energy, crying spells, suicidal ideation, anorexia with weight loss, and guilt), culminating in a refusal to eat or drink. He continues to refuse to eat or drink, is suicidal, and is probably experiencing auditory hallucinations. He has had episodes similar to this one in the past, although no episodes of mania have been described.

- **Most likely diagnosis:** Recurrent major depression with psychotic features

- **Best plan of action:** Close observation in the hospital, intravenous hydration, and consideration of electroconvulsive therapy (ECT) because of the severity of this episode of depression

Analysis

Objectives

1. Discern an episode of major depression based on the symptoms presented.
2. Understand that the major depression presented by this patient is severe and life-threatening.
3. Understand that the optimal treatment for severe major depression in a geriatric patient is ECT.

Considerations

The patient's history (per the family) offers a straightforward diagnosis of major depression. There is no evidence of medical problems that might have caused these symptoms, and the facts that the patient has had episodes of major depression in the past and that this one is similar (according to the family) are helpful in making a diagnosis of recurrent depression (Table 7–1). The mild hypertension experienced by this patient is expected based on his history and on the fact that he has not taken his medication for several days; otherwise, it is noncontributory in making the diagnosis. The patient's refusal to eat or drink anything, as well as his psychotic symptoms and his suicidal ideation, make him a prime candidate for ECT. Close observation in the hospital will be necessary because he is suicidal, and as his energy level improves following the ECT, he might have the energy to attempt suicide.

Table 7–1

DIAGNOSTIC CRITERIA FOR MAJOR DEPRESSIVE DISORDER, RECURRENT, WITH PSYCHOTIC FEATURES

- Occurrence of two or more episodes of major depression.
- Episodes of major depression are not better accounted for by schizoaffective disorder and are not superimposed on another psychotic disorder.
- No history of manic, hypomanic, or mixed episodes.
- Presence of delusions or hallucinations.

APPROACH TO MAJOR DEPRESSION WITH PSYCHOTIC FEATURES IN ELDERLY PATIENTS

Definitions

Electroconvulsive therapy (ECT): Treatment that involves the induction of generalized seizures. In order for this treatment to be effective, the seizures must last at least 25 seconds. After the patient is placed under general anesthesia, a seizure is induced by passing an electric current through the brain using either unilateral or bilateral electrodes on the forehead. After the procedure, the patient is awakened. This procedure is then repeated two to three times per week for a total of 6 to 12 treatments. The most common side effect is anterograde memory loss.

Electroconvulsive therapy is one of the safest and most effective treatments available for depression. It has become more widely accepted since the addition of modern-day anesthetics to the procedure. In addition to informed consent, the treatment requires thorough medical clearance. Seizure induction is thought to result in changes in neurotransmitter receptors and secondary messenger systems in the brain, creating an effect similar to that of antidepressant medications. For elderly patients who have difficulty tolerating antidepressants, and in cases where there are contraindications to their use, ECT is often an important treatment option.

Clinical Approach

Depression is very common in the geriatric population as a result of failing health, loss of a spouse or friends, and loss of autonomy or cognitive function. The **SIG: E** (nergy) **CAPS** mnemonic is useful (see Case 1). Each letter stands for a criterion (except for depressed mood) used in diagnosing an episode of major depression.

Differential Diagnosis

Although major depressive disorder is not uncommon in the elderly population, a new onset of a depressive illness should especially raise suspicion of an underlying nonpsychiatric cause, such as medication or a medical condition. Numerous medications can cause depressive symptoms, and geriatric patients are more sensitive to such side effects. Various medical conditions are also associated with depression. See Case 4 (Table 4–1) for a listing of various medications and medical illnesses that create depressive states. Given that elderly patients tend to focus on their somatic complaints when suffering from a depressive disorder, it is essential to obtain a complete history, a physical examination, and appropriate laboratory examinations in this patient population.

In developing the differential diagnosis, another condition to be considered unique to this age group is dementia, such as **Alzheimer** disease, which is also associated with depressive symptoms. There are several features that can help distinguish major depressive disorder from dementia. Patients with **depression** tend to display **transient cognitive impairments** that are reversible with treatment. When given cognitive testing, individuals with depression make little effort during the examination, whereas individuals with dementia usually make more of an effort. Patients with depression have considerable insight into their intellectual difficulties, whereas patients with dementia have little insight. In addition, major depressive disorder is not characterized by the cortical or neurologic signs seen in dementia.

Finally, adjustment disorder with depressed mood, bereavement, and general periods of sadness must be considered in preparing the differential diagnosis, as many significant life stressors occur in the geriatric population.

Treatment

The treatment options for major depression in elderly patients are the same as for younger patients. They include selective serotonin reuptake inhibitors (SSRIs), tricyclic antidepressants (TCAs), monoamine oxidase inhibitors (MAOIs), and ECT, as well as various psychotherapies. It is important to keep several pharmacologic issues in mind. **Older patients can require smaller doses to achieve therapeutic levels** because of decreased metabolism and clearance. Geriatric patients are more sensitive to side effects, especially orthostasis and anticholinergic symptoms. The adage, "start low and go slow" is particularly relevant here. Last, these individuals are often taking numerous medications, and so the clinician must be on the lookout for drug–drug interactions.

The treatment of major depressive disorder with psychotic features deserves special attention. Patients with this disorder require either antidepressant and antipsychotic medication *or* ECT. **ECT is a very efficacious, safe option in elderly patients, especially if they cannot tolerate medication.** It is also the optimal choice in situations where a rapid response is necessary, such as for patients who are imminently suicidal, catatonic, or refusing food or fluid.

Comprehension Questions

[7.1] An 80-year-old man undergoes an evaluation for dementia versus depression. His caregiver describes a history of gradually worsening depressed mood and confusion, with poor appetite, weight loss, poor self-care, and irritability. On his cognitive examination, he is alert and oriented to person and place but not to time. His concentration is impaired, and he displays poor short-term memory despite adequate recall. His effort is poor overall, and he often responds to questions stating, "I don't know." Which of the following features is more consistent with a depressive illness than with dementia?

A. Poor concentration
B. Poor effort during the interview
C. Poor self-care
D. Poor short-term memory

[7.2] Which of the following statements regarding the psychopharmacologic treatment of geriatric patients is most accurate?

A. Fewer side effects are reported.
B. Higher doses are used.
C. Lower blood levels are needed.
D. More drug–drug interactions are seen.

[7.3] Which of the following is the best indication for using ECT in an elderly patient with major depression?

A. Multiple medical problems
B. Psychotic symptoms
C. Recurrent episodes
D. Suicidal ideation without a plan

[7.4] You are consulted to evaluate an 84-year-old, widowed woman on the medical ward. She has a prior history of major depressive disorder, recurrent, and she was admitted for a syncopal episode. She was found to be extremely malnourished and has not been taking her antidepressant for many months. She describes having all the neurovegetative symptoms of depression and to not eating or drinking for days. When questioned about this, she admits to purposely "starving myself" as she believes that God is punishing her for directly causing the terrorist attacks of September 11, 2001. In fact, she has been "following God's instructions," which tell her to kill herself in atonement. Which of the following treatments would be the most appropriate for this patient?

A. Antidepressant only
B. Antipsychotic only
C. Electroconvulsive therapy only
D. Psychotherapy only
E. Psychotherapy plus antidepressant

Answers

[7.1] **B.** Difficulty concentrating, decreased self-care, and short-term memory deficits can be seen in both severe depression and dementia in elderly patients. However, during the cognitive examination, patients with depression usually make little effort but have considerable insight into their difficulties, whereas patients with dementia often make considerable effort but display confabulation and little insight into their mistakes.

[7.2] **D.** Geriatric patients are often taking multiple medications and therefore have a higher likelihood of being affected by drug–drug interactions. They are more likely to experience significant side effects from medications. Although the drug *levels* required to achieve efficacy are similar to those required in younger patients, because of the decreased clearance and metabolism seen in older patients, lower doses are required to reach the same levels.

[7.3] **B.** The most appropriate treatment for a patient with major depressive disorder with psychotic features (whether elderly or not) remains ECT or an antidepressant/antipsychotic combination. Other indications for ECT are when a rapid response is necessary, such as in an imminently suicidal patient, a catatonic patient, or a patient who is not ingesting adequate food or fluid. The treatment most likely to be of benefit to an individual with recurrent episodes is the one that was efficacious in the past.

[7.4] **C.** This woman's history and presentation are most consistent with major depression, severe, with psychotic features; the treatment of choice for this illness is either ECT *or* an antidepressant/antipsychotic combination. Given the medical urgency in this case and that medication would take several weeks for significant efficacy, ECT would be preferable. Neither antidepressants nor antipsychotics *alone* would be as efficacious in an episode of psychotic depression, and psychotherapy with or without medication would not be appropriate in someone with a severe depression as in this case.

CLINICAL PEARLS

- In the geriatric population, it is important to rule out an underlying substance, medication, or a medical condition as a cause of depression, especially if the patient does not have a history of this disorder.
- Elderly patients with depression can do poorly on cognitive tests; in general, they have more insight into their difficulties and make less effort during a cognitive examination in comparison to patients with dementia.
- The treatment options for major depression in geriatric patients are the same as for younger patients, although the doses of medication used are smaller and the side effects greater.
- Electroconvulsive therapy is the ideal treatment for major depression with psychotic features or where a rapid response is needed, such as when a patient is in imminent danger or has an inadequate nutritional/hydration status. It can be especially helpful in elderly patients, who can have trouble tolerating antidepressant medications and their side effects.

REFERENCES

American Psychiatric Association. Practice guidelines for the treatment of major depressive disorder. Available at: http://www.psych.org/clin_res/depression2e.book.cfm. Accessed July 14, 2005.

Kaplan H, Sadock B. Synopsis of psychiatry, 9th ed. Baltimore: Lippincott Williams & Wilkins, 2003:1138–1144, 1324, 1332–1333.

❖ CASE 8

A 35-year-old man visits a psychiatrist because he is overwhelmingly anxious about a speech he has to make. The man states that he was recently promoted to a position within his company that requires him to speak in front of an audience of approximately 100 people. He says that the first such speech is coming up in 2 weeks and that worrying about it keeps him from sleeping. He knows that his fear is out of proportion, but he is unable to control it. He explains that he has always had trouble with public speaking because he fears that he might "do something stupid" or otherwise embarrass himself. He has avoided public speaking in the past as much as possible or has spoken in public only before an audience of fewer than 10. Because he knows that he must make the presentation coming up in 2 weeks or he will not be able to keep his new job, he has visited the psychiatrist hoping to find a solution to the problem.

◆ **What is the most likely diagnosis?**

◆ **What are the treatment options open to this patient?**

ANSWERS TO CASE 8: Social Phobia

Summary: A 35-year-old man has a long history of being afraid to speak in public. He normally handles his fear by avoiding this activity or by keeping the size of the audience to a minimum. He is required to give a presentation in front of a large audience in 2 weeks and has been extremely anxious about it to the point where he cannot sleep. He is afraid he will somehow embarrass himself in front of the audience. Not being able to speak in front of this audience will negatively impact his job.

- **Most likely diagnosis:** Social phobia.
- **Treatment options:** Behavioral or cognitive-behavioral therapy is the treatment of choice. A typical treatment regimen involves relaxation training followed by progressive desensitization. Pharmacologic interventions include benzodiazepines or beta-blockers over the short term or an antidepressant such as imipramine.

Analysis

Objectives

1. Recognize social phobia in a patient.
2. Prescribe appropriate treatments for this disorder.

Considerations

This patient has had a long-standing **difficulty speaking in public.** He believes he will look stupid or otherwise embarrass himself. He usually handles this fear by avoiding speaking if possible or by speaking only before a small audience. Since his job promotion, he has been terrified by the thought of speaking to an audience of 100, although it is a necessary requirement of the new position. He has been unable to sleep because of his anxiety. He knows that this level of anxiety about public speaking is abnormal but is unable to quell his fears. His fear of speaking in public is consistent with social phobia (Table 8–1).

APPROACH TO SOCIAL PHOBIA

Definitions

Phobia: Persistent, irrational, exaggerated, and pathologic fear of a specific situation or stimulus that results in conscious avoidance of the dreaded circumstance.

Table 8–1
DIAGNOSTIC CRITERIA FOR SOCIAL PHOBIA

A. A marked, persistent fear of at least one social or performance situation in which exposure to unfamiliar people or possible scrutiny of others occurs. The person fears that he or she will act in a way or show anxiety symptoms that will be humiliating or embarrassing.
B. Exposure to the feared situation(s) invariably provokes anxiety that can take the form of a panic attack.
C. The person recognizes that the fear is unreasonable.
D. The avoidance of, anxious anticipation of, or distress in the feared situation(s) interferes with the person's normal routine, or there is marked anxiety about having the phobia.
E. The fear or avoidance is not related to a substance or a general medical condition.
F. If a general medical condition is present, the fear in criterion A is not related to it (e.g., the fear of stuttering, or trembling in a patient with Parkinson disease).

Relaxation training: Exercises to reduce arousal levels and increase one's sense of control; includes progressive muscle relaxation and imaging techniques to obtain this reduction in arousal.

Social phobia: Dread of being embarrassed in public, fear of speaking in public, or fear of eating in public.

Specific phobia: Dread of a particular object or situation, such as acrophobia (heights), agoraphobia (open places), algophobia (pain), claustrophobia (closed places), xenophobia (strangers), and zoophobia (animals).

Clinical Approach

Phobias are the single most common mental disorder in the United States, affecting 5% to 10% of the population. Specific phobias are more common than social phobias, and **women are more often affected** in both categories. Genetics can have a role in predisposing individuals to these disorders. **Specific phobias are often treated by exposure therapy,** a type of behavioral therapy in which **the individual is slowly desensitized with controlled "doses" of the feared stimulus.**

Differential Diagnosis

Individuals with social phobias are **distressed** about their fear, experience **anxiety,** and **recognize that their fright is unreasonable.** The most prominent disorders to rule out are also in the anxiety disorder group. Panic disorder with agoraphobia and agoraphobia without panic attacks are **more generalized** and are not focused just on situations where public scrutiny is possible. Generalized anxiety disorder is more global, and the focus of fear is not just about public performance. If the full criteria for a specific anxiety disorder are not met, anxiety disorder not otherwise specified can be used. Finally, anxiety associated with another major mental illness, performance anxiety, stage fright, or shyness must be considered prior to making a diagnosis.

Treatment

Psychotherapy is helpful in treating social phobia and usually involves a combination of behavioral and cognitive therapy using **desensitization** to the feared situation, **rehearsal** during sessions, and homework assignments in which patients are asked to place themselves in public situations in a graded fashion. In some cases, **psychopharmacotherapy** for severe social phobia has succeeded with the use **of selective serotonin uptake inhibitors (SSRIs), benzodiazepines, venlafaxine, and buspirone.** Buspirone has been shown to augment the treatment of this disorder when used adjunctively with SSRIs. Treating the **anxiety associated with performance situations** involves the use **of beta-adrenergic receptor antagonists just before the feared situation. Atenolol and propranolol** have been shown to be helpful in these instances and are the most commonly used.

Comprehension Questions

[8.1] Which of the following is a person with social phobia likely to experience?

A. Fear of heights
B. Fear of speaking in public
C. Fear of going to school
D. Fear of leaving his or her parents
E. Fear of leaving the house

[8.2] Which of the following is the treatment of choice for social phobia?

A. Behavior therapy
B. SSRIs
C. Electroconvulsive therapy
D. Psychoanalysis
E. Divalproex sodium (Depakote)

[8.3] A 24-year-old woman comes to a psychiatrist with the chief complaint, "I am afraid to go out of my house." She says that for the past 3 months she has become overwhelmingly anxious during discrete periods of time. The first such episode occurred when she was driving across a bridge, although she denies that anything stressful happened at that time. Since then, she has experienced similar episodes daily, up to three times a day. She says she is afraid to go out of the house and in public because she might have another episode. Prior to 3 months ago, the patient was functioning normally and had no complaints. Which of the following psychiatric disorders does this woman most likely have?

A. Social phobia
B. Panic disorder with agoraphobia
C. Generalized anxiety disorder
D. Avoidant personality disorder
E. Major depression

Answers

[8.1] **B.** Each of the other descriptions is more common in other anxiety disorders. Fear of heights is a specific phobia. Fear of going to school or leaving one's parents might be a symptom of separation anxiety disorder. Fear of leaving the house is agoraphobia, which can occur in panic disorder.

[8.2] **A.** Behavior therapy is the treatment of choice for social phobia. Benzodiazepines can be used to reduce the associated anxiety. A beta-blocker such as propranolol can also help reduce the autonomic hyperarousal that occurs in social settings.

[8.3] **B.** This patient has discrete panic attacks, which has resulted in a fear of going out in public because she may have another attack. This is a classic example of panic disorder with agoraphobia.

CLINICAL PEARLS

❖ Social phobia is one of the most common anxiety disorders, affecting approximately 3% of the general population. Onset usually occurs in late childhood or early adulthood, and the course is often chronic.

❖ Anxiety disorders have a high degree of comorbidity.

❖ Behavior therapy, a form of psychotherapy, is the treatment of choice for social phobia.

❖ Beta-blockers such as propranolol and atenolol are the agents of choice for treatment of the anxiety provoked by performance situations.

REFERENCES

Ebert M, Loosen P, Nurcombe B, eds. Current diagnosis and treatment in psychiatry. New York: McGraw-Hill, 2000:334–337.

Kaplan H, Sadock B. Synopsis of psychiatry, 9th ed. Baltimore: Lippincott Williams & Wilkins, 2004:674–677.

❖ CASE 9

An 18-year-old man is brought to the emergency department after he became belligerent at a party and started screaming and throwing punches at other guests. In the emergency department, the patient is unable to provide any kind of history and is so agitated, paranoid, and hostile that he is put in four-point leather restraints. One of the patient's friends who has accompanied him says that the patient "took something" given to him at the party but did not know what the substance was. He claims that the patient is normally "a really nice guy" and that his current behavior is completely out of character.

The mental status examination is limited because of the patient's extreme hostility and lack of cooperation. He struggles fiercely against the restraints, his speech is mildly slurred, and he appears to have vertical nystagmus. The patient refuses to answer questions about his mood, although he appears to be extremely angry. It is impossible to assess his thought process or thought content.

◆ **What is most likely diagnosis for this patient?**

◆ **What is the best treatment?**

ANSWERS TO CASE 9: Phencyclidine Intoxication

Summary: An 18-year-old man is brought to the emergency department after ingesting an unknown drug at a party. He is belligerent, paranoid, hostile, and violent and requires leather restraints. The patient's speech is slurred, and he has vertical nystagmus.

- **Most likely diagnosis:** Phencyclidine (PCP) intoxication.
- **Best treatment:** A PCP urine screening should be ordered to confirm the diagnosis. Medical monitoring is required, as is hospitalization for severe intoxication. Benzodiazepines can delay excretion of the drug and therefore should not be given unless absolutely necessary. Antipsychotics can worsen the symptoms because of their anticholinergic side effects but can be necessary nonetheless to control the violent behavior.

Analysis

Objectives

1. Recognize PCP intoxication in a patient.
2. Understand the emergency treatment for this disorder.

Considerations

This patient became hostile, paranoid, and violent after ingesting an unknown substance at a party. This behavior is not characteristic of the patient. The dysarthria and **nystagmus** observed are typical of **PCP intoxication.**

APPROACH TO PHENCYCLIDINE INTOXICATION

Definitions

Ataxia: A disturbance in gait; the patient cannot remain steady on his feet.

Dysarthria: A disturbance in speech, which appears slurred, garbled, or unclear.

Hyperacusis: Hearing that is especially sensitive.

Nystagmus: Rhythmic, oscillating motion of the eyes. This to-and-fro motion is generally involuntary and can occur in the vertical or horizontal plane.

Phencyclidine: Sometimes known as "angel dust," "horse tranquilizer," or "happy leaf" on the street, PCP is a piperidine similar to ketamine that was originally developed as an anesthetic agent. It is very potent, long-acting, and causes marked behavioral, physiologic, and neurologic toxic effects in humans, including agitation, disorientation, hallucinations, and delirium. Its effects are similar to those of lysergic acid diethylamide

(LSD), and it is often used in conjunction with other drugs of abuse such as marijuana (to which it is sometimes added), heroin, and cocaine. PCP can be smoked or injected intravenously and is easily synthesized and distributed.

Clinical Approach

Diagnostic Criteria

Phencyclidine intoxication is considered a psychiatric emergency because of the potential for psychosis and destructive behavior. The short-term effects last up to 6 hours, but the full effect of the drug can last for several days. Behavioral manifestations are very unpredictable; the individual can be sociable and cooperative one minute and hostile and extremely violent the next. Auditory and visual hallucinations are common, as are confused and disorganized thoughts. Common findings on a physical examination include hypertension, hyperthermia, and nystagmus, as well as muscle rigidity. The criteria for PCP intoxication are listed in Table 9–1.

Differential Diagnosis and Treatment

Laboratory evidence (a PCP assay) can confirm the diagnosis, but in the meantime other possible diagnoses must be considered. Psychotic disorders such as a manic episode of bipolar disorder, schizophrenia, or a brief episode of psychosis must be considered. Intoxication caused by other sedatives, stimulants, or narcotics should also be included, particularly those produced by hallucinogens, amphetamines, and ketamine.

Table 9–1
CRITERIA FOR PHENCYCLIDINE INTOXICATION

A. Recent use of phencyclidine (PCP) or a similar substance.
B. Disturbed behaviors such as hostility and violence, impulsivity, and psychomotor agitation after ingestion of PCP.
C. Two or more of the following signs within an hour of ingestion:
    1. Nystagmus
    2. Hypertension or tachycardia
    3. Numbness
    4. Ataxia
    5. Dysarthria
    6. Muscle rigidity
    7. Seizures or coma
    8. Hyperacusis
D. The symptoms are not secondary to a medical condition or to another mental illness.

The treatment of PCP intoxication must address the numerous aspects of the effects of PCP. Gastric lavage is contraindicated because of the risk of emesis. The patient should be kept in a room with minimal stimulation, that is, in the dark and away from the confusion of the usual emergency setting. Restraints should be avoided if possible because of the risk of muscle breakdown; benzodiazepines can be used for muscle spasms and seizures, as well as sedation. If agitation is marked, an antipsychotic medication can be indicated. Typical, low-potency antipsychotics should be avoided because their anticholinergic side effects can worsen symptoms. Hypertension can be treated with intravenous antihypertensive medications. Acidification of the urine (e.g., with cranberry juice) can promote excretion of the PCP. Most importantly, the patient might need to be hospitalized for 72 hours to allow the danger of violence or central nervous system complications to pass.

Comprehension Questions

[9.1] Which of the following signs or symptoms can most likely distinguish PCP intoxication from an episode of mania?

A. Disorganized thoughts
B. Hostile or violent behavior
C. Nystagmus
D. Hallucinations

[9.2] Phencyclidine is most closely related to which substance?

A. Alcohol
B. Ketamine
C. Amphetamines
D. Marijuana

[9.3] Which of the following sets of three symptoms is most indicative of PCP intoxication?

A. Nystagmus, muscle rigidity, numbness
B. Dilated pupils, bradycardia, excessive salivation
C. Pinpoint pupils, tachycardia, orthostatic hypotension
D. Ocular nerve palsy, cardiac arrhythmias, pseudobulbar palsy
E. Hallucinations, heart block, lower limb weakness

Answers

[9.1] **C.** Individuals with mania and PCP intoxication can have hallucinations, display hostility, and have disordered thoughts; nystagmus is commonly associated with PCP use but not with mania.

[9.2] **B.** Ketamine is also an anesthetic and is closely related to PCP; it also has some similar effects in humans.

[9.3] **A.** The triad of nystagmus, muscle rigidity, and numbness points strongly to PCP intoxication. Other symptoms that can occur include hypertension or tachycardia, ataxia, dysarthria, seizures or coma, and hyperacusis.

CLINICAL PEARLS

- Phencyclidine intoxication is an emergency; if it is suspected, the clinician must take precautions to protect both patient and staff from potential violent behavior.
- The patient can ingest PCP without knowing; it is a substance that is sometimes added to marijuana cigarettes.
- Nystagmus is commonly associated with PCP intoxication.
- Individuals with PCP intoxication often exhibit extraordinary physical strength.

REFERENCES

Baldridge EB, Bessen HA. Phencyclidine. Emerg Med Clin North Am 1990;8:541–550.

Gorelick DA, Wilkins JN. Inpatient treatment of PCP abusers. Am J Drug Alcohol Abuse 1989;15:1–12.

❖ CASE 10

A 32-year-old man comes to a psychiatrist with a chief complaint of being depressed since he broke up with his girlfriend 2 weeks previously. The patient explains that although he loves his ex-girlfriend, he broke up with her because his mother did not approve of her and would not allow him to marry her. He says that he cannot go against his mother because she "has taken care of me all these years." He states he could never fend for himself without his mother and alternates between being angry with her and feeling that "maybe she knows best." He has lived at home his entire life except for one semester away at college. He returned home at the end of the semester because he was homesick, and did not go back. The patient reports no loss of appetite, concentration, or energy.

The patient claims that he performs "adequately" at work and has no job-related problems. He works for an accounting firm in an entry-level position even though he has been there for several years. He says that he has turned down promotions in the past because he knows that he "couldn't possibly supervise anyone or make decisions for them." The patient has two close childhood friends whom he talks to on the telephone nearly every day and says he "feels lost without them." The results of his mental status examination are normal except for revealing a depressed mood (although the affect is full range).

◆ **What is the most likely diagnosis?**

 **What is the best treatment?**

ANSWERS TO CASE 10: Dependent Personality Disorder

Summary: The patient is a 32-year-old man who has been depressed since he broke up with his girlfriend 2 weeks ago. He has no vegetative signs or symptoms of major depression. He is overly reliant on his mother for major decisions and still lives at home. The patient does well at his job but has turned down any position that would require him to take responsibility for others. He seems to be very dependent on a few close friends as well.

- **Most likely diagnosis:** Dependent personality disorder.
- **Best treatment:** Insight-oriented therapies can often be helpful. Behavioral therapy, assertiveness training, family therapy, and group therapy have all proven useful with selected patients as well. Pharmacotherapy can be used to treat specific symptoms such as anxiety and depression as they arise.

Analysis

Objectives

1. Recognize dependent personality disorder in a patient.
2. Be familiar with the treatment recommendations appropriate for these patients.

Considerations

This patient exhibits what seems to be a **pervasive pattern** of an excessive need to be taken care of. He needs others to assume responsibility for him and does not disagree with them because he fears loss of their support. He feels uncomfortable and "lost" when alone and does not believe that he could fend for himself. He lacks self-confidence and does not initiate projects. He is preoccupied with a fear of being forced to take care of himself.

APPROACH TO DEPENDENT PERSONALITY DISORDER

Definitions

Idealization: A defense mechanism by which an individual deals with emotional conflict or stressors by attributing exaggerated positive qualities to others. For example, a woman being abused and neglected by her husband earnestly states, "He is the best thing that ever happened to me."

Reaction formation: A defense mechanism by which an individual deals with emotional conflict or stressors by substituting behavior, thoughts, or feelings that are diametrically opposed to his or her own unacceptable thoughts or feelings. For example, a woman who is very angry with her husband for having an affair cooks him a nice dinner and acts sweetly toward him.

Somatization: The expression of psychological difficulties as physical complaints. Somatization is considered a form of regression because being able to verbalize problems instead of making them physical complaints is considered a progressive step. For example, a woman who is upset about the death of her cat develops an intractable headache.

Clinical Approach

Patients with dependent personality disorder have a pervasive need to be taken care of by others. They are dependent and submissive and uncomfortable when alone. They are afraid of being left alone because they do not believe they can take care of themselves, and this leads to clinging behavior. They prefer to do things for others and have difficulty initiating projects on their own or disagreeing with others.

Dependence is a prominent factor in several personality disorders, including histrionic and borderline disorders. However, in these disorders, patients are generally dependent on a series of other people. Patients with dependent personality disorder tend to stick to one person, such as a parent or spouse, for the long term. Patients with this disorder also tend to be less labile and overtly manipulative than patients with histrionic or borderline personality disorders. Patients with agoraphobia can be dependent, but the dependent behavior usually does not start until the panic attacks or anxiety do—thus there is no pervasive, life-long pattern of dependency.

Dependent personality disorder, like all personality disorders, is difficult to treat. Patients can respond to psychosocial support groups in the face of loss of their usual support systems. Long-term psychodynamic psychotherapy might eventually help, but many patients do not have either the motivation or the insight needed to successfully undergo treatment.

Comprehension Questions

[10.1] To what cluster of personality disorders does dependent personality disorder belong?

A. Cluster A
B. Cluster B
C. Cluster C
D. Cluster D

[10.2] You are consulted to evaluate a 45-year-old, married woman who was admitted to the surgical service 2 days ago for an appendectomy. The procedure went well, but she was found to be tearful, stating "I wish I were dead." On obtaining further history, she is quite cooperative and talkative. She is questioned about her earlier comments, and she states that she "wanted attention, I guess." She is upset that her husband is not with her in the hospital; she has "never been away from him" for this long since they started dating when the patient was 16 years old. She feels helpless and is having a difficult time being active in her care. She feels overwhelmed regarding her postsurgical and discharge instructions, and the nursing staff has become frustrated with her constant "need for reassurance." Although at times she is tearful during the interview, she denies prior or recent pervasive depressive or neurovegetative symptoms and is not actively suicidal. Which of the following is the most appropriate approach to this patient?

A. Encourage her to learn more about her surgery and become more proactive in her care
B. Explain to her that she is overly attached to the hospital and should leave immediately
C. Persuade her to spend less time with her husband and develop other hobbies or interests
D. Spend regular, short periods of time with her to discuss discharge planning and aftercare

[10.3] Which of the following would be the most useful psychiatric treatment for the patient in question [10.2]?

A. Antianxiety medication
B. Antidepressant medication
C. Electroconvulsive therapy
D. Group psychotherapy

Answers

[10.1] **C.** Cluster C can also be remembered as the "sad" cluster (see Case 6). It includes dependent, avoidant, and obsessive-compulsive personality disorders. The clusters can be remembered by the words "mad" (cluster A—characterized by odd or eccentric behavior), "bad" (cluster B—characterized by dramatic or emotional behavior), and "sad" (cluster C—characterized by anxious or fearful behavior).

[10.2] **D.** This patient displays characteristics consistent with dependent personality disorder. The most effective approach in dealing with a patient with this disorder is to respect her need for attachment and schedule limited but regular appointments with her. Individuals with this illness wish to be taken care of, and therefore will not be proactive in their care; in circumstances such as these, it's helpful for the physician to be more active. Encouraging the patient to be less dependent in her primary relationship is not only *not* helpful, but can be damaging as she can feel rejected and become more regressed, upset, and helpless.

[10.3] **D.** Psychotherapies, such as insight-oriented, family, behavioral, and group therapy have been useful in patients with dependent personality disorder. Medications for depression and/or anxiety, or electroconvulsive therapy (ECT), would only be indicated if the patient had a comorbid psychiatric illness, not evident in the patient in question [10.2].

CLINICAL PEARLS

- Patients with dependent personality disorder have a pervasive need to be taken care of by others. They are dependent and submissive and are uncomfortable when alone because they do not believe they can take care of themselves.
- Physicians should reassure these patients of their availability but set limits as to how often the patient can contact them. If feeling "burned out" by the patient's extreme dependence, they should be careful not to reject the patient.
- Dependence is a prominent factor in several personality disorders, including histrionic and borderline disorders. Patients with dependent personality disorder tend to stick to one caregiver, such as a parent or spouse, for the long term and tend to be less manipulative.
- Patients with agoraphobia can be dependent, but the dependent behavior usually does not start until the panic attacks or anxiety do—thus there is no lifelong pattern of dependency.

REFERENCES

Ebert M, Loosen P, Nurcombe B, eds. Current diagnosis and treatment in psychiatry. New York: McGraw-Hill, 2000:481–482.

Kaplan H, Sadock B. Synopsis of psychiatry, 9th ed. Baltimore: Lippincott Williams & Wilkins, 2003:813–814.

❖ CASE 11

A 28-year-old woman comes to her internist with a chief complaint of muscle tension. She states that she has experienced a considerable amount of muscle tension during her entire life, but that it has become increasingly worse over the past 7 months. She describes herself as a worrier, and since her first child was born last year, her worrying has increased. She is unable to stop worrying even when she actively tries to do so. She worries about a whole host of issues—the status of U.S. relations with other countries, whether or not she and her husband can afford to put their child through college, her husband's health, and the stock market. The patient also reports symptoms of restlessness and insomnia. She can fall asleep without a problem but wakes up in the middle of the night and cannot fall asleep again. She describes her mood as "Okay" and denies any substance use other than an occasional glass of wine on the weekends. Both she and her husband work as lawyers, although the patient has had difficulty concentrating on her job since her child was born.

◆ **What is the most likely diagnosis?**

◆ **What is the best treatment?**

ANSWERS TO CASE 11: Generalized Anxiety Disorder

Summary: A 28-year-old patient presents with symptoms of chronic anxiety. These include worrying about a host of problems that are not specific to any one category. Her physical symptoms include muscle tension, insomnia, and restlessness. Her anxiety is interfering with her ability to work, and she is unable to control it.

- **Most likely diagnosis:** Generalized anxiety disorder (GAD).
- **Best treatment:** Benzodiazepines are effective treatments, although 25% to 30% of patients do not respond to this medication, become drowsy when taking it, or become addicted to it. Buspirone can also be prescribed, although it can be ineffective in patients previously exposed to benzodiazepines. Selective serotonin reuptake inhibitors (SSRIs) are effective in GAD, but they can take 2 to 3 weeks to work and can transiently increase anxiety.

Analysis

Objectives

1. Understand the diagnostic criteria for GAD (Table 11–1).
2. Be aware of the medications used to treat GAD and the problems associated with each.

Table 11–1

DIAGNOSTIC CRITERIA FOR GENERALIZED ANXIETY DISORDER

A. Excessive and uncontrollable anxiety persisting for at least 6 months.
B. The person struggles to control the worry.
C. Three of these six criteria:
   1. Restlessness or feeling keyed up or on edge
   2. Being easily fatigued
   3. Difficulty concentrating or mind going blank
   4. Irritability
   5. Muscle tension
   6. Sleep disturbance
D. The focus of the anxiety is not related to another axis I disorder such as somatization disorder.
E. The anxiety must cause clinically significant distress or impairment of functioning.
F. The anxiety is not caused by the direct effects of a substance of abuse or medication.

Considerations

This patient has a long history of being a worrier, and her worrying has increased over the past 7 months following the birth of her child. She worries about many problems in multiple categories. She has both cognitive (worry) as well as somatic (restlessness, insomnia, muscle tension) symptoms. She is unable to control her worrying, and it is interfering with her work. She denies medical or substance use/abuse problems. This clinical picture is classic for GAD.

APPROACH TO GENERALIZED ANXIETY DISORDER

Definitions

Anxiety: Worry or nervousness that can manifest as cognitive preoccupations (such as difficulty concentrating), emotional states (such as irritability), and somatic symptoms (such as muscle tension, restlessness, fatigue, or sleep problems).

Buspirone (Buspar): An azaspirone agent approved by the Food and Drug Administration for the treatment of anxiety disorders; it acts as an agonist on serotonin type 1A receptors. Two to four weeks are required for a successful therapeutic effect, and adverse effects include restlessness, insomnia, and nervousness.

Clinical Approach

Generalized anxiety disorder can be defined as anxiety and worry about several events and activities for a majority of the day over a 6-month time period. The anxiety and worry associated with GAD can be distinguished from normal anxiety by their excessive nature, the difficulty involved in controlling them, and their interference in everyday life. To establish a diagnosis of GAD, other etiologies of anxiety must be investigated, including hyperthyroidism, drug abuse, and even cardiovascular disease. Therefore, a thorough medical history and workup are essential.

Generalized anxiety disorder is **more common in women** than in men. The age of onset is often difficult to calculate, as most patients typically report a history of excessive worry throughout the duration of their lives. Somatic complaints can be prominent, and patients can present with symptoms of motor tension, autonomic hyperactivity, and cognitive vigilance. Symptoms of motor tension include shakiness, restlessness, and headaches. Patients with autonomic hyperactivity can have gastrointestinal, pulmonary, or cardiovascular complaints, whereas patients with cognitive vigilance are often irritable and easily frazzled. The etiology of GAD is unknown, but it is probably generated though the interaction of biological and psychosocial factors.

The course of GAD is variable. It is usually regarded as a **chronic condition** that worsens with life stressors and with the occurrence of negative life events. Approximately 50% to 90% of patients with GAD have an associated mental disorder such as major depressive disorder, panic disorder, and dysthymic disorder. Although GAD is a common psychiatric illness, only one third of patients actually seek treatment for it. Others seek help for somatic symptoms of this illness from various other physicians such as cardiologists, internists, and gastroenterologists.

Differential Diagnosis

It is important to distinguish GAD from other anxiety disorders, depression with comorbid anxiety, and anxiety secondary to medical conditions or substance use. A carefully constructed history and a urine toxicology study should distinguish these conditions from anxiety disorders. Several **medical conditions** are characterized by symptoms of anxiety: **Graves's disease, pulmonary embolism, hyperthyroidism, Sjögren syndrome, and certain seizures.** Typically, standard blood chemistry tests, an electrocardiogram, and thyroid function tests should be obtained.

Treatment

Individuals with GAD often initially seek treatment from primary care physicians or internists. Evidence-based treatments for GAD include pharmacotherapy and cognitive-behavioral therapy. The **three main agents** used in the treatment of GAD are **buspirone, benzodiazepines, and SSRIs;** beta-adrenergic blockers and tricyclic antidepressants have also been prescribed. Treatment length varies from 6 to 12 months to lifelong treatment. BuSpar (buspirone) is effective in the majority of patients with GAD (60% to 80%) but takes 2 to 3 weeks to become effective; it is not likely to be beneficial when instituted *after* benzodiazepines have been used. Benzodiazepines are effective immediately but are not efficacious in 25% to 30% of patients. Tolerance and dependence to benzodiazepines can develop in those patients with a history of substance dependence. Therefore, a mid–half-life benzodiazepine should be chosen and prescribed at the lowest effective dose. SSRIs are also effective but take 2 to 3 weeks to take effect; optimally they should be administered along with a benzodiazepine, and the latter tapered after a month or two.

Cognitive-behavioral therapy (CBT), which consists of methods to help the patient identify and change negative beliefs along with relaxation or biofeedback, has been shown to have both short- and long-term benefits. **Psychodynamic psychotherapy** aims at uncovering unconscious reasons for anxiety, such as **conflicts and fears;** there is some anecdotal evidence indicating that this form of therapy is effective in promoting improved mastery over anxiety.

Comprehension Questions

[11.1] A diagnosis of GAD is made for a 41-year-old female accountant who has had moderate but distressing symptoms for several years. She has strong negative feelings about taking any psychotropic medication, even after being educated about pharmacologic treatment options. Which of the following would be the most efficacious treatment option?

A. Cognitive-behavioral therapy
B. Psychoanalysis
C. Psychoeducation
D. Supportive psychotherapy

[11.2] A 38-year-old man without past medical history presents to his family physician with the chief complaint of "I'm having ulcers." His history, however does not appear to be consistent with gastritis, ulcers, or reflux. After further questioning, he describes ongoing headaches for eight months, along with difficulty sleeping. Although he denies any specific or recent stressors, he admits to "always being a worry-wart," worrying about many different aspects of his life. He only has been taking ranitidine over the counter as needed. He drinks one to two glasses of wine 1 to 2 days per week and denies drug use. Based on his likely diagnosis, which of the following additional psychiatric disorders are most likely to also be present in this patient?

A. Antisocial personality disorder
B. Dysthymic disorder
C. Factitious disorder
D. Schizophrenia
E. Somatization disorder

[11.3] A 45-year-old woman with alcohol dependence in full remission is referred to your practice. She has a history of GAD and was recently prescribed a benzodiazepine by her internist. Which of the following is the most appropriate treatment for her?

A. Add SSRI
B. Buspirone monotherapy
C. Continue benzodiazepine
D. Selective serotonin reuptake inhibitor monotherapy

Answers

[11.1] **A.** Because the patient's symptoms are moderate and she feels so negatively about medication, the best option for psychotherapy is CBT, the most studied evidence-based psychotherapy. Other interventions such as insight-oriented psychotherapy and supportive psychotherapy are less likely to be effective.

[11.2] **B.** This patient appears to suffer from generalized anxiety disorder. There is a high comorbidity in this illness, especially with other anxiety disorders, such as panic disorder and phobias. Dysthymic disorder and major depressive disorder are also very commonly associated conditions. Substance use disorders are also not uncommon in patients with GAD.

[11.3] **D.** SSRIs are a first-line treatment for GAD. Potentially addictive medications such as benzodiazepines should be avoided in patients with a history of substance dependence. Buspirone is not as effective in patients already exposed to benzodiazepines.

CLINICAL PEARLS

- Generalized anxiety disorder is almost always accompanied by another mental disorder; the physician should inquire about symptoms of depression, traumatic stressors, panic attacks, and substance abuse.
- Many medical conditions can mimic GAD, and so a full medical evaluation is mandatory in a workup for anxiety disorders.
- In anxiety disorders, genetic predisposition and environment are both etiologic factors; both biological and psychological explanations are pertinent in understanding these conditions.
- Buspirone, benzodiazepines, and SSRIs are the three most appropriate first-line medications for treating GAD.

REFERENCES

Rapee RM, Barlow DH. Generalized anxiety disorders, panic disorders, and phobias. In: Sutker PB, Adams HE, eds., Comprehensive handbook of psychopathology, 3rd ed. New York: Kluwer Academic/Plenum Publishers, 2001:131.

Thayer JF, Friedman BH, Borkevec TD. Autonomic characteristics of generalized anxiety disorder and worry. Biol Psychiatry 1996;39:255.

❖ CASE 12

A 27-year-old man is brought to the emergency department by his friends and his roommate. The friends state that the patient had not slept for the past 3 or 4 weeks. They have noticed that he stays up all night cleaning his apartment. He has bought new computer equipment and a digital video disc player, although his roommate claims that the patient cannot afford these kinds of items. The patient has also been bragging to his friends that he has slept with three different women in the past week, behavior very unlike his usual self, and he has been very irritable and explosive. He has been drinking a "lot of alcohol" for the past 2 weeks, which is uncharacteristic. The friends state that they have not seen the patient using drugs, and they do not think he has any medical problems or takes any prescription medication. They are not aware of any family history of medical or psychiatric disorders. They state that the patient is a graduate student in social work.

On a mental status examination, the patient is noted to be alternately irritable and elated. He is wearing a bright-orange top and red slacks, and his socks are mismatched. He paces the room and refuses to sit down when asked to do so by the examiner. His speech is rapid and loud, and it is hard to interrupt him. He claims that his mood is "great," and he is very angry with his friends for insisting that he come to the emergency department. He states that they have probably insisted that he come because "they are jealous of my success with women." He states that he is destined for greatness. His thought processes are tangential. He denies having any suicidal or homicidal ideation, hallucinations, or delusions.

- **What is the next diagnostic step?**
- **What is the most likely diagnosis?**
- **What is the best initial treatment?**

ANSWERS TO CASE 12: Bipolar Disorder, Manic (Adult)

Summary: A 27-year-old man presents to the emergency department with the classic signs and symptoms of mania. He has been abusing alcohol, but the abuse appears to have started *after* the onset of his manic symptoms. Whether he uses drugs is unknown and thus must be ruled out before a diagnosis of mania can be definitively established.

- ◆ **Next diagnostic step:** A urinalysis for drugs of abuse should be ordered, and a determination of alcohol blood level should be made as well.
- ◆ **Most likely diagnosis:** Bipolar disorder, manic.
- ◆ **Best initial treatment:** Admission to thc hospital should be recommended, although it is unclear whether the patient is committable at this point. At the least, he will need treatment with a mood stabilizer (lithium, carbamazepine, valproic acid) and perhaps with an antipsychotic (such as risperidone) as well.

Analysis

Objectives

1. Recognize the signs and/or symptoms of mania.
2. Realize that the use of drugs and/or alcohol must be ruled out before a diagnosis of mania can be made.
3. Understand the criteria for admission of a patient with mania.
4. Understand the criteria for involuntary admission of a psychiatric patient.

Considerations

This patient's history offers a rather straightforward description of manic behavior, and the results of his mental status examination are fairly classic as well. His lack of significant alcohol use (at least according to his friends) and his lack of medical problems make a diagnosis of mania more likely. Drug use, although denied by his friends, must be ruled out by a urine toxicology screening. Given the patient's irritability and lack of insight into his disease, it will probably be impossible to talk him into admitting himself to the hospital voluntarily, and he is not ill enough to be admitted involuntarily. At this stage, it is unlikely that the patient will agree to take medication either.

APPROACH TO BIPOLAR DISORDER, MANIC (ADULT)

Definitions

Involuntary commitment: Although their laws vary, all states have some sort of mechanism for placing a patient in a psychiatric hospital in the event of uncontrollable or imminently dangerous mental illness. Usually, patients must present an immediate danger to themselves (suicidality) or others (homicidality or extreme, violent, acting-out behavior) or be unable to care for themselves (e.g., walking outside unclothed in the middle of winter, walking in traffic). Commitment to a hospital involves the signing of commitment papers by a physician. The patient must then appear in court within a specified number of days so that it can be determined if the commitment should continue or the patient should be discharged.

Clinical Approach

Bipolar disorders are mood disorders with episodes of **depression and either mania or hypomania.** It has been estimated that bipolar I disorder has a lifetime prevalence of approximately 1%, and bipolar II disorder, a lifetime prevalence of approximately 0.5%. There is equal prevalence among men and women. The age of onset varies between 5 and 50 years of age, or older (in rare cases), with a mean of 30 years of age. Bipolar disorder usually presents with depression first.

Bipolar I disorder consists of **episodes of depression and episodes of full-blown mania.** Mania is indicated by an elevated, expansive, or irritable mood that deviates from the patient's normal mood. Patients are impulsive, grandiose, and distractible and participate in risky behaviors. The *Diagnostic and Statistical Manual of Mental Disorders, 4th edition (DSM-IV)* lists separate diagnoses for a single episode of mania and for a specific type of recurrent episode, based on the symptoms of the most recent episode (i.e., bipolar I disorder, most recent episode manic) (see Table 12–1).

Bipolar II disorder is characterized by episodes of depression and **episodes** of **hypomania,** which are symptoms that do not meet the full criteria for mania. For both disorders, the most recent episode can be described with certain specifiers such as "with psychotic features," "with melancholic features," "with atypical features," or "with catatonic features." Another classification is **rapid cycling,** which indicates that the patient has had at least **four episodes within a 12-month period.** In addition, patients with bipolar disorder can present with a "mixed state," with elements of both depression and mania or hypomania (for example, depressed mood with irritability and insomnia). Both bipolar disorders I and II should be differentiated from cyclothymic disorders.

Bipolar I disorder usually begins with an episode of depression and is a recurring disorder. After approximately five episodes, the time between

Table 12–1
DIAGNOSTIC CRITERIA FOR BIPOLAR DISORDER, MANIC (ADULT)

1. The patient must exhibit a continuously and abnormally elevated or irritable mood for at least 1 week.
2. During the period when their mood is disturbed, patients must exhibit three or more of the following:
   a. Inflated self-esteem or grandiosity
   b. Decreased need for sleep
   c. Increased talkativeness
   d. Racing thoughts
   e. Psychomotor agitation
   f. Excessive involvement in pleasurable activities that have a high potential for painful consequences (such as overspending or sexual indiscretions)
3. The symptoms do not meet the criteria for a mixed episode.
4. Social and/or occupational functioning is impaired.
5. The symptoms are not caused by a substance or by a general medical condition.

episodes stabilizes to approximately 6 to 9 months. The prognosis is worse for bipolar I disorder than for major depressive disorder. The disorder has a chronic course in approximately one third of all patients, and they experience significant social decline. The course of and prognosis for bipolar II disorder are currently being studied.

Differential Diagnosis

The differential diagnosis for mania is quite straightforward, but the diagnoses themselves can be difficult to establish. For example, identical clinical presentations can result from **substance-induced** mood disorder, mood disorder secondary to a general medical condition, and mania; hence, **illicit or prescribed agents must be ruled out** as well as medical conditions. Drugs such as **corticosteroids and levodopa** and stimulants such as **cocaine** have been known to cause manic-like behavior. General medical conditions such as metabolic disturbances caused by hemodialysis, infections, neoplastic diseases, and seizures can also cause these types of behavior. **Schizophrenia** must be on the differential list and must be ruled out by looking at secondary features such as family history, level of premorbid functioning, or a history of manic symptoms if the clinical features themselves do not set it apart. **Schizoaffective disorder** can be characterized by **psychotic behavior and manic features** and must be differentiated by the time courses of the two. In an episode of mania, an elevated mood and grandiosity can appear without psychotic symptoms, which in any case must not precede such symptoms. Patients with schizoaffective disorder can exhibit mood symptoms, but psychotic symptoms precede the mood symptoms and/or can continue after the mood reverts back to euthymia.

Treatment

Patients with bipolar disorder should be treated in a calm, structured environment. The patient and his or her family should be educated about the illness and treatment. Patients should be treated with mood stabilizers, alone or in combination with an atypical or second generation antipsychotic, first. **Mood stabilizers** such as **lithium, and valproic acid are generally the first-line mood stabilizers used. Carbamazepine or oxcarbazepine are second-line choices for mood stabilization. In patients with bipolar disorder presenting with depression, lamotrigine can be a more effective mood stabilizer. Risperidone and olanzapine are recommended as choices of antipsychotic medications. A benzodiazepine can be used short-term** until the mood stabilizer and antipsychotic take effect. **Antidepressants can be added to a mood stabilizer if depression does not respond to a mood stabilizer alone.** Supportive or insight-oriented psychotherapy can also be useful once patients have been stabilized, and they begin to work through the havoc this disorder usually produces in their lives.

Comprehension Questions

[12.1] A 62-year-old man presents to his primary care physician at the insistence of his wife. The man states that there is nothing wrong with him, but that he has not been sleeping nearly as much as he used to, often needing less than 2 hours of sleep a night. His wife notes that he has been exceedingly irritable, has been charging excessive amounts of money on their credit cards, and has been talking about running in a marathon, although he has never expressed such an interest before. The patient has no previous psychiatric or medical history. He denies the use of drugs or alcohol. Which of the following courses of action should the physician take first?

A. Request a urine toxicology screening for drugs of abuse
B. Perform a complete physical examination
C. Treat with a mood-stabilizing drug
D. Treat with an antipsychotic drug
E. Prescribe sleep medication

[12.2] An 18-year-old man is brought to the emergency department by his friends after he started a fight with one of them and subsequently was knocked unconscious. On awakening, the patient states that he was fighting for the "freedom of the world" and that he was told by "the voices in his head" that his friends held the key to winning the battle. The patient is irritable and restless and paces around in the emergency department. He is unable to sit still for the interview and prefers to stand up, keeping his back to the door as he speaks with the physician. The patient's friends state that he has been withdrawing from them and his schoolwork over the past 18 months and that they think he has become "odd." They report that his mood has become irritable only over the past several days. They say that he hoards random scraps of paper in his room and that his grades have dropped dramatically over the past 6 months. The results of a toxicology screening are negative, as are those of a physical examination, although the examination was limited because of poor cooperation on the part of the patient. Which of the following is the most likely diagnosis?

A. Schizophrenia
B. Bipolar disorder, manic
C. Schizoaffective disorder
D. Mood disorder secondary to a general medical condition
E. Substance-induced mood disorder

[12.3] A 24-year-old woman with a diagnosis of bipolar disorder, manic, is treated with a mood stabilizer (lithium) and haloperidol, an antipsychotic. Which of these medications should be discontinued first once her condition has been stabilized?

A. Lithium because of the risk of renal damage
B. Lithium because of the risk of weight gain
C. Haloperidol because of the risk of habituation
D. Haloperidol because of the risk of extra pyramidal side effects
E. Both should be discontinued simultaneously once the patient's condition is stable.

[12.4] A 33-year-old woman with bipolar disorder is 22 weeks pregnant. She has been taking valproic acid for her symptoms. Which of the following is the most likely abnormality that an ultrasound examination would show?

A. Fetal microcephaly
B. Fetal spina bifida
C. Fetal abdominal wall defect
D. Fetal renal dysplasia

Answers

[12.1] **B.** In a patient of this age, with no psychiatric or medical history, general medical conditions responsible for his behavior should be ruled out before an episode of bipolar mania is considered.

[12.2] **A.** This patient is currently experiencing a frank episode of psychosis, which appears to be quite manic. However, he has a history of a disturbance in premorbid functioning that predates the mood symptoms by 18 months. He is also in the prime age range for new-onset schizophrenia, making this the more likely diagnosis.

[12.3] **C.** Because tardive dyskinesia is irreversible, antipsychotics with a potential for causing this disorder should be discontinued as soon as the patient's psychotic symptoms remit, and the patient's condition is stable.

[12.4] **B.** Maternal use of valproic acid is associated with a 1% to 2% risk of fetal neural tube defects such as spina bifida.

CLINICAL PEARLS

- Patients in the midst of an episode of mania are often quite irritable and have very little insight into their own disease, making compliance with treatment difficult.
- Schizoaffective disorder can be differentiated from acute mania by obtaining a longitudinal history and finding the presence of psychosis in the absence of mood symptoms, which confirms the former.
- Mood stabilizers such as lithium and valproic acid are generally the first-line drugs used to treat this disorder. Psychotherapy or other agents (antidepressants or antipsychotics) should be used only after therapeutic mood stabilizer levels.
- During the course of an episode of acute mania, patients almost always require an antipsychotic in addition to a mood stabilizer, at least for the short term.

REFERENCES

American Psychiatric Association. Treating bipolar disorder. In: Compendium of APA Practice Guidelines. Arlington, VA: American Psychiatric Press Inc., 2004.

Ebert M, Loosen P, Nurcombe B, eds. Current diagnosis and treatment in psychiatry. New York: McGraw-Hill, 2000:311–322.

Goldman HH. Review of general psychiatry, 5th ed. New York: McGraw-Hill, 2000:263–283.

❖ CASE 13

A 13-year-old girl is brought to a psychiatrist by her mother. The patient states that for the past 6 months she has been showering for long periods, up to 5 hours at a time. She says she is unable to stop this behavior although it is distressing to her and causes her skin to crack and bleed. She reports that the symptoms started after she began to have recurrent thoughts of being dirty or unclean. These thoughts occur many times a day. She states that she grows increasingly anxious until she is able to take a shower and clean herself. The patient claims that the amount of time she spends in the shower is increasing because she must wash herself in a particular order to avoid getting the "clean suds" mixed up with the "dirty suds." If this happens, she must start the whole showering process over again. The patient states that she knows that she "must be crazy," but she seems unable to stop herself. The patient's mother verifies the patient's history. She claims that her daughter has always been popular in school and has many friends. She emphatically states that her daughter has never used drugs or alcohol. The patient's only medical problem is a history of asthma, which is treated with an albuterol inhaler. The patient's mental status examination is otherwise unremarkable except as noted earlier.

◆ **What is the most likely diagnosis for this patient?**

◆ **What would be the best type of psychotherapy for this condition?**

◆ **What would be the best type of pharmacotherapy for this patient?**

ANSWERS TO CASE 13: Obsessive-Compulsive Disorder (Child)

Summary: A 13-year-old girl has a 6-month history of excessive showering, up to 5 hours at a time. This showering is preceded by recurrent thoughts of being dirty or unclean. The patient becomes increasingly anxious because of these thoughts unless she is able to shower. She has a particular order of showering that must be followed or she must start over again. The patient is aware of the abnormal nature of her thoughts and behavior and is distressed by them.

- **Most likely diagnosis:** Obsessive-compulsive disorder (OCD)
- **Best psychotherapy:** Behavioral therapy involving exposure and response prevention
- **Best pharmacotherapy:** A selective serotonin reuptake inhibitor (SSRI)

Analysis

Objectives

1. Understand the diagnostic criteria of obsessive-compulsive disorder.
2. Know the psychotherapeutic treatment of choice for this disorder.
3. Know the pharmacologic treatment of choice for this disorder.

Considerations

This patient has a classic history of OCD. She has recurrent thoughts of being dirty or unclean (obsessions) and must shower (the compulsion), or she becomes increasingly anxious. The thoughts she has are not simply excessive worries about real-life problems. She has tried to ignore these thoughts but is unable to do so and is distressed by them. (Note that the ability to see that the obsessions and/or compulsions are unreasonable is a prerequisite for the diagnosis in adults, although not in children.) There is no evidence that this patient is abusing drugs or alcohol or has a medical disorder that might be causing her symptoms.

APPROACH TO OBSESSIVE-COMPULSIVE DISORDER (CHILD)

Definitions

Clomipramine: A serotonin and dopaminergic neurotransmitter inhibitor in the class of tricyclic and tetracyclic agents that is effective in the treatment of OCD. The main adverse effects are sedation, anticholinergic side effects, and at toxic levels, cardiac dysrhythmias. (Because of the side effects, many clinicians use SSRIs for this disorder; higher doses than those used for depression are required.)

Compulsions: Repetitive behaviors or mental acts that a person feels driven to perform in response to an obsession according to a rigid set of rules. These behaviors or mental acts are aimed at preventing or reducing distress or preventing a feared event or situation. Typically, there is no realistic connection between the feared event or situation and the behavior or mental act.

Exposure: Presenting the patient with the feared object or situation. Exposure to the feared object or situation, coupled with relaxation training and response prevention, constitutes a behavior modification program proven successful in patients with OCD.

Obsessions: Recurrent and persistent thoughts or images that are experienced as intrusive and inappropriate and cause marked anxiety or distress. They are not simply excessive worries about real-life problems.

Clinical Approach

According to the *Diagnostic and Statistical Manual of Mental Disorders, text revision (DSM-IV-TR)* the hallmark of **OCD** is recurrent obsessions and/or compulsions (Table 13–1). The obsessions are persistent in the conscious awareness of the patient, who typically recognizes them as being absurd and irrational and often has a desire to resist them. However, half of all patients offer little resistance to compulsions. Overall, OCD is a disabling, time-consuming, distressing disorder that interferes with one's normal routine, occupational function, social activities, and/or relationships.

The lifetime prevalence of OCD is approximately 2% to 3% across all ethnicities. Obsessive-compulsive disorder accounts for up to 10% of outpatient psychiatric clinic visits, making it the fourth most common psychiatric diagnosis after phobias, substance-related disorders, and major depressive disorder. Men and women are affected equally; however, adolescent males are more

Table 13–1
DIAGNOSTIC CRITERIA FOR OBSESSIVE-COMPULSIVE DISORDER

A. The presence of either obsessions or compulsions.
B. The person realizes that the obsessions or compulsions are excessive and unreasonable; this requirement need not apply to children.
C. The obsessions or compulsions cause marked distress, are time-consuming, or interfere with the person's normal routine.
D. If another major mental illness is present, the contents of the obsessions or compulsions are not restricted to it.

commonly affected than adolescent females. The mean age of presentation is 20 years of age. Onset can occur in childhood, and case reports describe children as young as 2 years old with the disorder. Individuals affected with OCD often have additional psychiatric disorders; these include major depressive disorder, social phobia, generalized anxiety disorder, alcohol use disorders, specific phobia, panic disorder, and eating disorders. Interestingly, 20% to 30% of OCD patients have a history of tics, with Tourette's disorder comorbid in 5% to 7% of patients.

Differential Diagnosis

The differential diagnosis for OCD must include other anxiety disorders that could cause a person to behave outside his or her normal behavior patterns. Persons with obsessive-compulsive personality disorder do not meet the criteria for the disorder, and they have a lesser degree of impairment. Patients with phobias (specific phobia or social phobia) attempt to avoid the feared object but do not obsessively ruminate about it unless directly presented with it. Patients with generalized anxiety disorder worry excessively, and their anxiety is spread across many areas, not on just one aspect of the obsession. They also do not develop compulsions. Care must be taken to rule out any medical conditions or the use of any substances with effects that might mimic symptoms of OCD. Thoughts and behavior must be carefully evaluated to ensure that they are not overtly bizarre or psychotic, and thus, indicating that the patient is suffering from a psychotic disorder such as schizophrenia.

Treatment

The treatment of OCD in children and adolescents can involve psychotherapeutic and psychopharmacologic interventions. Both have been shown to be helpful in controlled clinical trials. The greatest efficacy can be seen when psychotherapy is combined with SSRIs. The primary psychotherapeutic treatment involves behavior therapy referred to as **exposure/response prevention.** In this type of treatment, the therapist and patient develop a list of triggers for the compulsive behavior. The items on this list are arranged into a hierarchy, which is the key to the treatment. The **child is exposed to the least anxiety-provoking trigger first and then, using anxiety-reducing techniques, is gradually moved to higher levels** of the hierarchy until tolerance is developed. Repeated exposure to the triggers is associated with decreased anxiety. This type of treatment requires a good relationship with the therapist as well as a moderate to high degree of motivation on the part of the patient.

The second type of treatment shown to be effective for OCD in clinical trials is psychopharmacologic intervention. The class of medications found to be most effective in treating OCD includes **SSRIs.** The first medication used was the **nonselective agent, clomipramine.** In appropriate doses, it has been found to be significantly superior to a placebo in reducing OCD symptoms. It can require several weeks to become effective at appropriate dose levels. The more recent and specific **SSRIs (fluoxetine, sertraline, and fluvoxamine)** have been shown to significantly reduce both obsessions and compulsions in children and adolescents compared to a placebo.

Comprehension Questions

[13.1] A 17-year-old high school senior is referred to a psychiatrist by his counselor because of academic difficulty. Although he had always been an honors student, this past year his grades have quickly dropped, especially in mathematics. When questioned, he reveals the new onset of "superstitions" involving numbers. When presented with certain numbers, he feels compelled to count forwards and then backwards to and from that number. He becomes anxious about not completing this task, although he is unable to state a particular consequence. If interrupted, he must begin all over again. He realizes that there is "no good reason" for his behavior, but is unable to stop it. As a result of this, he not only feels "tortured," but he may need to repeat this year in school. He denies any past psychiatric history. He had an appendectomy at age 15 and takes no medications. He does not drink alcohol or use tobacco products or illicit drugs. Which of the following would be the most efficacious treatment for his condition?

A. Behavioral therapy alone
B. Behavioral therapy plus pharmacotherapy
C. Pharmacotherapy alone
D. Psychodynamic psychotherapy alone
E. Psychodynamic psychotherapy plus pharmacotherapy

[13.2] The patient in question [13.1] begins exposure and response prevention therapy with some improvement. It is decided to begin a psychotropic medication to further decrease his symptomatology. Which of the following neurotransmitter systems should be targeted in order to achieve the most efficacy?

A. Adrenergic
B. Cholinergic
C. Dopaminergic
D. Serotonergic

[13.3] The patient in questions [13.1] and [13.2] is subsequently started on clomipramine. Which of the following side effects would he most likely develop as a result of the medication?

A. Activation
B. Diarrhea
C. Dry mouth
D. Frequent urination
E. Hypertension

Answers

[13.1] **B.** This individual suffers from OCD with his obsessions, compulsions, significant anxiety, and interference in his academic functioning. Whereas behavioral therapy and medications such as clomipramine and SSRIs are helpful in treating OCD, there is evidence that a combination of the two provides the greatest efficacy. There is an absence of studies documenting improvement in OCD solely with psychodynamic psychotherapy.

[13.2] **D.** The serotonergic system appears to be involved in both the genesis and treatment of OCD. This is supported by the fact that medications specific in affecting serotonin, such as clomipramine and SSRIs, are more effective in treating OCD when compared with less-specific antidepressants.

[13.3] **C.** Clomipramine, being in the class of tricyclic and tetracyclic antidepressants, blocks several different receptors, thereby causing a host of side effects. These include cholinergic (causing dry mouth, constipation, and urinary retention), histaminic (causing sedation and weight gain), and adrenergic (causing orthostatic hypotension). Because of these various side effects, SSRIs are generally better tolerated as first-line medications for treating OCD.

CLINICAL PEARLS

❖ Some children with OCD do not understand that the symptoms are unreasonable because they have not yet achieved the necessary developmental capacity.

❖ Behavior therapy has proven effective for the treatment of OCD.

❖ Clomipramine was considered the gold standard for the treatment of OCD, although SSRIs are more frequently used given their improved specificity and tolerability.

❖ The combination of SSRIs with behavior therapy can provide the best outcomes for treating OCD.

REFERENCE

Kaplan H, Sadock B. Synopsis of psychiatry, 9th ed. Baltimore: Lippincott Williams & Wilkins, 2003:616–623.

❖ CASE 14

A 45-year-old man comes to see his primary care physician with a chief complaint of fatigue lasting for the past 6 months. The man states that he goes to sleep easily enough but then wakes up repeatedly throughout the night. He has had this problem with sleep since his wife left him 6 months ago. On questioning, he reports drinking 6 to 12 beers a day, as well as several ounces of hard liquor. He says that it takes more alcohol than it used to "to get me relaxed." The patient claims he has experienced several blackouts caused by drinking during the past month. He admits that he often has a drink of alcohol first thing in the morning to keep him from feeling shaky. Despite his wife leaving him and his receiving several reprimands at work for tardiness and poor performance, he has been unable to stop drinking.

On mental status examination, the patient is alert and oriented to person, place, and time. He appears rather haggard, but his hygiene is good. His speech is of normal rate and tone, and he is cooperative with the physician. His mood is noted to be depressed, and his affect is congruent, although full-range. Otherwise, no abnormalities are noted.

◆ **What is the most likely diagnosis for this patient?**

◆ **What are some of the medical complications resulting from this disorder?**

ANSWERS TO CASE 14: Alcohol Dependence

Summary: A 45-year-old man comes to see his physician with a chief complaint of fatigue. Because of his heavy drinking, his wife left him 6 months ago, and he has not been sleeping well since then. He drinks 6 to 12 beers a day plus several ounces of hard liquor. He reports blackouts, an inability to quit drinking, tolerance for alcohol, and likely withdrawal symptoms. He has tried to quit on several occasions but has been unable to do so.

- **Most likely diagnosis:** Alcohol dependence.
- **Commonly associated medical complications:** Withdrawal seizures, delirium tremens, Wernicke-Korsakoff syndrome, cerebellar degeneration, peripheral neuropathy, fetal alcohol syndrome, hepatic encephalopathy, malabsorption syndromes, pancreatitis, cardiomyopathy, anemia, and an increased incidence of trauma (all types).

Analysis

Objectives

1. Recognize alcohol dependence in a patient.
2. Be familiar with the many medical complications that can be caused by the excessive use of alcohol.

Considerations

A 45-year-old man comes to see his physician with a chief complaint of fatigue. He has not been sleeping well for 6 months, and the pattern he describes is characteristic of alcohol dependence. His wife has left him, and his job is in jeopardy, but he is still unable to quit drinking. He drinks 6 to 12 beers a day plus several ounces of hard liquor. He reports blackouts, an inability to quit drinking, tolerance (it takes more alcohol to "make him relaxed"), and withdrawal symptoms (shakes).

APPROACH TO ALCOHOL DEPENDENCE

Definition

Delirium tremens: A delirium characterized by disorientation, fluctuation in the level of consciousness, elevated vital signs, and tremors as the result of an abrupt reduction in or cessation of heavy alcohol use that has lasted for a prolonged period of time.

Korsakoff syndrome (psychosis): Not actually a psychotic state but amnesia, especially anterograde amnesia (inability to learn new information), that develops after chronic alcohol use. It is usually **irreversible** and is also caused by a **thiamine deficiency.**

Wernicke syndrome: An acute, usually **reversible,** encephalopathy resulting from a **thiamine deficiency** and characterized by the **triad of delirium, ophthalmoplegia, and ataxia.**

Clinical Approach

In the United States, alcohol-related disorders are the third largest health problem (after heart disease and cancer) and the most common substance-related disorders. Furthermore, alcohol is associated with increased rates of cancer, heart disease, and hepatic disease. In the United States, 30% to 45% of all adults have had at least one episode of an alcohol-related problem (e.g., a blackout, driving while intoxicated [DWI], missing work, an automotive accident), whereas 3% to 5% of women and 10% of men will meet the diagnostic criteria for alcohol dependence during their lifetime. Alcohol is associated with 50% of all homicides and 25% of suicides. Yearly, 200,000 deaths are attributed to alcohol abuse. Alcohol use is also strongly associated with illicit drug use.

Alcohol dependence can be characterized by different drinking patterns. For instance, some individuals require a large amount of alcohol each day, others drink heavily only on weekends, and some binge heavily for days followed by days of no alcoholic intake at all. Alcohol dependence is also associated with behaviors such as an inability to cut down or stop drinking, repeated attempts to curb drinking ("going on the wagon"), binging (intoxication throughout the day for a minimum of 2 days), episodes of amnesia (blackouts), and drinking despite a known medical disorder that is exacerbated by the intake of alcohol (Table 14–1). Individuals with alcohol dependence show impairment in social and occupational functions. This behavior can be manifested by violence toward others, absence from work, legal difficulties (DWI, intoxicated behavior), and finally, strained relationships with friends and family.

Table 14–1

DIAGNOSTIC CRITERIA FOR ALCOHOL DEPENDENCE*

Three or more of the following are present:

1. Tolerance for alcohol
2. Withdrawal symptoms (e.g., elevated vital signs, tremors, delirium tremens, seizures)
3. Alcohol taken in larger amounts or over a longer period of time than was intended
4. Persistent desire or unsuccessful efforts to cut down or control alcohol use
5. A great deal of time spent obtaining alcohol, using alcohol, or recovering from the effects of alcohol
6. Important social, occupational, or recreational activities given up or reduced in frequency because of alcohol use
7. Alcohol use continued despite the knowledge that it causes or worsens physical or psychological problems (e.g., ulcer disease, depression)

*It is helpful to note that these are the same general criteria for all substances of abuse.

Differential Diagnosis

An important distinction is the difference between alcohol dependence and alcohol abuse. Alcohol abuse (like the abuse of all substances) is characterized by a pattern of use resulting in at least one of the following:

1. Failure to fulfill obligations at work, school, or home
2. Continued use in dangerous situations (e.g., DWI, operating heavy machinery)
3. Alcohol-related legal problems (e.g., driving while under the influence [DUI], DWI)
4. Social or interpersonal problems (e.g., arguments about alcohol, spousal abuse)

The previous criteria for *misuse* (abuse) of alcohol differ from the criteria for alcohol dependence, which demonstrate an *inability to control alcohol use* (physical and/or psychological dependence).

Treatment

The essential treatment of alcohol dependence rests with the patient controlling his or her alcohol use, which is usually best achieved through total abstinence. Twelve-step programs such as the one sponsored by Alcoholics Anonymous (AA) are extremely helpful, as they address important issues necessary for recovery. These issues include denial that one has an addiction (prevalent in all addictive disorders), feelings of responsibility and blame, discouraging the enabling behavior of loved ones, establishing social support systems (through a sponsor), and a sense of hope within a community. Membership in these groups is free; they often meet daily and are located throughout the United States.

Antabuse (disulfiram) is a medication that blocks the enzyme acetaldehyde dehydrogenase. The purpose of taking this drug is to deter a patient from consuming alcohol, as concurrent use with alcohol (or alcohol-containing products such as foods and aftershave) causes extremely uncomfortable (and in high doses potentially fatal) physical symptoms. For this reason, the patient needs to be motivated, responsible, and without significant cognitive deficits, so that compliance with treatment instructions can be ensured. Another pharmacologic option is ReVia (naltrexone), an opioid antagonist. Studies have shown this medication to decrease craving for alcohol, believed to be caused by blocking the rewarding effects of alcohol.

The third, but least studied medication is Campral (acamprosate). The precise mechanism is unknown, but it has shown promise in improving abstinence when used in conjunction with psychological and behavioral treatment regimens.

Chronic alcohol use results in the depletion of many vitamins, most notably **thiamine.** This condition occurs because of decreased absorption as well as because of the poor nutrition often seen in individuals with alcohol dependence. It is therefore important for any individual with a pattern of heavy, chronic alcohol consumption to receive vitamin supplements. **Acute thiamine depletion causes Wernicke encephalopathy, and chronic thiamine depletion is thought to cause Korsakoff syndrome.** Wernicke encephalopathy is not an uncommon presentation in the emergency department setting. Intravenous administration of thiamine should be given to all patients suspected of alcoholism, because the combined Wernicke-Korsakoff syndrome has been precipitated in these patients after the administration of thiamine-free intravenous solution containing glucose.

Comprehension Questions

[14.1] A 28-year-old man presents with a 12-year history of regular alcohol use. Although he has been able to maintain employment as a truck driver, he often drives when "buzzed" in order to make his deadlines. He has been reprimanded on numerous occasions for failure to perform his job adequately, and this has led to increasing conflict with his wife. He denies any recent increase in drinking or any withdrawal symptoms, but he does admit to not getting "as drunk as I used to" following consumption of the same amount of alcohol. Which of the following factors in his history is the most specific for alcohol *dependence?*

A. Driving while intoxicated
B. Marital conflicts
C. Not becoming intoxicated as easily
D. Occupational problems
E. 12-year history of regular alcohol use

[14.2] Which of the following questions is the most sensitive in screening a patient for alcohol dependence?

A. Have you ever attempted to cut down on your drinking?
B. How frequently do you drink?
C. How much do you drink per day?
D. When did you start drinking regularly?
E. Do you drink hard liquor, or beer and wine only?

[14.3] A 48-year-old woman is brought to the emergency department. She is unresponsive to questions, stumbles around the room, and is agitated. On physical examination, you notice that she smells of alcohol, and she is not cooperative during the remainder of the examination. Administration of what medicine would be the most appropriate initial treatment?

A. Benzodiazepine
B. Disulfiram
C. Glucose
D. Thiamine
E. An antipsychotic agent

[14.4] A 60-year-old man is brought into the emergency room by his wife for "confusion." She reluctantly confides to the staff that he is a "heavy drinker," that he had drunk up to a case of beer almost every day for the past 30 years. Although he has not changed his alcohol intake significantly, over the past year he has eaten less, preferring alcohol to large meals. She has noticed a gradual weight loss as a result. His last drink was earlier this day. Which of the following would be the most likely finding on the mental status examination of this patient?

A. Confabulation
B. Delusions
C. Elevated affect
D. Fluctuating consciousness
E. Loose associations

Answers

[14.1] **C.** Although DWI, marital conflicts, and occupational problems are all criteria for alcohol abuse, only not becoming intoxicated as easily as in the past is a criterion for alcohol dependence. Tolerance for alcohol (experiencing either the same effect with an increased amount or a decreased effect with the same amount), withdrawal from alcohol, and an inability to control alcohol use are the characteristics of alcohol dependence.

[14.2] **A.** Although questions regarding the specific frequency, kind of alcohol, amount, and initial use of alcohol are important in establishing a history and pattern of abuse, only asking about attempts to cut back is specific for alcohol dependence, as this question addresses the inability to control alcohol use. The CAGE questionnaire (Ewing, 1984) has been validated in screening for alcohol dependence. It uses the mnemonic **CAGE.** A yes answer to two or more of the following questions is a sensitive indicator in diagnosing alcohol dependence.

Have you ever felt you should **C**ut down on your drinking?
Have you ever felt **A**nnoyed by someone criticizing your drinking?
Have you ever felt **G**uilty about your drinking?
Have you ever had an **E**ye opener (a drink first thing in the morning)?

[14.3] **D.** The most appropriate treatment is administration of thiamine. This patient presents with Wernicke encephalopathy, characterized by the triad of delirium, ataxia, and ophthalmoplegia. Thiamine must be given prior to glucose in patients suspected of having this disorder.

[14.4] **A.** This patient has a long history of heavy, regular alcohol use and likely malnutrition. A common sequela of this is chronic thiamine deficiency, resulting in Korsakoff syndrome. Korsakoff syndrome is characterized by an anterograde amnesia; this memory impairment is often (poorly) compensated for by the patient's confabulation, or filling in the missing memories with false information.

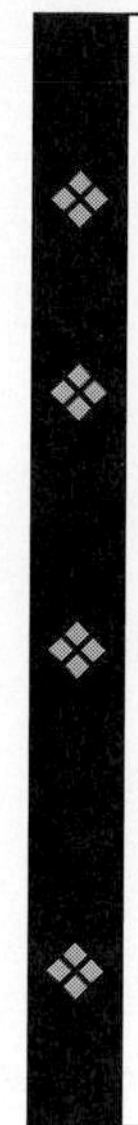

CLINICAL PEARLS

- Alcohol abuse is characterized by the recurrent *misuse* of alcohol, resulting in occupational, academic, interpersonal, or legal problems or in potentially dangerous situations.
- Alcohol dependence is characterized by a recurrent physical or psychological *dependence* on alcohol resulting in a tolerance for alcohol, withdrawal from alcohol, or an *inability to control alcohol use*.
- Both Wernicke and Korsakoff syndromes are thought to be caused by a thiamine deficiency. Wernicke syndrome classically features the triad of encephalopathy, ataxia, and ophthalmoplegia. A hallmark of Korsakoff syndrome is amnesia, especially anterograde amnesia.
- In a patient with suspected Wernicke encephalopathy, thiamine should be administered intravenously *prior to* glucose.

REFERENCES

Ebert M, Loosen P, Nurcombe B, eds. Current diagnosis and treatment in psychiatry. New York: McGraw-Hill, 2000:233–259.

Ewing JA. Detecting alcoholism: The CAGE questionnaire. JAMA 1984;252: 1905–1907.

Kaplan H, Sadock B. Synopsis of psychiatry, 9th ed. Baltimore: Lippincott Williams & Wilkins, 2003:412–413.

❖ CASE 15

A 24-year-old woman was admitted to the obstetrical service for the delivery of a full-term baby boy. One day after the delivery, the obstetrics service requested a consultation from the psychiatrist on duty to "rule out schizophrenia."

The psychiatrist interviews the patient and finds out that the pregnancy was the result of a rape the patient suffered 9 months previously. The patient is planning to give the baby up for adoption. She claims that she has never seen a psychiatrist and has never felt a need to do so. She speaks at length about how the rape was "written in the stars" for all to see; she is an avid astrologer. She denies having recurrent thoughts or nightmares about the rape itself. She states that she has very few close friends, preferring to study astrology and astral projection at home by herself. She believes strongly in reincarnation, although she knows that her family thinks this belief is strange. She admits that she has worked intermittently as a "crystal ball gazer" but has never held a steady, full-time, paying job.

During the mental status examination the patient sits upright in her hospital bed dressed in three hospital gowns and a robe, which she is wearing backward. Her hair is neatly combed, although one side is in braids and the other is not. She is cooperative with the interviewer. She states that her mood is good, and her affect is congruent although constricted. She has tangential thought processes and ideas of reference but no suicidal or homicidal ideation, hallucinations, or delusions.

◆ **What is the most likely diagnosis?**

◆ **What should your recommendations to the obstetrics service be?**

ANSWERS TO CASE 15: Schizotypal Personality Disorder

Summary: A 24-year-old immediately postpartum woman is referred to a psychiatrist by the obstetrics service because staff members believe she might be schizophrenic. The patient has odd beliefs and thinking, ideas of reference, and a constricted affect. She also dresses in a peculiar manner. She does not have close friends. Her thinking is tangential, but her thought content is within normal limits.

- **Most likely diagnosis:** Schizotypal personality disorder (SPD).
- **Recommendations to the obstetrics service:** Outpatient psychiatric follow-up. The patient does not have schizophrenia. Although transient psychotic episodes can occur in response to stress in patients with SPD, the patient is not having psychotic symptoms currently. The patient's odd beliefs and magical thinking should be conceptualized as a **nonpsychotic thought disorder or partial loss of reality testing.** If she develops an acute psychosis (hallucinations, thought disorganization, loose association) then treatment with a typical or atypical antipsychotic medication in the hospital is indicated. Otherwise, medication is not started in the hospital in the absence of acute psychosis because the patient will be unlikely to comply with medication unless she has a good therapeutic relationship with a psychiatrist.

  Ideally the psychiatrist who will follow her as an outpatient will see her briefly before discharge to increase the likelihood that she will follow through. Once a therapeutic relationship has been developed, there is a growing body of evidence to suggest that a low dose neuroleptic can impact the magical thinking and odd beliefs. Studies show that only 10% of patients with SPD have ever received antipsychotic medication. The same studies show that in their lifetimes, patients with SPD spend approximately 44 months involved in psychotherapy, countering the belief that these patients will not seek treatment.

Analysis

Objectives

1. Recognize schizotypal personality disorder in a patient.
2. Understand the relationship of schizotypal personality disorder and schizophrenia.

Considerations

This patient is viewed by members of the obstetrics team as odd, but she does not see herself in this manner. Although several abnormalities are observed during her mental status examination, including ideas of reference (not delusions of reference), unusual beliefs, unconventional thinking, a constricted affect, and an odd appearance, she does not exhibit any signs of a true psychosis. **She does not have hallucinations or fixed delusions,** and therefore her symptoms do not meet the diagnostic criteria for schizophrenia. She does not appear to have any psychological sequelae resulting from the rape (no symptoms of posttraumatic stress disorder), although she does seem to have incorporated its meaning into her unusual beliefs about the world.

Currently conceptualized as being a biologically-based disorder that is related to schizophrenia, SPD is a milder disorder on the schizophrenia spectrum. Family and adoptive studies suggest a greater prevalence of SPD in the relatives of patients with schizophrenia than in the general population. Interestingly, a greater prevalence of chronic schizophrenia in the relatives of patients with SPD is not as consistently found. It is thought that this means that susceptibility genes for psychosis is less prevalent in families of patients with SPD than those with schizophrenia. It appears that there are at least two inherited sets of genetic factors in SPD: One related to the bizarre thinking (nonpsychotic thought disorder) and one related to the social isolation and lack of comfort with other people seen in individuals with SPD.

APPROACH TO SCHIZOTYPAL PERSONALITY DISORDER

Definitions

Denial: A defense mechanism in which an individual deals with emotional conflict or stressors by refusing to acknowledge some painful aspect of external reality or subjective experience that is apparent to others. The term "psychotic denial" is used when there is gross impairment in reality testing.

Derealization: A feeling that the world, or reality, has changed. The environment feels unreal or strange.

Dysphoria: A state of mood that is unpleasant, often sad.

Idealization: A defense mechanism in which an individual deals with emotional conflict or stressors by attributing exaggerated positive qualities to others. Use of this mechanism can alternate with devaluation, its opposite.

Magical thinking: Thinking similar to that seen in young children in which the patient's thoughts, words, or actions are seen to have power over external events. (For example: It snows in the winter because I buy sidewalk salt every fall.)

Clinical Approach

Diagnostic Criteria

Patients with SPD have deficits in their abilities to have interpersonal relationships and **peculiarities in ideation, appearance, and behavior.** There is a pattern of acute discomfort when in close relationships, cognitive or perceptual distortions, and **eccentricities in behavior.** They **usually do not have close friends.** A patient can experience anxiety, depression, or other dysphoric mood states and can be suspicious or paranoid. Under stress, these patients can become **transiently psychotic.** Occurring in approximately 3% of the population, SPD is frequently diagnosed in females with fragile X syndrome.

Differential Diagnosis

Although both schizoid and SPD patients have discomfort with interpersonal relationships, patients with SPD can be differentiated from those with schizoid personality disorder by their peculiar behavior, thinking, and speech. Individuals with paranoid personality deal with the world as a hostile place and are suspicious that others will take advantage of them, but their suspiciousness never gets a delusional quality, and they do not have the odd behavior seen in SPD. Individuals with SPD are not frankly psychotic (i.e., do not have delusions and hallucinations), except perhaps transiently when under stress, which differentiates them from those with schizophrenia. More than 50% of individuals with SPD have at least one lifetime episode of major depression, and this should be treated with antidepressants when it occurs with SPD.

Treatment

Although these patients often exhibit bizarre speech, behavior, or beliefs, it is important for physicians not to ridicule their beliefs or to be judgmental about them, as this disrupts any alliance that is to be built. Low-dose antipsychotic agents can be helpful if transient psychoses appear. Group therapy can sometimes help alleviate the social anxiety and awkwardness common to such patients. Supportive individual psychotherapy can be beneficial.

Comprehension Questions

[15.1] Which of the following is an associated disorder in the family histories of patients with schizotypal personality disorder?

A. Bipolar disorder
B. Schizophrenia
C. Alcohol dependence
D. Panic disorder
E. Hypochondriasis

[15.2] Which of the following features must be present in a patient's history for schizotypal personality disorder to be diagnosed?

A. The patient must have a history of active substance use.
B. The patient must have a history of intense, short-lived friendships.
C. The patient must have auditory hallucinations.
D. The patient must have a history of suicidal ideation.
E. The patient must have a history of cognitive and perceptual distortions.

[15.3] A 25-year-old man with schizotypal personality disorder comes to his psychiatrist with a chief complaint of a depressed mood. He notes that since losing his job as an astrologer, he has been depressed and unable to sleep. He states that although his mood is usually fairly low (4 out of a possible 10), it has lately been a constant 2. The patient also notes problems with concentration and energy level and has experienced several crying spells. A mental status examination reveals ideas of reference and some mild paranoia. Which of the following medications is most likely to be helpful to this patient?

A. Ambien for insomnia
B. Ziprasidone for ideas of reference
C. Escitalopram for depressive symptoms
D. Divalproex for mood disturbance
E. Risperidone for paranoia

Answers

[15.1] **B.** There is a greater association of cases of schizotypal personality disorder among biological relatives of patients with schizophrenia than among controls.

[15.2] **E.** The odd quality of the way in which these patients perceive and think about the world is one of the diagnostic criteria for schizotypal personality disorder.

[15.3] **C.** Escitalopram is a selective serotonin reuptake inhibitor (SSRI) useful in the treatment of depression. Patients with schizotypal personality disorder who have either a depressive component to their illness or a secondary superimposed major depression (as can be the case with this patient) should be treated with antidepressants. Geodon (ziprasidone) and Risperdal (risperidone) are atypical antipsychotics that would be effective if the patient was having a transient psychotic episode, but he is not. Divalproex is an antiepileptic agent used as a mood stabilizer to treat conditions such as mania.

CLINICAL PEARLS

- Patients with schizotypal personality disorder show a pervasive, stable pattern of social and interpersonal deficits, a reduced capacity for (and discomfort with) interpersonal relationships, cognitive or perceptual distortions, and odd behavior.
- Schizotypal personality disorder is currently conceptualized as being a biologically based disorder that is related to schizophrenia but is a milder disorder on the schizophrenia spectrum.
- Individuals with SPD can be differentiated from those with paranoid personality in that the latter deal with the world as a hostile place and are suspicious that others will take advantage of them, but their suspiciousness never gets a delusional quality.
- Patients with this disorder can be differentiated from patients with schizoid personality disorder by their family history of schizophrenia, rarely successful work careers, and odd behavior, speech, and beliefs.
- Physicians do well in dealing with these patients when they can remain nonjudgmental about the patient's peculiar speech, beliefs, and behavior.

REFERENCES

Bender DS, Dolan RT, Skodal AE, et al. Treatment utilization by patients with personality disorders. Am J Psychiatry 2001;158(2):295–302.

Cloninger CR, Svrakic DM. Personality disorders. In: Sadock BJ, Sadock VA, eds. Kaplan and Sadock's comprehensive textbook of psychiatry, 7th ed. Philadelphia: Lippincott Williams & Wilkins, 2000:1723–1764.

Siever LJ, Davis KL. The pathophysiology of schizophrenia disorders: Perspectives from the spectrum. Am J Psychiatry 2004;161(3):398–413.

❖ CASE 16

A 29-year-old woman is brought to the emergency department by the police after they picked her up attempting to break into a grocery store. When they apprehended her, they noticed that her pupils were widely dilated and that she seemed "high." The patient states that she has been "smoking" for the majority of the past year. She claims that her habit now costs more than $100 per day, although she used to get the "same high" for $10. Without her "smokes," she craves the drug, becomes very sleepy, is depressed, and has a huge appetite. She has lost 30 lb in the past 6 months. When using this drug, she feels "really good" and has a lot of energy. She has tried to quit on numerous occasions, even entering an inpatient treatment program at one point, but has always gone back to using drugs. The patient used to be a secretary but lost her job because she was chronically late and stole money to pay for her habit; this is the reason why she was trying to rob the grocery store.

◆ **What is the most likely diagnosis?**

ANSWERS TO CASE 16: Cocaine Intoxication

Summary: A 29-year-old woman was arrested while attempting to rob a grocery store. She lost her job because she was always late and stole from her employer to support her habit. The patient has needed increased amounts of her drug of choice to get high, and she suffers from cravings, sleepiness, depression, and hyperphagia when she is unable to obtain it. When high, the patient notes a feeling of euphoria and heightened energy. She has tried to quit "smoking" but has been unsuccessful. Her pupils are widely dilated, and she has lost 30 lb in 6 months.

◆ **Most likely diagnosis:** Cocaine intoxication.

Analysis

Objectives

1. Recognize drug dependence in a patient.
2. Identify, based on a patient's history and a physical examination, the likely drug.

Considerations

This patient exhibits the classic signs of addiction—she has a tolerance for the drug (requires more and more to achieve the same effect) and goes into withdrawal without it. She has tried to stop using cocaine but is unable to do so despite the negative effects it has had on her life. Her drug use results in her feeling euphoric and energetic when high, and depressed, hungry, and sleepy during withdrawal.

APPROACH TO COCAINE DEPENDENCE

Clinical Approach

The criteria for cocaine dependence are the same as for all substance dependencies (see Table 14–1). Cocaine intoxication can produce numerous behavioral and physiologic changes (Table 16–1). Individuals using this drug can also develop hallucinations (both auditory and visual), paranoid delusions, and bizarre behavior (including participation in sexual and violent activities). There can be serious physical health risks associated with cocaine use and dependence, including cerebral infarctions, transient ischemic attacks, seizures (including status epilepticus), myocardial infarctions, and cardiomyopathies.

Cocaine withdrawal can last 2 to 4 days, and even longer in heavy users. The **"crash"** is commonly accompanied by **dysphoria,** irritability, anxiety,

Table 16–1
COCAINE-ASSOCIATED BEHAVIORAL AND PHYSICAL CHANGES

Behavioral changes include:
1. Euphoria or blunting of feelings
2. Hypervigilance or hypersensitivity
3. Heightened anxiety or irritability/anger
4. Impaired judgment

Physical changes in cocaine intoxication may include:
1. Dilated pupils
2. Signs of autonomic instability such as elevated blood pressure, tachycardia, or bradycardia
3. Chills or sweating
4. Nausea/vomiting
5. Psychomotor agitation
6. Chest pain/arrhythmias
7. Confusion, seizures, stupor, or coma
8. Evidence of weight loss

and hypersomnia. Patients can develop marked depressive symptoms with suicidal ideation and can require hospitalization. They frequently experience strong cravings for the drug during the withdrawal period.

Differential Diagnosis

There are numerous psychiatric syndromes and conditions comorbid with cocaine dependence. Some disorders, such as a broad spectrum of anxiety disorders, antisocial personality disorder, and attention-deficit/hyperactivity disorder, can predate the development of cocaine dependence. Patients with cocaine dependence can also have major depressive disorder, bipolar disorder, cyclothymia, or various anxiety disorders. Because cocaine can also produce mood, anxiety, and even psychotic symptoms, diagnosis of the latter can be difficult if an individual is actively using cocaine. Therefore, a period of several months of abstinence can be required before an accurate diagnosis of other disorders can be made. In addition, cocaine dependence is often accompanied by other substance abuse or dependence disorders, especially those associated with opiates and alcohol. The latter substances are often used to temper the irritability and hypervigilance that can follow cocaine intoxication and withdrawal.

Treatment

Because cocaine delivers a particularly positive and reinforcing high, most users do not seek treatment voluntarily until the behavioral patterns have resulted in significant impairment in function (job and relationship losses, legal consequences) or health problems. Craving for cocaine is often so intense that an individual needs to be initially entered into residential treatment in order to establish abstinence from the drug.

Treatment must be multimodal, including medical, psychological, and social strategies to help the patient establish and maintain abstinence. Frequent unscheduled urine toxicology screenings are essential in both short- and long-term treatment of cocaine dependence, as denial is a prominent aspect of *all* addictions. Individual and group therapies can focus on support, education, and reduction of denial, as well as on building skills to avoid further drug use. Narcotics Anonymous sponsors a well-known, widely available, and free group therapy that offers all of the previously mentioned components. Family therapy can also be helpful in confronting both the patient with the effects of his or her drug-related behavior, and the family with ways they enable or reinforce the addictive behavior. Social interventions can include abstinence-focused housing programs and vocational training. Psychotropic medications such as antidepressants, anxiolytics, or mood stabilizers are indicated for treating any comorbid psychiatric illnesses in patients with cocaine dependence. Unlike in alcohol and opiate addictions, there are no pharmacologic agents definitively shown to reduce cocaine craving; research in this area continues to be pursued, however.

Comprehension Questions

[16.1] A 30-year-old man is brought to the emergency department by companions; he is not sure why he is there. He is clearly euphoric but also agitated and somewhat paranoid; he says he "feels fantastic" but is wary of answering any questions. On physical examination, the patient exhibits a moderately elevated blood pressure and pulse rate. Intoxication with which of the following substances is most likely in this individual?

A. Alcohol
B. Barbiturates
C. Benzodiazepines
D. Cocaine
E. Opiates

[16.2] Which of the following physical findings would be most likely present in the patient in question [16.1]?

A. Anorexia
B. Decreased temperature
C. Hypersomnia
D. Myosis
E. Bradycardia

[16.3] The patient in questions [16.1] and [16.2] is subsequently admitted to a detoxification unit in the hospital. After his euphoria and paranoia resolve, he is able to give a more complete history. He describes a 5-year history of almost daily crack cocaine use, with no periods of sobriety lasting for greater than one to two weeks. During those times, he felt "depressed," with an increased appetite and fatigue. He denies alcohol or other drug use, and his psychiatric review of systems is otherwise negative. Which of the following is the most appropriate treatment for this patient?

A. Antabuse
B. Bupropion
C. Naltrexone
D. Narcotics Anonymous
E. Selective serotonin reuptake inhibitor

Answers

[16.1] **D.** Cocaine intoxication can present with euphoria, irritability, anxiety, and psychosis such as paranoia, as well as with elevated vital signs. Conversely, intoxication with alcohol, barbiturates, benzodiazepines, and opiates generally causes depression, somnolence, and depressed vitals signs.

[16.2] **A.** Cocaine use causes decreased appetite and eventual weight loss. Also similar to a stimulant, cocaine intoxication can cause fever, insomnia, and mydriasis.

[16.3] **D.** The most beneficial approach to cocaine addiction without additional psychopathology is to stress abstinence and relapse-prevention. Narcotics Anonymous meetings are easily accessible, approachable, and provide ongoing group and individual support. Antabuse and naltrexone have not been shown to prevent cocaine cravings or relapse. Other psychotropics such as antidepressants would only be indicated if there was a clear comorbid mental illness.

CLINICAL PEARLS

❖ Cocaine acts like a stimulant, causing euphoria, anxiety, increased energy/activity, and psychotic symptoms, as well as elevated vital signs, dilated pupils, weight loss, chest pain, and seizures.

❖ Denial is more the rule than the exception in regard to a patient's awareness and acknowledgment of cocaine use.

❖ On average, cocaine is cleared from the body within 72 hours, and so a 3-day waiting period following its use is necessary for a patient to produce negative results from urine toxicology screening.

REFERENCES

Galanter M, Egelko S, DeLeon G, Rohrs C, Franco H. Crack-cocaine abusers in the general hospital: assessment and initiation of care. Am J Psychiatry 1992;149:810–815.

Withers NW, Pulvirenti L, Koob GF, Gillin JC. Cocaine abuse and dependence. J Clin Psychopharmacol 1995;15:63.

❖ CASE 17

A psychiatrist is called to see a 64-year-old man after he began screaming that there were strange men in his hospital room. The patient underwent a coronary artery bypass graft (CABG) 3 days previously and appeared to be recovering without complications. He claims that the previous evening he had seen several men standing in his room by the windows. The patient states that they did not say anything to him but that he was "sure that they were going to hurt [him]." He has never seen anything unusual before, and has no prior history of psychiatric difficulties. The nurses' notes from the late shift indicate that the patient became agitated and restless, although at times during the evening he was also noted to be disoriented and stuporous. He was not observed in this condition on previous evenings. On a mental status examination, the patient was alert and oriented to person and place, but he thought that the date was several months earlier than it actually was. Otherwise, the results of his mental status examination were normal. No hallucinations or delusions were noted at the time of the examination.

◆ **What is the most likely diagnosis for this patient?**

◆ **What is the next step in the treatment of this patient?**

ANSWERS TO CASE 17: Delirium

Summary: The patient is a 64-year-old man who underwent surgery 3 days previously. The night prior to the psychiatric consultation he experienced visual hallucinations and paranoia, as well as being alternately disoriented and stuporous. On examination the following morning, the patient is oriented to person and place but not to time. Otherwise, the results of his mental status examination are normal. He has no prior history of psychiatric illness.

- **Most likely diagnosis:** Delirium.
- **Next step in treatment:** A cause of the delirium should be sought. The patient's medication list should be examined. He should undergo laboratory testing and a physical examination to determine the medical causes of the delirium, for example, hypoxia, an electrolyte imbalance, or infection.

Analysis

Objectives

1. Recognize and diagnose delirium in a patient.
2. Be familiar with the steps to be followed in the case of new-onset delirium.

Considerations

This patient, who has no history of psychosis, began having visual hallucinations and paranoia 3 days after undergoing a CABG. Intensive care settings and/or major surgical procedures are risk factors for delirium, especially for geriatric patients. He also experienced waxing and waning of consciousness and was disoriented. Most of the symptoms resolve during the day, but presumably worsen in the evening (sundowning). The short-term nature of the event and the fluctuations in cognition and consciousness observed are consistent with delirium (Table 17–1).

APPROACH TO DELIRIUM

Definitions

Hypoxia: A condition defined by a low supply of oxygen
Orthostasis: A decrease in systolic blood pressure of 20 mm Hg on a change in position
Stuporous: A state of diminished alertness or awareness
Sundowning: Worsening of a delirium at night

Table 17–1
DIAGNOSTIC CRITERIA FOR DELIRIUM*

- Disturbance of consciousness with a reduced ability to focus, sustain, or shift attention
- A change in cognition (a memory deficit, disorientation, a language disturbance) or a perceptual disturbance not better accounted for by dementia
- The disturbance develops over a short period of time (hours to days) and tends to fluctuate over the day
- There is evidence from the patient's history, a physical examination, or laboratory findings that the disturbance is caused by a general medical condition, substance intoxication or withdrawal, a medication, or multiple etiologies

*Note that the criteria are essentially the same regardless of the etiology.

Clinical Approach

As noted, **the hallmark of delirium is a fluctuation in the level of consciousness.** Any disease process, substance of abuse, or medication that affects the central nervous system can produce delirium, especially in individuals who are elderly, medically ill, taking multiple medications, have recently undergone surgery, or are demented. Table 17–2 lists many of the causes of delirium. It is important to remember that it is quite common for several potential causes of a delirium to be present simultaneously in the same patient. Along with a fluctuation in the level of consciousness, there is usually disorientation and/or perceptual disturbances, commonly visual hallucinations or paranoia. These result in behavioral problems that can interfere with the patient's care, such as yelling, agitation, wandering, and pulling out intravenous lines.

Table 17–2
CAUSES OF DELIRIUM

Acute intermittent porphyria
Cardiovascular diseases: Arrhythmias, congestive heart failure
Central nervous system disorders: Brain trauma, epilepsy, infections, neoplasm, stroke, subdural hematoma, vasculitis
Drugs of abuse (in intoxication or withdrawal): Alcohol, barbiturates, benzodiazepines, narcotics
Electrolyte imbalances
Endocrine disorders: Adrenal insufficiency, hypoglycemia, parathyroid dysfunction
Medications: Anticholinergics, anticonvulsants, antihypertensive agents, antiparkinsonian agents, cimetidine, digitalis, ranitidine, steroids
Pulmonary disorders: hypercarbia, hypoxemia
Sepsis
Uremia
Vasculitis
Vitamin deficiencies: B_{12}, folic acid, thiamine

Table 17–3
CHARACTERISTIC OF DELIRIUM AND DEMENTIA

CHARACTERISTIC	DELIRIUM	DEMENTIA
Onset	Short	Long
Course	Fluctuating	Stable
Level of alertness	Reduced	Stable
Prognosis	Reversible	Irreversible

Differential Diagnosis

Having dementia increases the risk of developing delirium, but delirium cannot be diagnosed if the condition is better explained by dementia. This difficulty is compounded because both delirium and dementia can exhibit very similar symptoms (e.g., memory impairment, cognitive disturbances, and behavioral problems). Several characteristics help to distinguish between these two illnesses: the onset of **delirium** is **short** (hours to days), whereas that for **dementia is longer** (months to years); **the course of delirium fluctuates** over the day, whereas **that of dementia remains relatively stable;** the level of consciousness is reduced in delirium, whereas in dementia it is not; delirium is usually reversible, whereas dementia is usually irreversible (Table 17–3).

Other diseases in the differential diagnosis for delirium include psychotic disorders such as schizophrenia. However, individuals with delirium display a fluctuating level of consciousness, and patients with schizophrenia usually maintain an alert level of consciousness. Delirious patients often have visual hallucinations, but primary psychotic disorders are more frequently characterized by auditory hallucinations and delusions.

Treatment

The cornerstone of treatment for delirium is identification and correction of the underlying abnormality. This approach results in reversal of the delirious state, usually over several days to a week. Pharmacologic management of the behavioral disturbances can be accomplished with low doses of high potency antipsychotics (such as droperidol or haloperidol), given their lower incidence of orthostasis and anticholinergic side effects, which can worsen the patient's condition. Atypical antipsychotics (such as risperidone, olanzapine, and quetiapine) are also receiving attention as therapeutic agents to manage behavioral disturbance. A low dose of a short-acting benzodiazepine such as lorazepam can also be helpful, but it can have the unwanted result of disinhibition, oversedation, or paradoxical excitation, particularly in the case of elderly individuals. In situations where the delirium is caused by withdrawal from benzodiazepines or alcohol (delirium tremens), administration of benzodiazepines is the treatment of choice. Other nonpharmacologic approaches involve strategies to help facilitate the orientation of the patient, such as a calendar or clock, access to a window during the day, a television set or a radio playing during the day, family pictures, and familiar faces such as those of relatives or friends.

Comprehension Questions

[17.1] Which of the following is the most sensitive in diagnosing delirium?

A. Chest radiograph
B. Computerized tomography scan of the brain
C. Electrocardiogram
D. Electroencephalogram (EEG)

[17.2] Which of the following neurotransmitters is most likely involved in delirium?

A. Acetylcholine
B. Dopamine
C. Norepinephrine
D. Serotonin

[17.3] Which of the following features most distinguishes delirium from dementia?

A. Altered level of consciousness
B. Behavioral disturbances
C. Cognitive deficits
D. Disorientation

[17.4] Which of the following is the most important treatment approach in patients with delirium?

A. Detection and correction of the underlying abnormality
B. Environmental strategies to help with orientation
C. Pharmacotherapy for behavioral problems and hallucinations
D. Physical restraint to protect the patient from injury

Answers

[17.1] **D.** Although the other studies are all helpful in determining the etiology of delirium, only an EEG is sensitive in diagnosing this disorder. In almost all cases of delirium, an EEG shows generalized slowing. In cases where alcohol or sedative-hypnotic withdrawal is causing delirium, an EEG can show fast low-voltage activity. In hepatic encephalopathy, an EEG characteristically displays triphasic delta waves.

[17.2] **A.** Acetylcholine is the neurotransmitter most implicated in cases of delirium, as most notably demonstrated by the fact that anticholinergics are notorious for causing delirium.

[17.3] **A.** Both delirium and dementia can result in behavioral disturbances, cognitive deficits, and poor orientation. However, in all cases of delirium there is an alteration (reduction) in the level of consciousness, whereas in dementia (in the early stages) there is an alert, stable level of consciousness.

[17.4] **A.** Although environmental strategies and pharmacologic and physical interventions can be helpful and necessary to help orient patients or protect them from harm, the most essential treatment approach in all cases of delirium is to detect and correct the underlying cause of the disorder. The occurrence of an episode of delirium itself suggests a poor prognosis, meaning these patients have a significantly elevated future incidence of mortality.

CLINICAL PEARLS

- The hallmark of delirium is a fluctuation in the level of consciousness.
- Medications are a significant cause of delirium.
- An EEG is very sensitive in detecting delirium.
- The most important treatment approach for a patient with delirium is to detect and correct the underlying condition. Behavioral management can be accomplished with a low dose of a high-potency antipsychotic or a short-acting benzodiazepine.

REFERENCES

American Psychiatric Association. Quick reference to the American Psychiatric Association practice guidelines for the treatment of psychiatric disorders, compendium 2002 First MD, ed. Washington, DC: American Psychiatric Publishing, 2002:1–12.

Ebert M, Loosen P, Nurcombe B, eds. Current diagnosis and treatment in psychiatry. New York: McGraw-Hill, 2000:197–202.

Stoudemire A, ed. Clinical psychiatry for medical students, 3rd ed. Philadelphia: Lippincott Williams & Wilkins, 1998:112–114.

❖ CASE 18

A 16-year-old student is brought to the emergency department by her parents. She says that for the past 6 weeks, she feels as if she "just can't cope with all the pressure at school." She broke up with her boyfriend 6 weeks ago. Since that time, she cannot sleep more than 3 or 4 hours a night. She lost 15 lb without trying to, and her appetite decreased. She says that nothing interests her and that she cannot even concentrate long enough to read a magazine, much less her textbooks. Her energy level is very low. She is not doing things with her friends like she was in the past and says that when she is with them "things just aren't fun like they used to be." She tends to be irritable and gets angry with slight provocations.

On a mental status examination, she is observed to be a well-dressed teenager with good hygiene. She notes that her mood is very depressed, 2 on a scale of 1 to 10. Her affect is dysphoric and constricted. She admits to hearing a voice telling her that she is "no good." She has heard this voice at least daily for the past week. She admits to having had thoughts of suicide frequently over the past several days but denies that she would act on these thoughts because it would be a "sin." She does not have a suicide plan. No delusions are present, and she is alert and oriented to person, place, and time.

◆ **What is the most likely diagnosis?**

 **What is the next step?**

ANSWERS TO CASE 18: Major Depression with Psychotic Features

Summary: A 16-year-old woman experienced a depressed mood with anhedonia, anergia, insomnia, and a decreased appetite with weight loss since her boyfriend left her 6 weeks previously. She also has decreased energy, suicidal ideation, and **mood-congruent auditory hallucinations.** Even with all these symptoms, however, she is well dressed and has good hygiene. Her mood and affect are dysphoric, and she has noted an increase in her irritability. She is suicidal but does not have a specific intent or plan.

- **Most likely diagnosis:** Major depression with psychotic features (auditory hallucinations).

- What is the best plan of treatment? She should be **offered a psychiatric admission** because her major depression is severe. Although she is not committable; she could still be hospitalized by her parents because she is a minor. She should be started on a selective serotonin reuptake inhibitor (SSRI) and an atypical antipsychotic medication. When stabilized, the patient should be seen weekly for a least 4 weeks by the physician or qualified mental health professional to assess for any increase in suicidal thinking in compliance with current Food and Drug Administration (FDA) warnings for antidepressant use in children.

Analysis

Objectives

1. Recognize major depression in a patient.
2. Understand admission criteria for a patient with major depression with psychotic features.

Considerations

This patient has clear-cut major depression with psychotic features. Although the depression seems to have been precipitated by her break-up with her boyfriend, the combination of **vegetative symptoms, suicidal ideation,** and auditory hallucinations points to major depression. An adjustment disorder probably would not have all these features. Children and adolescents with major depression often report their mood as angry or mad as opposed to sad or depressed. She is obviously quite depressed, reporting suicidal ideation and auditory hallucinations; thus hospital admission is a reasonable decision choice. However, she does not appear to be in imminent danger to herself or to others, nor is there evidence that she cannot take care of herself; therefore she is not committable. However, a minor can be hospitalized with a parent's permission, and this certainly should be sought.

Table 18–1
DIAGNOSTIC CRITERIA FOR MAJOR DEPRESSION WITH PSYCHOTIC FEATURES

A. The patient must have five or more of the following symptoms, which should be present during a 2-week period; this symptom picture must be significantly different from the patient's usual functioning:
   a. Depressed mood nearly every day for most of the day
   b. Significantly decreased pleasure or interest in usual activities during most of the day for several days
   c. A significant decrease or increase in appetite; weight loss (without dieting) or weight gain (more than 5% of body weight)
   d. Daily insomnia or excessive sleeping
   e. Psychomotor slowing (retardation) or agitation
   f. Decreased or absent energy for most of the day for several days
   g. A sense of worthlessness or unusual feelings of guilt most of the day for most days
   h. Decreased ability to concentrate or slowed thinking
   i. Thoughts of death (not just fear of death) or suicide
B. The symptoms are not those of an episode of bipolar disorder, mixed.
C. The symptoms must cause the patient considerable distress or a decrease in functioning (social life, job, activities of daily living).
D. The symptoms are not the effects of a medical illness or a substance (prescription or street drug).
E. The symptoms are not part of normal bereavement following a loss.

In this patient's case, the description of the disorder is major depression, *severe with psychotic features* (Table 18–1).

APPROACH TO MAJOR DEPRESSIVE DISORDER WITH PSYCHOTIC FEATURES

Definitions

Anhedonia: Loss of a subjective sense of pleasure.

Mood-congruent delusions or hallucinations: The content of the delusions or hallucinations reflects the nature of the illness. For example, in major depression, delusions and hallucinations are often about being defective, deficient, diseased, or guilty and deserving of punishment.

Psychosis: A syndrome characterized by hallucinations and/or delusions (fixed, false beliefs). The individual's ability to assess reality is impaired.

Somatic delusions: False beliefs about one's body; in depression, these are beliefs regarding illness, for example, that one has cancer and is about to die.

Vegetative symptoms: Symptoms of depression that are physiologic or are related to body functions, such as sleep, appetite, energy, and sexual interest. Other symptom categories for depression are cognitive (poor concentration, low self-esteem) and emotional (crying spells).

Clinical Approach

Differential Diagnosis

Studies suggest the prevalence of major depression is 0.3% in preschoolers, 3% in elementary school children, and 6% to 7% in adolescents. Genetic factors, loss of a parent at an early age (before the age of 11), and adverse early life experiences are significant predictors for major depression in childhood and adulthood. Depressed youth often present first to their pediatrician with complaints of sudden onset of anger and irritability, lack of interest in fun activities, decreased energy, sudden poor grades (caused by decreased ability to concentrate), staying up late (under the claim of wanting to watch TV but really because the patient has trouble falling asleep), and withdrawal from friends and family. It is then important to inquire about psychotic symptoms and suicidal thoughts. Suicide rates in 15- to 19-year-olds have quadrupled over the last four decades and are usually in the top three or four causes of death in adolescents. The rate is 18.25/100,000 in males and 3.48/100,000 in females. Females attempt more often, but males use more lethal means. Diagnosis is often complex because there are many comorbid disorders such as anxiety disorders, disruptive behavior disorders, or substance abuse that can confuse the picture. Similarly, many personality disorders can begin to be seen in adolescence and need to be considered as well. In adults, many medical conditions and substances can cause mood disorders. (See Tables 4–1 and 4–2 for a listing of the general medical illnesses and substances that can cause mood symptoms.)

Other mood disorders such as bipolar illness and dysthymia can be difficult to differentiate from major depression. Sometimes a patient with bipolar disorder has several episodes of depression before the first episode of mania; and examining a carefully recorded family history and a clinical history can raise the clinician's suspicion of bipolar disorder. Sometimes a patient has an episode of major depression superimposed on lifelong dysthymia, making the diagnosis difficult. Schizoaffective disorder includes both depressive and psychotic symptoms; knowledge of the history and course of the illness is often necessary to make a diagnosis. Patients with schizophrenia can experience episodes of depression, but they usually develop later in the course of the illness, and the predominant picture is one of psychosis and negative symptoms. An active substance dependence makes the diagnosis of depression difficult because depressive and psychotic symptoms accompany the use of many substances (such as alcohol or cocaine); these can be indistinguishable from major depression. Often a patient must abstain from the substance for several weeks before the diagnosis can be confirmed.

In normal bereavement, especially during the first 2 months after the loss of a significant other, an individual can have symptoms of major depression. However, these gradually diminish with time. Indications that a bereaved person can be developing major depression include a preoccupation with guilt, feeling that one has caused the death of the loved one, and suicidal thoughts. It is important to remember that in children and adolescents with normal bereavement, they will often have hallucinatory phenomena where they will see or hear the deceased loved one, often with messages that are reassuring and comforting. These are not usually signs of a psychotic depression. Hostile accusatory hallucinations are more typical of major depression with psychotic features.

Treatment

The Texas Children's Medication Algorithm Project (CMAP) is a data driven, expert consensus decision tree for making treatment decisions. When compared to children whose doctors are not following any type of treatment algorithm, children whose doctors follow CMAP show a greater magnitude of improvement. According to CMAP, this patient should initially be started on a SSRI and an atypical neuroleptic with doses of both increased gradually until a therapeutic response is achieved, a maximum dose for body size is reached with no response, or the patient is experiencing side effects. If the patient's depression has no response or only a partial response to an adequate trial of the first SSRI, an alternative SSRI should be tried. If that fails to produce a response, consideration should be given to (1) augmentation with lithium or buspirone or (2) switching to a different class of antidepressant. For youth who don't respond to these options, CMAP gives additional options. Similarly, if one atypical antipsychotic does not control the psychotic symptoms with adequate dosing, a switch to another should be considered.

If the child suffering from major depression with psychotic features responds to the combination of antidepressant and atypical antipsychotic, the atypical antipsychotic should be continued for 3 months and then tapered off. The antidepressant should be continued for 6 to 9 months and then tapered over 2 to 3 months by 33% per month.

Comprehension Questions

[18.1] A 10-year-old girl is brought in for treatment by her father following the death of her mother 6 weeks previously because of an unexpected heart attack. The father is worried because the child is not sleeping well, has lost 7 lb because of a decreased appetite, seems to be tired much of the time, and is preoccupied with memories of her mother. He notes that she cannot concentrate on her usual favorite television shows and has lost interest in many of her previous social activities. The patient reports that she deeply misses her mother, but she also smiles in recalling many pleasant memories of their life together. Which of the following is the most likely diagnosis?

A. Adjustment disorder with depressed mood
B. Major depression
C. Normal bereavement
D. Sleep disorder
E. Dysthymic disorder

[18.2] A 17-year-old honors student is brought to the emergency department by his parents. In the last academic quarter, his grades have suddenly dropped, he is irritable with friends and family, he has no energy, he doesn't go to bed until 1 AM, and he has a poor appetite. He also has auditory hallucinations in which a man's voice tells him that he is a "lazy bastard" and that his family "would be better off with him dead." Which of the following would be the most appropriate pharmacologic treatment plan?

A. Benzodiazepine
B. Antidepressant and antipsychotic medications
C. Antidepressant medication
D. Antipsychotic medication and a benzodiazepine
E. Antidepressant medication and lithium

[18.3] Psychotic depression is diagnosed in a 14-year-old boy, and he is treated with an antipsychotic agent, risperidone, and an antidepressant. Three months later, his mood symptoms have resolved, and he is no longer psychotic. Which of the following best describes the next step?

A. Both medications should be discontinued via a taper.
B. The antipsychotic medication should be discontinued via a taper.
C. The antidepressant medication should be discontinued via a taper.
D. Both agents should be continued for 6 to 9 months.
E. The antipsychotic medication should be stopped immediately.

Answers

[18.1] **C.** Normal bereavement. This patient's symptoms fulfill the criteria for major depression, but she is in the very early stages of bereavement when such behavior is considered normal. Her sleep problems are part of bereavement. If her symptoms do not diminish in the subsequent 4 months, the clinician should make a reassessment for major depression.

[18.2] **B.** An antidepressant combined with an antipsychotic agent is needed for this patient who has major depression with psychotic symptoms. A benzodiazepine can address neither the depressive nor the psychotic symptoms. Lithium is an augmenting agent that can be considered later.

[18.3] **B.** The antipsychotic agent should be discontinued because the psychotic symptoms have abated. The antidepressant should be continued for approximately 6 to 9 months in a patient with the first onset of major depression, and for longer (perhaps indefinitely) for a patient with recurrent depression.

CLINICAL PEARLS

- Psychotic symptoms indicate severe depression and should prompt a serious consideration of hospitalization.
- Children and adolescents with major depression often report their mood as angry or mad as opposed to sad or depressed.
- Patients with depression are relieved when the clinician inquires about suicidality; asking about suicidal thoughts *does not* increase the risk that patient will kill themselves. Suicide rates in 15- to 19-year-olds have quadrupled over the last four decades and are usually in the top three or four causes of death in adolescents. Always ask about suicide in depressed children and adolescents. (Have you ever wanted to die? Have you ever thought about or tried to kill yourself?)
- According to CMAP, youth suffering from major depression with psychosis should initially be started on an SSRI and an atypical neuroleptic with doses of both increased gradually until a therapeutic response is achieved, a maximum dose for body size is reached with no response, or the patient is experiencing side effects.
- If the child suffering from major depression with psychotic features responds to the combination of antidepressant and atypical antipsychotic, the atypical antipsychotic should be continued for 3 months and then tapered off. The antidepressant should be continued for 6 to 9 months and then tapered over 2 to 3 months by 33% per month.

REFERENCES

Emslie GJ, Hughes CW, Crismon ML, et al. A feasibility study of the childhood depression medication algorithm project (CMAP). J Am Acad Child Adolesc Psychiatry 2004;43(5):519–527.

Hughes CW, Emslie GJ, Crismon ML, et al., and the Texas Consensus Conference Panel on Medication Treatment of Childhood Major Depressive Disorder. The Texas children's medication algorithm project: report of the Texas consensus conference panel on medication treatment of childhood major depressive disorder. J Am Acad Child Adolesc Psychiatry 1999;38(11):1442–1454.

Pataki CS. Mood Disorders and suicide in children and adolescents. In: Sadock BJ, Sadock VA, eds. Kaplan and Sadock's comprehensive textbook of psychiatry, 7th ed. Philadelphia: Lippincott Williams & Wilkins, 2000:2740–2757.

CASE 19

A 15-year-old girl is brought to a psychiatrist by her parents because they are concerned that she might be depressed. The parents had no complaints until 2 or 3 years ago. The patient's grades have fallen because she cuts classes. She gets into fights, and her parents claim that she hangs out with the "wrong crowd"; some nights she does not come home until well past her curfew.

The patient says that there is "nothing wrong" with her and that she wants her parents to "butt out of her life." She claims that she is sleeping and eating well. She says she skips school to hang out with her friends and admits that they frequently steal food from a convenience store and spend time watching movies at one of their homes. She claims that she fights only to prove that she is as tough as her friends but admits that she often picks on younger students. She is not concerned about her grades and just wants her parents to "lay off" and let her enjoy her youth. She denies the use of drugs or alcohol other than occasionally at parties. Her blood alcohol level is zero, and the results of a urinalysis are negative for drugs of abuse.

What is the most likely diagnosis?

What treatment should be started?

ANSWERS TO CASE 19: Conduct Disorder

Summary: A 15-year-old girl gets into fights, intimidates others, steals, skips school (resulting in falling grades), and breaks her curfew regularly. She does not exhibit any remorse for her behavior. She denies having any depressive symptoms such as sleep or appetite disturbances and says she feels pretty good about herself. She does not report any suicidal or homicidal thoughts.

- **Most likely diagnosis:** Conduct disorder (CD).

- **Best treatment:** Multisystemic treatment (MST) approach with involvement of parents and teachers. The treatment of CD can be difficult. There are few studies that look at CD systematically and study various treatment techniques. Over the last few years, a number of new studies have begun to look at how to treat CD. In terms of behavioral interventions, multisystemic-based therapeutic approaches are quite helpful. These approaches combine a well-coordinated plan to help parents develop new skills at home, such as parent-child interaction training, to help the relationship between parents/caregivers and the child. In addition, it is helpful to teach classroom social skills, institute playground behavior programs, and facilitate and encourage communication between teachers and parents. Psychopharmacologic interventions also show some promise. Many children with CD have a comorbid diagnosis of attention-deficit/hyperactivity disorder (ADHD). This needs to be identified and treated. Even if a child does not meet full diagnostic criteria for ADHD, there is evidence that CD is amenable to treatment with stimulants—often leading to less aggression and impulsiveness. There are also a few studies showing that the use of newer antipsychotics, such as risperidone, may be useful with CD.

Analysis

Objectives

1. Understand the diagnostic criteria for CD.
2. Understand when medications should be used in CD.

Considerations

This patient presents with a pattern of aggression, truancy, deceitfulness, theft, and serious violations of the rules of expected behavior for her age that fits the criteria for CD (Table 19–1). This behavior has been ongoing for 2 or 3 years and appears to be at least in part peer-mediated. Although her parents are concerned that she might be depressed, she appears engaged and nonchalant. It is important to collect information about substance use or abuse as well. This often requires gathering information from sources outside of the

Table 19–1
DIAGNOSTIC CRITERIA FOR CONDUCT DISORDER

A. Persistent, repetitive pattern of behavior that infringes on the basic rights of others or violates major age-appropriate societal norms: This pattern is manifested by the presence of at least three of the following symptoms in the last 12 months with at least one occurring in the last 6 months. The symptom categories are
   1. Aggression toward people or animals
   2. Destruction of property
   3. Deceitfulness or theft
   4. A serious rule violation

The person can have more than one symptom in a category.

B. The disturbance causes clinically significant impairment.

C. If the patient is older than age 18, the criteria for antisocial personality disorder are not met.

child, such as teachers, parents, siblings, and so on. It is important to remember that CD is a mental illness that is amenable to treatment. Without treatment, a large percentage of these children will go on to develop antisocial personality disorder and possible imprisonment. Treatment as children reduces the likelihood of this.

APPROACH TO CONDUCT DISORDER

Definitions

Antisocial personality disorder: Pervasive disregard for and violation of rights of others starting by age 15

Wraparound: A framework for organizing services in high-needs, mentally ill children involving a number of core values including cultural sensitivity, strengths focus, creativity, natural supports, and team approaches

Clinical Approach

Differential Diagnosis

Oppositional defiant disorder also is characterized by a negative behavior pattern; however, the offenses **do not typically cause significant harm to others** or involve violations of major societal norms. The behavior cannot occur exclusively in the context of an episode of mania or as a reaction to some stressor (in which case, adjustment disorder with disturbance of conduct is diagnosed instead). Finally, **antisocial personality disorder** is diagnosed if the symptoms appear **after the age of 18.**

Working with Children and Their Families

Conduct disorder is a very difficult disorder to treat, requiring participation from a number of systems involved with the child. The recommended interventions require considerable effort and change on the part of the parents who are often frustrated and feel hopeless. By the time the family comes in for evaluation, many years of maladaptive behavior and parental responses to this behavior have already passed. **The parents have lost control of their home and their child, and a great effort will be required to make an impact on the situation.** The child has also learned that even if the parents change for a while, the change is not likely to last. He or she **can simply outlast the latest parental efforts** or "up the ante" on the problematic behavior. However, it is important to note that with appropriate community interventions and support, such as with wraparound programs or MST, the outcome of this disorder can be hopeful. More than just about any other psychiatric illness in children, the prognosis is related to the degree in which one can organize a community-oriented intervention.

Comprehension Questions

[19.1] Which of the following is most appropriate in treating individuals with CD?

A. Parents should be encouraged to give their child some slack and ease up on their demands.
B. Store owners should be encouraged not to press legal charges against youthful offenders.
C. Patients should be allowed to drop out of school if they choose.
D. Patients should receive jail sentences in keeping with their behavior.
E. Patients should be removed from their friends.

[19.2] Which of the following treatment is best employed to treat the co-morbid depressive symptoms of an adolescent with CD?

A. Multisystemic therapy
B. Attendance in group therapy
C. An antidepressant medication
D. Treatment of the family to address the underlying reasons for the depression
E. Helping the adolescent change schools

[19.3] Which of the following epidemiologic statements about CD is correct?

A. Patients are more likely to have parents with a history of schizophrenia.
B. Patients are more likely to be female.
C. Patients are more likely to have parents who have antisocial personality disorder and alcohol dependence.
D. The prevalence of CD is independent of socioeconomic class.

Answers

[19.1] **D.** Natural consequences (the legal consequences of criminal activity) is one of the most effective treatments for young people with CD. Avoiding consequences (as in answer B) is counterproductive and serves only to reinforce the negative behavior. Parents need to be encouraged to regain control of their homes by setting firm limits with their child.

[19.2] **C.** If the criteria for a comorbid condition are met, this disorder should be the first target of psychopharmacologic intervention.

[19.3] **C.** Conduct disorder is more common in children of parents with antisocial personality disorder and alcohol dependence than it is in the general population.

CLINICAL PEARLS

- Conduct disorder can be a predecessor of antisocial personality disorder.
- Treatment of CD is very difficult and typically involves a community-oriented and highly organized treatment approach.
- When there are comorbid psychiatric conditions, they should be the target of psychopharmacologic interventions.
- Conduct disorder can be diagnosed prior to age 18, whereas antisocial disorder cannot be diagnosed until after age 18.

REFERENCES

Ebert M, Loosen P, Nurcombe B, eds. Current diagnosis and treatment in psychiatry. New York: McGraw-Hill, 2000:570–576.

Kaplan H, Sadock B. Synopsis of psychiatry, 8th ed. Baltimore: Lippincott Williams & Wilkins, 1998:1205–1209.

Siennick, SE, Findling RL, Guelzow, BT. Conduct disorder/aggression. Emotional and Behavioral Disorders in Youth 2005;5(2):35.

CASE 20

A 36-year-old man is referred to his employment assistance agency because he has trouble making timely decisions and is often late with important work. The patient has angrily complied with this request although he does not believe that anything is wrong with him. He describes himself as "so devoted to my work that I make others look bad," believing that this is why he has been singled out for attention. The patient says that he has worked at the company for 4 years and during that time has put in anywhere from 10 to 12 hours of work per day. He admits that he often misses deadlines but claims that "they are unreasonable deadlines for the quality of work that I provide." He states, "If more people in the country were like me, we would get a lot more done—there are too many lazy slobs and people who don't follow the rules." He points out that his office is always perfectly neat, and he says, "I know where every dollar I ever spent went."

On a mental status examination, the patient does not reveal any abnormalities in mood, thought processes, or thought content. His manner is notable for its rigidity and stubbornness.

- **What is the most likely diagnosis?**

- **What other psychiatric disorder is this condition often confused with, and how does one tell them apart?**

ANSWERS TO CASE 20: Obsessive-Compulsive Personality Disorder

Summary: A 36-year-old man has a lifetime preoccupation with rules, work, order, and stinginess. Even so, he is in trouble at work because he keeps missing deadlines and has difficulty making decisions. The patient does not realize that he is the cause of his problems—rather, he blames them on others. He comes across as rigid and stubborn in manner.

- **Most likely diagnosis:** Obsessive-compulsive personality disorder.
- **Differential diagnosis:** Obsessive-compulsive disorder (OCD). When recurrent obsessions or compulsions (checking rituals, washing hands repeatedly, etc.) are present, OCD should be diagnosed on axis I.

Analysis

Objectives

1. Recognize obsessive-compulsive personality disorder.
2. Understand the difference between obsessive-compulsive personality disorder and OCD itself.

Considerations

This patient's difficulties fit a personality disorder in that he is inflexible in his thinking or behavior, which causes problems in social or work settings. This man came into the employee assistance program because of problems he was having at work: rigidity, stubbornness, and difficulty in making decisions and keeping to deadlines. Typically (as in this case) the patient's disorder is egosyntonic; that is, he does not recognize his problems as originating from within himself but rather blames them on others in the outside world. Also, he is stingy with his money, although he works many hours a week. He seems somewhat moralistic about others and about their work habits, especially when they are compared to his own. **No obsessions (intrusive, repetitive thoughts) or compulsions (ritualistic behaviors)** are noted that are typical of **OCD;** the results of his mental status examination are otherwise normal.

APPROACH TO OBSESSIVE-COMPULSIVE PERSONALITY DISORDER

Definitions

Compulsion: The pathologic need to act on an impulse. If the action is not performed, anxiety results. Usually, the compulsion has no true end in itself other than to prevent some imagined disaster from occurring. For example, a patient has an obsession about being dirty, and the compulsion associated with it is ritualistic washing.

Defense mechanisms: A psychodynamic term that defines various means that an individual might use to psychologically cope with a difficult situation. These defense mechanisms range from relatively mature ones such as humor to quite immature ones such as often seen with borderline personality disorder. These might include mechanisms such as devaluation, idealization, projection, projective identification, and splitting. Commonly used defense mechanisms with obsessive personality disorder are intellectualization, rationalization, undoing, and isolation of affect.

Intellectualization: A defense mechanism by which an individual deals with emotional conflict or stressors by the excessive use of abstract thinking to control or minimize disturbing feelings. For example, a man is involved in a car accident that causes him to be paralyzed. He spends hours in the hospital brooding over the details of the accident and the treatment he has received in the hospital but does so in an emotionally barren manner.

Isolation of affect: A defense mechanism by which an individual deals with emotional conflict or stressors by separating ideas from the feelings originally associated with them. The individual loses touch with the feelings associated with the given idea (e.g., the traumatic event) although remaining aware of the cognitive elements of it (e.g., descriptive details). For example, a man comes home to find his wife in bed with another man. Later, describing the scene to a friend, the man can relate specific details of the scene but appears emotionally unmoved by the whole event.

Obsession: An intrusive, repetitive thought that comes unbidden and cannot be eliminated from consciousness by effort or logic. It is usually anxiety-producing.

Personality disorder: An enduring pattern of inner experience and behavior that deviates markedly from the expectations of the individual's culture, is pervasive and inflexible, has an onset in adolescent or early adulthood, is stable over time, and leads to distress or impairment.

Rationalization: A defense mechanism by which an individual deals with emotional conflict or stressors by concealing the true motivations for thoughts, actions, or feelings through the elaboration of reassuring or self-serving but incorrect explanations. For example, a woman steals a coat from a local department store although she can afford to pay for it. She tells herself, "It's okay—that department store has plenty of money, and they won't miss one coat!"

Undoing: A defense mechanism by which an individual deals with emotional conflict or stressors with words or behavior designed to negate or to symbolically make amends for unacceptable thoughts, feelings, or actions. Undoing can be realistically or magically associated with the conflict and serves to reduce anxiety and control the underlying impulse. An example of undoing is seen in the child's game in which one avoids stepping on cracks in the sidewalk to avoid "breaking your mother's back."

Clinical Approach

Diagnostic Criteria

The essential feature of this condition is a pervasive pattern of perfectionism and inflexibility. Patients with this disorder are emotionally constricted. They are excessively orderly and stubborn and often have trouble making decisions because their perfectionism interferes. These patients usually lack spontaneity and appear very serious. They are often misers when it comes to spending and frequently cannot discard worn-out or worthless objects that have no sentimental value. They tend to be overdevoted to work to the exclusion of involvement in leisure activities and friendships.

Differential Diagnosis

Patients with OCD have repetitive obsessions and compulsions, whereas those with the personality disorder tend to be rigid, stubborn, and preoccupied with details. Individuals with the personality disorder can brood over imagined insults or slights, which one could interpret as being obsessive, but they do not perform the compulsory, anxiety-reducing acts, such as ritual hand washing, that characterize people with OCD. It is also sometimes difficult to differentiate individuals with obsessive-compulsive personality traits from those with the diagnosable disorder. The occupational or social lives of patients with the personality disorder are significantly impaired as a result of this condition—the question is to what degree.

Interviewing Tips and Treatment

Individuals with this disorder do best when treated with a scientific approach and should be provided with documentary evidence and details. They can be among the most compliant patients because their own thoroughness can be used to self-monitor whatever condition is being observed. (For example, patients with obsessive-compulsive personality disorder and insulin-dependent diabetes can be asked to self-monitor their blood glucose level at exact times during the day, and physicians can be sure this will be done.)

The definitive treatment for obsessive-compulsive personality disorder is long-term, insight-oriented psychodynamic psychotherapy, but as in all patients with personality disorders, insight and motivation are usually lacking, rendering the treatment impossible to carry out. At times, cognitive interventions can be very well received, leading to a lessening of some maladaptive behavior. For example, a patient can be confronted with a key assumption such as "I must be perfectly in control at all times," and this assumption can then be discussed and ways created to refute it.

Comprehension Questions

[20.1] A 24-year-old woman is called into the head office of the agency where she works and told that her chronic lateness in completing her assignments will result in her dismissal if she does not change her behavior. The patient really loves her job, and the news comes as a major blow. That night at home, she tells her boyfriend in great detail about each and every step of the meeting and spends the entire night thinking about her job. The boyfriend tells her that she does not "look" particularly upset. Which of the following defense mechanisms is being used by this woman?

A. Undoing
B. Displacement
C. Intellectualization
D. Rationalization
E. Splitting

[20.2] A 23-year-old medical student makes lists of all the tasks that he must accomplish each day. He spends hours studying and refuses to go out with his colleagues even when there are no tests on the immediate horizon, preferring to spend his time looking at specimens in the laboratory. He keeps meticulous notes during all his classes and prefers to attend every lecture, not trusting his colleagues to take notes for him. He is doing well in school and has a girlfriend who is also a medical student. Which of the following disorders does this student most likely have?

A. OCD
B. Obsessive-compulsive personality disorder
C. Obsessive-compulsive traits
D. Schizoid personality disorder
E. Paranoid personality disorder

[20.3] A 26-year-old woman comes to see a psychiatrist because she has been taking showers for 6 to 7 hours every day. She explains, "It all starts when I wake up. I am sure I am covered in germs, and if I don't wash, I will get sick. If I don't wash, I get paralyzed with anxiety. Once I'm in the shower, I have to shower in a particular order. If I mess up, I have to start over, and this takes hours and hours. My skin is cracking and bleeding because I spend so much time in the water." Which of the following disorders does this patient most likely have?

A. Obsessive-compulsive disorder
B. Obsessive-compulsive personality disorder
C. Obsessive-compulsive traits
D. Paranoid personality disorder
E. Schizoid personality disorder

[20.4] For the patient described in question [20.3], which of the following treatments might best be used by the psychiatrist?

A. Lithium
B. Interpersonal psychotherapy
C. Buspirone
D. Cognitive behavioral therapy (CBT)-evoked response prevention
E. Parent assertiveness training

Answers

[20.1] **C.** Intellectualization is a defense mechanism by which an individual deals with emotional conflict or stressors with an excessive use of abstract thinking to control or minimize disturbing feelings. Because the stressors have been successfully defended against in this instance, the patient does not appear particularly distressed.

[20.2] **C.** Although this student clearly demonstrates some traits of obsessive-compulsive behavior, his social and occupational functioning are both good, which rules out the personality disorder.

[20.3] **A.** This patient demonstrates the classic obsessions, followed by compulsions, of OCD.

[20.4] **D.** The standard pharmacologic approach to the treatment of OCD is to prescribe a selective serotonin reuptake inhibitor (SSRI) or clomipramine, although these are not answer choices. The best psychotherapeutic choice would involve gradually exposing the patient to the anxiety-provoking circumstance and teaching her how to manage that anxiety through CBT techniques.

CLINICAL PEARLS

- Patients with obsessive-compulsive personality disorder are characterized by their rigidity, stubbornness, and perfectionism so that they often have trouble meeting deadlines at work or making choices. They tend to be work-centered to the exclusion of enjoying social activities and leisure time. They are often miserly with money and hoard possessions excessively.
- Physicians can use the preoccupation with rules and order shown by these patients to teach them to self-monitor their own conditions. These individuals can be extremely compliant. They need to know the details of their condition in scientific language.
- Patients with OCD have prominent obsessions and compulsions that alternately create anxiety and reduce it (through the compulsive behavior).
- Patients with obsessive-compulsive personality disorder have pervasive patterns of behavior that include rigidity and perfectionism but not true obsessions and compulsions.
- Patients with obsessive-compulsive personality traits often resemble patients with the personality disorder. The difference is one of degree and impairment of function. Individuals who are significantly impaired can exhibit symptoms that meet the requirements for the personality disorder.
- Defense mechanisms include rationalization, intellectualization, undoing, isolation of affect, and displacement.

REFERENCES

American Psychiatric Association. Diagnostic and statistical manual of mental disorders, 4th ed. Washington, DC: American Psychiatric Publishing, 1994:113–115.

Ebert M, Loosen P, Nurcombe B, eds. Current diagnosis and treatment in psychiatry. New York: McGraw-Hill, 2000:482–484.

Kaplan H, Sadock B. Synopsis of psychiatry, 9th ed. Baltimore: Lippincott Williams & Wilkins, 2003:111–114.

❖ CASE 21

A 34-year-old woman comes to a psychiatrist with a chief complaint of a depressed mood. She states that she was raped 1 year previously by an unknown assailant in the parking lot of a grocery store, and since that time, "things just [have not been] the same." She notes that she becomes irritable and angry with her spouse for no apparent reason and feels disconnected from him emotionally. Her sleep is restless, and she is having trouble concentrating on her work as a laboratory technician. She has nightmares about the rape in which the event is replayed. The patient states that she has told very few people about the rape and tries "not to think about it" as much as possible. She avoids going anywhere near the location where the event occurred.

On a mental status examination, her appearance, behavior, and speech are all observed to be normal. Her mood is described as depressed, and her affect is congruent and restricted. Her thought process is linear and logical. She denies any psychotic symptoms or suicidal or homicidal ideation, although she says that she wishes her attacker would "die a horrible death."

◆ **What is the most likely diagnosis?**

◆ **Should this patient be hospitalized?**

ANSWERS TO CASE 21: Posttraumatic Stress Disorder

Summary: A 34-year-old woman suffered a traumatic event 1 year ago. Since that time, she has been depressed, irritable, angry, and disconnected emotionally. She has trouble sleeping and concentrating. She has nightmares about the rape, tries not to think about it, and avoids going near the place where it occurred. On a mental status examination she shows a depressed mood that is congruent with her affect, which is also restricted. She has passive homicidal ideation.

- **Most likely diagnosis:** Posttraumatic stress disorder (PTSD).
- **Should this patient be hospitalized:** No. Although she has passive homicidal ideation (which is fairly typical in this kind of circumstance), she has no specific intent or plan to cause "something terrible to happen" and does not know her attacker or his location. This patient is not committable. Admission to the hospital should not be offered on a voluntary basis either, as she would probably do well on an outpatient basis.

Analysis

Objectives

1. Recognize PTSD in a patient.
2. Be aware of the need to hospitalize such a patient (or not).

Considerations

This patient shows several of the characteristic signs and symptoms of PTSD. After a significant traumatic event, she finds herself responding emotionally (depression, anger, irritability) and withdrawing from those she cares about. She has recurrent intrusive thoughts about the event and tries not to think about it (by pushing it out of her mind and avoiding the location where she was raped). She has trouble sleeping and concentrating, which is interfering with her ability to work. The results of a mental status examination are consonant with this picture as well.

APPROACH TO POSTTRAUMATIC STRESS DISORDER

Definition

Posttraumatic stress disorder: A syndrome that develops after a person witnesses, experiences, or hears of a traumatic event; the person reacts with feelings of helplessness, fear, and horror.

Clinical Approach

The identification of PTSD in a patient involves investigating the traumatic event and the patient characteristics. The trauma itself can be a single event or multiple events occurring over several weeks, months, or even years (such as in cases of domestic violence). The context of the trauma is also important: The experience of an auto accident is quite different from that of torture or rape. If the trauma occurs when the individual is very young or very old, the effects can be much more severe. For individuals exposed to a trauma, risk factors for developing PTSD include female gender, previous psychiatric illness, lower educational level, and lower socioeconomic status. Resilience in the face of trauma is increased by the presence of strong social support and a previous successful mastery of traumatic events.

Differential Diagnosis

Posttraumatic stress disorder is frequently accompanied by a comorbid condition, such as major depression, another anxiety disorder, or substance dependence; this must be kept in mind when reviewing the differential diagnosis (Table 21–1). Patients can suffer injuries during traumatic events, and

Table 21–1

DIAGNOSTIC CRITERIA FOR POSTTRAUMATIC STRESS DISORDER

A. The individual has been exposed to a situation in which he or she witnessed, experienced, or was confronted with event(s) that involved actual or threatened death or serious injury or a similar threat to others.
B. The individual persistently reexperiences the event in the form of distressing and repeated memories, which can be in the form of images, thoughts, perceptions, dreams and/or nightmares or flashbacks. The individual can experience intense distress when exposed to cues or reminders of the original trauma, and these reactions can take the form of strong physiologic responses.
C. The individual repeatedly avoids reminders of the traumatic event (including people, places, and activities), avoids thoughts of the event, and may be unable to recall certain aspects of the event. In addition, the patient can display numbness or diminished interest in normal activities and feel estranged or detached from other people. Individuals can exhibit a restricted range of affect and sense that their future will be foreshortened.
D. The individual experiences persistent symptoms of hyperarousal, such as insomnia (difficulty falling or staying asleep), irritability or angry outbursts, difficulty concentrating, hypervigilance, and/or a pronounced startle response.
E. The symptoms cause significant distress or a disturbance in social or occupational functioning.
F. Posttraumatic stress syndrome is considered acute if the duration is less than 3 months, and chronic if it is more than 3 months.

symptoms and sequelae of head injuries, particularly partial complex seizures can mimic symptoms of PTSD. If the patient is not questioned about the occurrence of a trauma or about intrusive memories, other symptoms of PTSD can resemble those of generalized anxiety or panic disorder. The social withdrawal and numbing exhibited by some individuals with PTSD can be confused with depressive symptoms. Patients with borderline personality disorder can also have a history of trauma, especially trauma related to events occurring in early childhood, and can exhibit posttraumatic symptoms such as intrusive memories and hyperarousal. Many patients with dissociative disorders also have a history of trauma and can experience posttraumatic symptoms. However, these patients describe and/or exhibit prominent dissociative symptoms such as episodes of amnesia. An individual with acute intoxication or undergoing withdrawal can display many of the symptoms of PTSD. In addition, these conditions can exacerbate chronic PTSD symptoms. Malingering is rare, but when compensation is involved, there is a potential for false claims of illness.

Treatment

The **treatment of PTSD** is usually **multimodal, including pharmacotherapy, psychotherapy, and social interventions.** Currently, selective serotonin reuptake inhibitors (SSRIs) such as **sertraline and paroxetine** are very effective in reducing most symptom clusters in PTSD; in addition, there were successful trials of tricyclic medications and phenelzine (a monoamine oxidase inhibitor [MAOI]). Selective serotonin reuptake inhibitors are usually first administered at a low dose and titrated up to maximum dose, as tolerated by the patient. Some response can be noted by 2 to 4 weeks, but a full response to medication can take up to 24 weeks. Initially, a hypnotic medication (such as trazodone) can be used at night to facilitate sleep.

Adrenergic inhibiting agents, such as the beta-blocker, propranolol, and alpha 2 adrenergic agonists, clonidine and prazosin, can be very effective in targeting the hyperarousal and hypervigilance of PTSD. These medications can afford immediate relief of symptoms in the early stages of treatment. Benzodiazepines, although they can improve sleep, are not helpful in reducing the symptoms of PTSD.

The psychotherapies that have been used most successfully in PTSD include various forms of cognitive-behavioral therapy (CBT) and supportive therapies. Some examples of CBT used in PTSD are prolonged exposure therapy, in which the patient is encouraged to relive the traumatic event(s) in his or her imagination, and cognitive processing therapy, in which various thoughts and beliefs generated by the trauma are explored and reframed. These types of therapies require significant training and should be conducted only by experienced clinicians.

Social interventions can be of primary importance following a traumatic event: Providing shelter, food, clothing, and housing can be the first necessary tasks. Restoring a sense of safety and security is crucial after a traumatic event; for example, increasing social support to individuals and groups who have suffered a natural or accidental disaster can be the first order of business. For many individuals, joining a support group of fellow survivors (rape, combat) is very helpful.

Comprehension Questions

[21.1] Which of the following conditions is most commonly associated with PTSD?

A. Major depression
B. Dementia
C. Schizophrenia
D. Narcissistic personality disorder

[21.2] A 36-year-old businessman who survived a serious car accident 4 months ago complains of "jitteriness" when driving to work and is currently using public transportation because of his anxiety. He has found himself "spacing out" for several minutes at a time at work and having difficulty concentrating on his job. He has trouble sleeping at night, has lost 4 lb because of a decreased appetite, and admits that his job performance is slipping. Which of the following is the most likely diagnosis?

A. Major depression
B. Panic disorder
C. Social phobia
D. Hyperthyroidism
E. Grand mal seizures

[21.3] Which of the following medications is most likely to be helpful for patients with PTSD?

A. Buspirone
B. Risperidone
C. Alprazolam
D. Paroxetine
E. Valproic acid

Answers

[21.1] **A.** Major depression, other anxiety disorders, and substance dependence commonly occur with PTSD as comorbid conditions.

[21.2] **A.** This patient exhibits the features of major depression, which commonly occurs with PTSD as a comorbid condition. Also, this patient exhibits two of the three symptom clusters for PTSD, and a clearly traumatic event has preceded his symptoms. He also complains of several symptoms consistent with depression, which often accompanies PTSD. It would be unlikely for him to suddenly develop an anxiety disorder such as panic disorder or social phobia. Nevertheless, the "spacing-out" periods can be episodes of dissociation occurring as a result of the trauma, but possible neurologic injury should be considered, especially because of his history and the change in his job performance. In addition, the patient can be using alcohol to aid in sleeping or to decrease the hypervigilance he has experienced since the accident.

[21.3] **D.** Individuals with PTSD often respond to SSRIs such as paroxetine. Although alprazolam might assist in decreasing the patient's anxiety, the incidence of substance abuse is high among patients with PTSD; thus, addictive medications should be avoided in these individuals.

CLINICAL PEARLS

❖ Stress symptoms exist along a continuum similar to that existing between an upper respiratory infection and pneumonia. The milder forms require only a "tincture of time" to resolve; symptoms that persist 3 months after the trauma are unlikely to resolve without treatment.

❖ Establishing safety should be the first treatment intervention in trauma-related disorders.

❖ A diagnosis of PTSD rests on exposure to an event associated with real or threatened death or serious injury, reexperiencing the event, avoidance of and distress about the event, and persistent symptoms such as insomnia.

❖ Selective serotonin reuptake inhibitors are generally helpful in the treatment of PTSD, and adrenergic inhibitors can reduce hyperarousal symptoms.

REFERENCES

Foa EB, Davidson JRT, Francis A. The expert consensus guideline series: treatment of posttraumatic stress disorder. J Clin Psychiatry 1999;60(suppl 16):3–76.

Foa EB, Keane TM, Friedman MJ, eds. Effective treatments for PTSD. New York: Guilford Press, 2000:135–164.

Ursano RJ, et al. Practice guidelines for the treatment of patients with acute stress disorder and posttraumatic stress disorder. Am J Psychiatry 2004;161 (Nov suppl):11.

CASE 22

A 34-year-old man visits a psychiatrist with a chief complaint of a depressed mood lasting "for as long as [he] can remember." The patient states that he never feels as if his mood is good. He describes it as being 4 on a scale of 1 to 10 (10 being the best the patient has ever felt). He states that he does not sleep well but has a "decent" energy level. His appetite fluctuated for the past several years, although he did not lose any weight. He feels distracted much of the time and has trouble making decisions at his job as a computer operator. He notes that his self-esteem is low, although he denies thoughts of suicide. He notes that he was hospitalized once 5 years ago for major depression and was treated successfully with an antidepressant, although he does not remember which one. He notes that he has felt depressed for at least the last 10 years and that the feeling is constant and unwavering. He denies manic symptoms, psychotic symptoms, or drug or alcohol abuse. He has no medical problems.

- **What is the most likely diagnosis for this patient?**
- **Should this patient be given any medication?**

ANSWERS TO CASE 22: Dysthymic Disorder

Summary: A 34-year-old man suffered from major depression in the past and, according to his history, a 10-year-period of depressed mood with insomnia, a fluctuating appetite, and a decreased ability to concentrate. He also notes that his self-esteem is low. He is experiencing no suicidal ideation, psychotic symptoms, or weight loss and is able to continue working. He denies any other psychiatric symptoms or medical problems.

- **Most likely diagnosis:** Dysthymic disorder.
- **Best medical therapy:** Selective serotonin reuptake inhibitors (SSRIs) as well as other antidepressants such as bupropion can be helpful in many patients with this disorder. Although other antidepressants such as tricyclic antidepressants (TCAs) and monoamine oxidase inhibitors (MAOIs) can be effective, SSRIs have a better side effect profile and are usually the first choice.

Analysis

Objectives

1. Understand the diagnostic criteria for dysthymic disorder (Table 22–1).
2. Be aware of the pharmacologic treatment options available for this disorder.

Table 22–1

DIAGNOSTIC CRITERIA FOR DYSTHYMIC DISORDER

A. A subjective or objective depressed mood most of the day for more days than not for at least 2 years; can be only 1 year for children and adolescents.
B. The presence of two or more depressive symptoms such as appetite changes, sleep changes, a low energy level, low self-esteem, poor concentration or indecisiveness, or feelings of hopelessness.
C. During the 2-year time period the person has never been without the depressive symptoms for more than 2 months.
D. The criteria for major depression are not met during the first 2 years of the mood disturbance.
E. No manic, hypomanic, or mixed episodes or cyclothymic disorder have ever been present.
F. Not related to a psychotic disorder exclusively.
G. Symptoms are not caused by substances or by a general medical condition and must cause clinically significant impairment.

Considerations

This patient has at least a 10-year history of a depressed mood; this duration fulfills the **2-year requirement** for diagnosis. Although he experiences a fluctuating appetite and insomnia, neither appears to be severe. (The patient is able to continue to work and has not lost any weight.) He complains of other symptoms consistent with dysthymic disorder, such as poor concentration and low self-esteem. He **does not have psychotic symptoms or suicidal ideation,** either of which suggest a more severe disorder. He experienced major depression in the past, but does not currently meet criteria, and his prior episode did not occur during the first 2 years of the dysthymic disorder. The patient denies alcohol, drug abuse, or medical problems, all of which can mimic dysthymic disorder; therefore, a complete history, physical examination, and laboratory studies should be performed.

APPROACH TO DYSTHYMIC DISORDER

Clinical Approach

Dysthymic disorder is fairly common, affecting approximately 5% to 6% of the population. Whereas major depression is typically characterized by discrete episodes, dysthymia is usually chronic and nonepisodic. Other mental disorders often coexist with dysthymia, such as major depressive disorder, anxiety disorders (particularly panic disorder), substance abuse, and borderline personality disorder.

Differential Diagnosis

As in all affective disorders, substances of abuse (such as alcohol), medications (such as beta-blockers), and medical conditions (such as hypothyroidism) must be ruled out as potential causes of the depressive symptoms. Often, it can be difficult to make the distinction between dysthymic disorder and major depressive disorder (Table 22–2). Although there is a **significant overlap between the two,** there are important differences. **Dysthymic disorder tends to have an earlier onset** (in the teenage years and in early adulthood) and a **more chronic course** than major depressive disorder, which tends to be more episodic. In other words, **dysthymic disorder can be viewed as a less intense, longer-lasting depressive illness** compared to major depressive disorder. When an individual with dysthymic disorder develops an episode of major depression (after 2 years in adults), the condition is often referred to as "double depression," which has a poorer prognosis than either illness alone.

Table 22–2
CHARACTERISTICS OF VARIOUS AFFECTIVE DISORDERS

DISORDER	CRITERIA
Major depression	Five or more SIG: E CAPS criteria for at least 2 weeks
Bipolar I disorder, manic	Meets critieria for **mania** (three or more criteria for at least 1 week causing **marked impairment or psychosis**) with or without depression (if present, major)
Bipolar II disorder (hypomania)	Meets critieria for **hypomania** (three or more criteria for at least 4 days **not** causing marked impairment or psychosis) with or without depression (if present, major)
Dysthymia	Depressed mood for most of the day on more days than not, for 2 years (1 year for adolescents and children), no mania or hypomania, no major depression during the first 2 years
Cyclothymia	Numerous episodes of hypomania and dysthymia for 2 years (1 year for adolescents and children)

Treatment

Although psychotropic medications were previously viewed as not being effective in individuals with dysthymic disorder, more recent research demonstrates a significant benefit from antidepressants. As in major depressive disorder, **SSRIs, bupropion, TCAs, and MAOIs can all be useful in treating dysthymic disorder.** Because of its chronic nature, a significant therapeutic effect can require up to 8 weeks, and treatment is often continued for many years or even for life. Other modalities useful in treating dysthymic disorder include various psychotherapies. Whereas **cognitive-behavioral therapy** is the best studied, insight-oriented therapy and interpersonal therapy are also likely to be of benefit. Because of the pervasive nature of this illness, it is not unusual for patients to be treated with both pharmacotherapy and psychotherapy. This combination can be more efficacious than either treatment alone.

Comprehension Questions

[22.1] A 22-year-old woman is referred to your office from her family physician for evaluation of "depression." Her primary care doctor is unsure whether she is suffering from dysthymic disorder or a major depressive disorder. Which of the following characteristics is more consistent with dysthymic disorder versus major depression?

A. Early onset of illness
B. Episodic course
C. Numerous neurovegetative symptoms
D. Presence of psychotic symptoms
E. Severe impairment in functioning

[22.2] The patient in question [22.1] is evaluated fully and determined to have dysthymic disorder. Which of the following medications is the most appropriate first-line treatment for her?

A. Desipramine
B. Lithium
C. Lorazepam
D. Phenelzine
E. Sertraline

[22.3] The patient in questions [22.1] and [22.2] decides that she does not want medications at this time, but she would still like her depression treated. What would your recommendation be for the next best, evidence-based treatment modality?

A. Cognitive-behavioral therapy
B. Interpersonal therapy
C. Psychoanalysis
D. Supportive therapy

Answers

[22.1] **A.** Although the distinction between dysthymic disorder and major depressive disorder can sometimes be challenging (especially if the major depressive illness is chronic and/or recurrent), patients with dysthymic disorder tend to have an earlier onset of symptoms, a more chronic course, fewer neurovegetative symptoms, lack of psychosis, and less severe psychosocial or occupational impairment when compared to individuals with major depression.

[22.2] **E.** SSRIs (such as sertraline) and bupropion have demonstrated efficacy in treating dysthymia. Although TCAs and MAOIs are also beneficial, newer antidepressants such as SSRIs are better tolerated and safer in overdose. Neither lithium nor lorazepam are indicated for dysthymic disorder.

[22.3] **A.** If medications are not beneficial, poorly tolerated, or not preferred in patients with dysthymic disorder, there are various types of psychotherapy that can be pursued. Although interpersonal therapy and insight-oriented therapies such as psychoanalysis are likely efficacious, cognitive-behavioral therapy has the most research supporting its use in treating dysthymia.

CLINICAL PEARLS

❖ Patients with dysthymic disorder can function relatively well in their lives but experience subjective symptoms of a depressed mood and mild vegetative symptoms.

❖ Dysthymic disorder can be diagnosed in children if they are symptomatic over a 1-year time period (instead of the 2 years required for adults).

❖ Dysthymic disorder can be successfully treated with antidepressant medication, psychotherapy, or a combination of the two.

REFERENCES

Ebert M, Loosen P, Nurcombe B, eds. Current diagnosis and treatment in psychiatry. New York: McGraw-Hill, 2000:307–311.

Kaplan H, Sadock B. Synopsis of psychiatry, 9th ed. Baltimore: Lippincott Williams & Wilkins, 2003:572–576.

❖ CASE 23

A 69-year-old man is brought to his primary care physician by his wife, who complains that his memory has been failing for the past several months. The patient states that he forgets the names of friends and family members and loses his way back home from the grocery store, and that in general he is unable to remember much of the information he acquired earlier. Previously, the man was "meticulous" about remembering his appointments and taking his medication. Now, he has to be reminded each and every time by his wife. The wife also reports that the patient's behavior is much more disorganized—he recently put his cell phone in the freezer and his shoes in the bathtub.

On a mental status examination, the patient is alert but oriented only to person and place. He does not remember his physician's name, although he has seen the same physician for more than 12 years for treatment of mild hypertension (well-controlled). Some mild aphasia is noted, and the patient can recall only two out of three objects at 5 minutes.

◆ **What is most likely diagnosis for this patient?**

◆ **What is the next step?**

ANSWERS TO CASE 23: Dementia

Summary: A 69-year-old man has been having problems with memory and disorganized behavior for the last few months. Previously, he functioned at a much higher level than he currently does. Mild aphasia and memory impairment are noted on a mental status examination.

 **Most likely diagnosis:** Dementia

◆ **Next step:** Reversible causes of dementia should be ruled out.

Analysis

Objectives

1. Recognize dementia in a patient.
2. Initiate further steps in the diagnosis and treatment of dementia.

Considerations

The patient is a reasonably healthy elderly gentleman. He is experiencing an insidious onset of problems with his memory and his organizational ability, which worsened markedly over the past few months. Previously (according to his history), the patient functioned at a much higher level. Mild aphasia and memory impairment, noted on the mental status examination, lend further credence to the diagnosis. See Table 23–1 for the diagnostic criteria.

Table 23–1
DIAGNOSTIC CRITERIA FOR DEMENTIA*

- Multiple cognitive deficits involving both
  1. Memory impairment and
  2. One or more of the following:
     - A. Aphasia
     - B. Apraxia
     - C. Agnosia
     - D. Disturbance in executive functioning (i.e., planning, organizing, sequencing, abstracting)
- The cognitive deficits cause significant impairment in functioning that represents a considerable decline from a previous level of functioning
- The deficits do not appear exclusively during the course of a delirium

*Note that the criteria for dementia are essentially the same regardless of the different etiologies, with the exception of evidence from a history, a physical examination, or laboratory studies indicating a specific cause.

APPROACH TO DEMENTIA

Definitions

Agnosia: Failure to recognize or identify objects despite intact sensory function

Aphasia: Language impairment

Apraxia: Impaired ability to carry out motor activities despite intact motor function

Executive functioning: Planning, organizing, sequencing, abstracting

Clinical Approach

The essential features of dementia **are memory impairment coupled with at least one other cognitive deficit, such as aphasia, apraxia, agnosia, or disturbance in executive functioning.** In most cases, the development of dementia is **gradual,** occurring over months to years. Infections (as in a case of meningitis) can occur with a somewhat more rapid onset. The **most common cause of dementia is Alzheimer** disease, followed by vascular dementia (formerly referred to as multi-infarct dementia). Although dementia cannot be newly diagnosed in a delirious patient, many of the same underlying diseases can create both conditions. Table 23–2 lists many of the etiologies for dementia.

Table 23–2
CAUSES OF DEMENTIA

Alzheimer disease	Huntington's chorea
Vascular (multi-infarct)	Folic acid deficiency
Parkinson disease	Vitamin B_{12} deficiency
Head trauma	Tertiary (neuro) syphilis
Multiple sclerosis	Chronic granulomatous meningitis (tuberculosis, fungal)
Pick disease	Neoplasms
Alcohol and other substances of abuse	Creutzfeldt-Jakob disease
Human immunodeficiency virus	Postanoxic states
Normal-pressure hydrocephalus	Progressive supranuclear palsy
Hypothyroidism	Wilson disease

A complete, thorough evaluation is necessary with a patient suspected of having dementia. This process includes obtaining a detailed history, including collateral sources, and performing a physical examination (with a full neurologic evaluation), a mental status examination (including cognitive testing), appropriate laboratory studies, and computed tomography (CT) or magnetic resonance imaging (MRI) (Figure 23–1). Various cognitive tests are available, and one of the most common is the Mini-Mental State Examination (MMSE). Table 23–3 shows the complete test. The final score ranges from 0 to a perfect score of 30. A score of less than 20 is strongly indicative of significant cognitive impairment. The MMSE is useful not only as a screening tool but also as a means of monitoring change, that is, either improvement or worsening of the dementing process.

Table 23–3
MINI-MENTAL STATE EXAMINATION

1. Questions (total of 30 points)
   A. Orientation (10 points)
      1. Year, season, date, day of week, month
      2. State, county, town or city
      3. Hospital or clinic, floor
   B. Registration (3 points)
      1. Name three objects: apple, table, penny
      2. Each must be spoken distinctly and with a brief pause
      3. Patient repeats all three (1 point for each)
      4. Repeat process until all three objects have been learned
      5. Record the number of trials needed to learn all three objects
   C. Attention and calculation (5 points)
      1. Spell WORLD backward: DLROW
      2. Points are given up to the first misplaced letter
      3. Example: DLORW scores as only 2 points
   D. Recall (3 points)
      1. Recite the three objects memorized in B.
   E. Language (9 points)
      1. Patient names two objects when they are displayed
         Example: pencil and watch (1 point each)
      2. Repeat a sentence: No ifs, ands, or buts
      3. Follow a three-stage command:
         a. Take a paper in your right hand
         b. Fold it in half
         c. Put it on the floor
      4. Read and obey the following:
         a. Close your eyes
         b. Write a sentence
         c. Copy the design

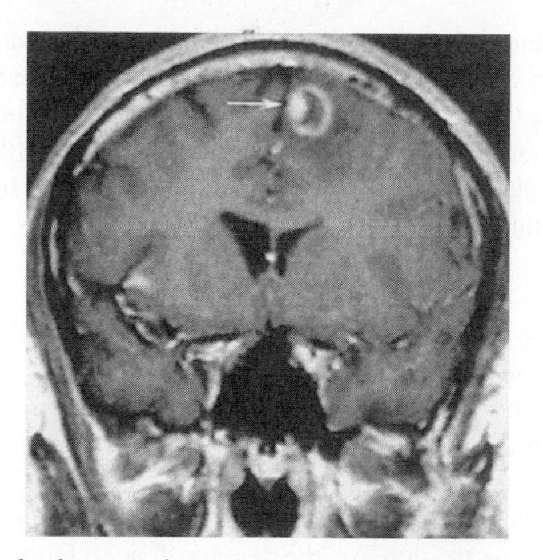

Figure 23–1. Cerebral magnetic resonance image showing an enhanced lesion suggestive of toxoplasmosis. (Reproduced, with permission, from Fauci A, et al. Harrison's Principles of Internal Medicine, 15th ed. New York, NY: McGraw-Hill, 2001:1893.)

Clinical Approach

Differential Diagnosis

Both dementias and amnestic disorders feature a memory deficit. Several factors can be used to distinguish between the two conditions, however. One of the most important is that dementia requires not only impairment of memory but also one or more other cognitive deficits such as aphasia, apraxia, agnosia, or difficulty with executive functioning. Patients with amnestic disorders do not have these problems. In addition, **dementias are generally progressive diseases of older individuals,** whereas amnestic disorders are often acute conditions arising in patients of varying ages. Amnestic episodes generally follow head trauma or the use of a psychoactive substance.

Dementias can also be confused with deliriums, as both can result in marked cognitive impairment. However, except in the very late stages of the disease, patients with dementia maintain an alert level of consciousness, whereas in **delirium, patients always demonstrate a fluctuating level of consciousness.** The course of dementia is more often over months to years, whereas the onset of delirium usually occurs over hours to days. Most dementias are irreversible conditions, but delirious states are usually reversible.

Dementing illnesses can often be mistaken for depressive illnesses in older individuals. Both can result in a decline in overall cognitive functioning and self-care. During the cognitive examination, however, patients with dementia usually make a considerable effort to minimize their disability, whereas those with depression characteristically make little effort, easily become frustrated, and complain bitterly about their perceived deficits.

Treatment

In cases where the dementia is reversible (e.g., hypothyroidism, infection, normal-pressure hydrocephalus), the approach is to treat the underlying condition. Medications can slow down (but not stop) the progression of dementias such as Alzheimer and Parkinson diseases. In Alzheimer dementia, acetylcholine is the neurotransmitter most affected, and **acetylcholinesterase inhibitors** are used to increase the levels of acetylcholine in the central nervous system in mild to moderate cases. These agents (including donepezil, galantamine, rivastigmine, and tacrine) act as reversible nonacetylating inhibitors of acetylcholinesterase, the enzyme that catabolizes acetylcholine. Although tacrine was the first of these agents, it was largely replaced by the other agents (particularly donepezil) as a first-line agent, given tacrine's hepatoxic effects and dosing schedule. Memantine (an *N*-methyl-d-aspartate [NMDA] receptor antagonist) is indicated in moderate to severe Alzheimer dementia, often in combination with acetylcholinesterase inhibitors. In Parkinson disease, dopamine agonists are used in conjunction with medications that decrease the breakdown of endogenous dopamine. The side effects of many of these agents include extrapyramidal movement disorders.

Other pharmacologic interventions address the behavioral difficulties that plague patients with dementia and their families and caregivers. A low dose of a high-potency or atypical antipsychotic medication can decrease the agitation and aggressiveness that often occurs. Although these drugs have the advantage of not causing as much orthostasis, oversedation, or worsening cognition like lower-potency antipsychotics, they can worsen movement disorders in certain dementias, most notably Parkinson and Lewy-body dementias. Another alternative is a low dose of a short-acting benzodiazepine such as lorazepam, but the potential for disinhibition and further violence must be monitored closely.

Just as important as pharmacologic treatment is the provision of adequate structure, stimulation, and supportive medical care to patients, as well as education and empathic support to their family members, who are often overwhelmed by the financial, physical, and emotional burden of caring for them.

Comprehension Questions

[23.1] A 75-year-old man is brought in by his daughter to have his mental condition evaluated. He has become increasingly forgetful over the past year, missing engagements with his children and grandchildren. He is also unable to remember directions, resulting in his becoming lost when driving alone. He has no psychiatric history, although his wife died 14 months ago. His medical history is significant for poorly controlled hypertension. Which of the following additional features is necessary in order to diagnose dementia?

A. Another cognitive deficit
B. Fluctuation in consciousness
C. Radiographic findings
D. Hallucinations

[23.2] Given the loss of a spouse suffered by the patient in question [23.1], a depressive disorder as a cause of his memory problems (pseudodementia) should be considered in the differential diagnosis. Which of the following findings on cognitive testing would be most consistent with dementia rather than a depressive illness?

A. Decreased effort with decreased insight
B. Decreased effort with increased insight
C. Increased effort with decreased insight
D. Increased effort with increased insight

[23.3] A provisional diagnosis of Alzheimer disease versus vascular (multi-infarct) dementia is made for the patient in question [23.1]. Which of the following best describes the likely progression of vascular dementia?

A. No change
B. Gradual worsening
C. Stepwise deterioration
D. Rapid progression

[23.4] As the dementia in the patient in question [23.1] progresses further, he becomes more agitated and aggressive. Which class of medication would be the most appropriate management for his behavior?

A. Acetylcholinesterase inhibitor
B. High-potency antipsychotic
C. Long-acting benzodiazepine
D. Low-dose antidepressant

Answers

[23.1] **A.** For a diagnosis of dementia, one or more additional cognitive deficits must be present in addition to memory impairment. They can include aphasia, apraxia, agnosia, or a disturbance in executive functioning. Individuals with vascular dementia can demonstrate findings on a CT or MRI scan, such as evidence of past strokes. Patients with Alzheimer disease, however, do not necessarily show any significant findings on radiologic studies. Individuals with dementia usually remain alert, whereas those with delirium display a fluctuation in consciousness. Hallucinations can be seen in dementia and in many other psychiatric disorders as well.

[23.2] **C.** On cognitive testing, patients with dementia generally put forth considerable effort, display poor insight into their deficits, and minimize their problems. In contrast, those with depressive disorders often are apathetic, make little effort, and complain about their memory problems.

[23.3] **C.** Vascular dementias characteristically cause a stepwise deterioration in cognitive functioning corresponding to either small ischemic events or emboli causing strokes. Alzheimer disease progresses gradually over many years, whereas dementias caused by head trauma or anoxia are generally sudden in onset and have a subsequently stable course. Dementias with certain infectious etiologies, such as Creutzfeldt–Jakob disease, have a fairly rapid rate of progression.

[23.4] **B.** Treatment with a low dose of a high-potency antipsychotic is an appropriate pharmacologic approach to decreasing agitation and aggression in individuals with dementia. High-potency medications have an advantage over lower-potency antipsychotics in minimizing anticholinergic and orthostatic side effects. Short-acting benzodiazepines can also be used but can disinhibit patients and worsen their behavior. Long-acting benzodiazepines should be avoided because they can build up in elderly patients and cause oversedation or ataxia. Antidepressants can be useful in treating the depressive and neurovegetative symptoms that are common in dementia. Acetylcholinesterase inhibitors can be helpful in improving cognition in the early and mid stages of Alzheimer disease.

CLINICAL PEARLS

❖ A diagnosis of dementia requires both memory impairment *and* another cognitive deficit.

❖ The MMSE is a very sensitive screening tool for diagnosing dementia.

❖ Alzheimer disease is the most common form of dementia; vascular disease is the next most common.

❖ Most dementias have a slow rate of onset, are irreversible, and are progressive.

❖ A low-dose, high-potency antipsychotic or a low-dose, short-acting benzodiazepine can be helpful in decreasing the agitation seen in patients with dementia.

REFERENCES

Cummings JL, Frank JC, Cherry D, et al. Guidelines for managing Alzheimer's disease: part II. Treatment. Am Fam Physician 2002;65(12):2525–2534.

Ebert M, Loosen P, Nurcombe B, eds. Current diagnosis and treatment in psychiatry. New York: McGraw-Hill, 2000:220–221.

Folstein MF, Folstein SE, McHugh PR. Mini-mental state: a practical method for grading the state of patients for the clinician. J Psychiatr Res 1975;12:189–198.

Kaplan H, Sadock B. Synopsis of psychiatry, 9th ed. Baltimore: Lippincott Williams & Wilkins, 2004:1232–1234.

❖ CASE 24

A 54-year old woman is referred to a psychiatrist by her primary care practitioner. The patient tells the psychiatrist that she has come only to "appease my doctor, who thinks this is all in my head." She reports that she saw the same primary care practitioner for the past year, during which time she made more than 20 appointments. She believes that she has some kind of serious medical disease because she "just doesn't feel right." The patient complains of vague stomach rumblings, aches and pains in her ankles and wrists, and occasional headaches. She scours the Internet for articles about serious, life-threatening diseases and brings these articles in when she visits her physician, convinced that she has a variety of the diseases listed. She states that she feels relieved and "safe" for a short period of time after every negative test result but then becomes convinced that she is ill again and makes another doctor's appointment. In the past year, she took off so much time from work for doctors' visits that she was put on probation. Other than noting that she is depressed and anxious about having a serious disease, the results of her mental status examination are unremarkable.

◆ **What is most likely diagnosis for this patient?**

◆ **What should the psychiatrist tell the primary care practitioner to do for this patient?**

ANSWERS TO CASE 24: Hypochondriasis

Summary: A 54-year-old woman is sent to a psychiatrist by her physician. She complains of numerous vague symptoms and believes that they are caused by a serious illness. These problems resulted in her scheduling numerous appointments with the physician in the past year. She is depressed and anxious about the prospect of having a serious disease, although she is temporarily relieved when test results come back negative. Her behavior has serious ramifications in her work life.

- **Most likely diagnosis:** Hypochondriasis.
- **Best approach:** Schedule frequent, regular physical examinations with the patient to assure her that her complaints are being taken seriously. Invasive diagnostic techniques or procedures should be avoided unless there is convincing objective evidence that they are necessary.

Analysis

Objectives

1. Recognize hypochondriasis in a patient.
2. Understand the treatment recommendations for the primary physician treating the patient.

Considerations

This patient clearly meets the criteria for hypochondriasis (Table 24–1). She is preoccupied with the idea that she has a serious medical illness. Despite appropriate medical evaluation, the fear persists, although it is temporarily alleviated when test results come back negative. Her preoccupation with illness is impairing other aspects of her life. There are no other signs or symptoms suggesting another psychiatric disorder that might account for this behavior (such as generalized anxiety disorder or panic disorder).

Table 24–1

DIAGNOSTIC CRITERIA FOR HYPOCHONDRIASIS

- Preoccupation with fears of having a serious illness based on a misinterpretation of bodily symptoms
- Preoccupation persists despite medical evaluation and reassurance
- Belief is not delusional or limited to a specific concern about appearance
- Preoccupation causes distress or impairment in functioning
- Duration of 6 months
- Preoccupation is not better accounted for by another mental disorder

APPROACH TO HYPOCHONDRIASIS

Definitions

Dysmorphia: A condition in which one body part is perceived to be out of proportion to the rest of the body. (For example, the nose is much too large or an arm is much too small.)

Somatoform disorder: A condition in which physical symptoms seem as if they are part of a general medical disorder although no general medical condition, other mental disorder, or substance is present. In this case, psychological conflicts can be translated into physical problems or complaints. With the number one complaint of patients being about some type of physical symptom, it is no wonder that this disorder is often observed in a general medical setting.

Clinical Approach

Differential Diagnosis

As in other somatoform disorders, it is important to rule out medical conditions that can be the cause of chronic complaints, especially those that do not present an obvious diagnosis, for example, autoimmune diseases, occult malignancies, neurodegenerative diseases, and human immunodeficiency virus (HIV) disease. On the *initial* presentation of a patient suspected of having hypochondriasis, obtaining a thorough history, review of systems, and performing a physical examination are necessary in order to assure both clinician and patient that a serious illness is not likely present.

Given the degree of preoccupation with having an illness, the symptoms of hypochondriasis can be mistaken for the delusions present in a psychotic disorder such as schizophrenia or delusional disorder, somatic type. In psychotic disorders such as schizophrenia and schizoaffective disorder, however, other associated symptoms and signs are part of the picture, including hallucinations, paranoia, ideas of reference, a flat affect, loose associations, and disorganized behavior. In delusional disorder, somatic type, the specific illness is always the same, and the patient cannot be reassured and will *not* consider other alternatives. In **hypochondriasis,** however, the **bodily complaints or disease can change over time,** and the **patient can usually be reassured,** albeit temporarily, when presented with medical evidence. In individuals with poor insight, making this distinction can be quite difficult.

Finally, other somatoform disorders should be considered in the differential diagnosis. In hypochondriasis, the focus is on the fear of having a serious illness because of misinterpreted bodily sensations. In somatization disorder, the focus is on having multiple physical complaints involving several different systems rather than an actual disease. In conversion disorder, a sensory or motor deficit is present and is usually transient. Although pain disorder (like hypochondriasis) is a chronic illness, the symptoms are limited to the sensation of pain. In body dysmorphic disorder, the preoccupation is not with having a serious illness but with an imagined defect in appearance or excessive concern about a minor physical anomaly.

Treatment

There is no *treatment* for hypochondriasis per se, although if comorbid depressive or anxiety disorders are present, they should be treated appropriately. *Management* of hypochondriasis is a more realistic goal, and this is usually accomplished by the primary care physician, as patients are often reluctant to see a psychiatrist given their belief about having a *medical* illness. **Regularly scheduled appointments** are much more helpful than "as needed" visits, as this establishes a trusting relationship, minimizes doctor shopping, and avoids repeated and unnecessary tests and procedures. **The complaints and concerns of patients should be taken seriously,** and they should be assured that they will be well cared for. This is not to say that inappropriate or unnecessary tests should be performed in order to reassure a patient; only when there is a high level of suspicion of or a clear clinical indication of a disease should an extensive evaluation or invasive procedure be pursued. Although individuals with hypochondriasis can be reassured when presented with evidence, the effect is usually only temporary, and they usually return with the same fear or the belief that they have a different disease.

Comprehension Questions

[24.1] A 42-year-old woman describes a 20-year history of numerous physical complaints, including joint pain, dysuria, headaches, chest pain, nausea, vomiting, irregular menses, and double vision. Although they do not all occur at the same time, she has been suffering from one or more of these problems throughout her adult life. Many workups have been done for her, and she has undergone repeated hospitalizations, but no specific cause has yet been found. She is extremely anxious and has become significantly disabled as a result. Which of the following is the most likely diagnosis?

A. Body dysmorphic disorder
B. Hypochondriasis
C. Pain disorder
D. Somatization disorder

[24.2] A 26-year-old woman presents to her physician with the chief complaint of, "I have epilepsy." She states that for the past 3 weeks she has had almost daily seizures. She describes the episodes as falling on the ground, followed by shaking her arms and legs uncontrollably. These events last for approximately 10 minutes. She is unable to otherwise move during the time, although she denies any loss of consciousness, bladder, or bowel functions. She has never injured herself during these, but as a result she has been unable to continue her job. She is somewhat bothered as she received a promotion 1 month ago. Which of the following is the most likely diagnosis?

A. Body dysmorphic disorder
B. Conversion disorder
C. Hypochondriasis
D. Seizure disorder
E. Somatization disorder

[24.3] A 36-year-old male is referred to a primary care physician for evaluation of his complaints. He is convinced that he has colon cancer despite being told that it is unlikely because of his young age. He occasionally notices blood on the toilet paper and has abdominal cramps when he eats too much. A review of the records demonstrates numerous prior appointments in connection with the same or similar complaints, including repeatedly negative results from tests for occult fecal blood and normal results from colonoscopies. He continues to be worried about dying of cancer and requests another colonoscopy. Which of the following is the most likely diagnosis?

A. Body dysmorphic disorder
B. Hypochondriasis
C. Pain disorder
D. Somatization disorder

[24.4] Which of the following strategies by the primary care doctor would be the most effective in treating the patient in question [24.3]?

A. Antianxiety medication
B. Extensive medical workups to provide reassurance
C. Referral for psychotherapy
D. Regularly scheduled appointments

Answers

[24.1] **D.** The most likely diagnosis for this woman is somatization disorder. She presents with numerous somatic complaints, related to several bodily areas, which are not fully explained by a medical cause. The focus is on the *symptoms* themselves, **not** on a perceived physical defect (as in body dysmorphic disorder), on the fear of having a specific disease (as in hypochondriasis), or on symptoms of pain (as in pain disorder).

[24.2] **B.** The most likely diagnosis in this woman is conversion disorder ("pseudo seizures"). Conversion disorder patients present with neurological symptoms (e.g., sensory deficit, motor weakness, seizures) that are felt to be unconsciously produced and believed to be caused by a psychological conflict or stressor. It is unlikely a seizure disorder given her retention of consciousness and lack of incontinence or injury. Her focus is not on an imagined defect in appearance, on the fear of having a serious illness caused by misperceived body sensations, or on multiple physical complaints.

[24.3] **B.** The most likely diagnosis for this man is hypochondriasis. His chief complaint is a concern that he has colon cancer. He remains focused on this illness despite prior evaluations with negative results and reassurance from his physician. Although he has several gastrointestinal symptoms (blood in stools and abdominal cramps), he is probably misinterpreting them. His worry is caused by fears of having colon cancer, not about a distorted body image, pain sensations, or numerous physical symptoms.

[24.4] **D.** The most effective strategy for treating individuals with hypochondriasis is to schedule regular appointments. In this way, any physical complaints are addressed, and reassurance is provided, albeit temporarily. This approach also minimizes both doctor shopping and unnecessary testing. Treatment with an antianxiety (or antidepressant) agent is not helpful in hypochondriasis, unless a comorbid anxiety (or depressive) disorder is present. Because individuals with this disorder are fearful of having a medical illness, they usually resist seeing a psychiatrist.

CLINICAL PEARLS

- The distinctive feature of hypochondriasis is a fear of having a serious illness based on a misinterpretation of bodily sensations.
- Extensive, repetitive, or invasive tests or procedures should be avoided in individuals with hypochondriasis unless a clear clinical indication is present.
- Antidepressants and antianxiety medications are not indicated unless comorbid depressive or anxiety disorders are present.
- The most effective treatment for patients with hypochondriasis is to schedule frequent, regular appointments with the same primary care physician, coupled with education and reassurance.

REFERENCES

Ebert M, Loosen P, Nurcombe B, eds. Current diagnosis and treatment in psychiatry. New York: McGraw-Hill, 2000:371–373.

Kaplan H, Sadock B. Synopsis of psychiatry, 9th ed. Baltimore: Lippincott Williams & Wilkins, 2003:651–653.

❖ CASE 25

A 32-year-old man is seen by a jail psychiatrist after getting into a fight with another inmate over a $5 bet. Jailed for forging bad checks, this is the patient's fourth incarceration. Previous incarcerations were for assaulting a police officer, stealing from a department store, and, at age 13, stealing a car. The patient states that he fought with another inmate because "I was bored and felt like it." He admits that the $5 was not really his to begin with, but he shows no remorse either about trying to take the money or about getting into a physical altercation with the other inmate. The patient states that he has seen psychiatrists in the past (always reluctantly and always because of demands made either by his mother or by the courts) but states, "There isn't anything wrong with me so why should I bother?" He denies using drugs or alcohol currently but admits that if he were not in jail, he would probably be using both, at least intermittently.

On a mental status examination, the patient is alert and oriented to person, place, and time. He cooperates with the examiner, although he is obviously irritated with the process. At times, he is rude and disrespectful. He is dressed in jail garb. His speech is normal in rate, rhythm, and tone. His mood is described as "fine," and his affect is congruent. He shows no disorders of thought processes or thought content.

◆ **What is the most likely diagnosis?**

◆ **What other psychiatric disorders might one suspect in this patient?**

ANSWERS TO CASE 25: Antisocial Personality Disorder

Summary: A 32-year-old man who is incarcerated is seen by a psychiatrist after he gets into a fight with a fellow inmate. He has a long history of incarcerations and an inability to conform to social norms, which began at least as early as age 13. He appears to be irritated by the examiner and does not seem to be remorseful about his actions.

- **Most likely diagnosis:** Antisocial personality disorder.
- **Other suspected psychiatric disorders:** High on the list of comorbid psychiatric disorders is any kind of substance abuse or dependence.

Analysis

Objectives

1. Know the diagnostic criteria for antisocial personality disorder.
2. Understand the common comorbidities found in patients with this disorder.

Considerations

This patient presents a typical case of antisocial personality disorder. He clearly does not conform to societal norms (multiple arrests), nor does he show any remorse for his actions. He is deceitful (forging checks), impulsive (stealing cars and from department stores), and irresponsible. His behavior appears to be a lifelong pattern, beginning in his adolescence. The fact that he freely admits to drug and alcohol abuse makes it even more likely that some kind of substance abuse or dependence is comorbid in this patient.

APPROACH TO ANTISOCIAL PERSONALITY DISORDER

Definitions

Acting out: A defense mechanism in which an individual guards against uncomfortable emotional conflicts or stressors through actions rather than reflections or feelings. For example, a man who has a hard day at work and is humiliated by his boss goes out that night and starts a fight at a local bar.

Projective identification: Projective identification is a defense mechanism that helps an individual deal with emotional conflict or stressors by falsely attributing to another person the individual's own unacceptable feelings, impulses, or thoughts—just as in projection. However, unlike the situation in projection, the individual remains aware of his or her own feelings and impulses and considers them justifiable reactions to another person. Not infrequently, the individual induces in others the very feelings that he or she first mistakenly believed to be there. For example, a paranoid patient has uncomfortable hostile emotions and projects them onto another person—"He is hostile to me." He then behaves *as if* the other person is going to be hostile to him. The other person, seeing the suspiciousness and the withdrawal of the patient, eventually acts in a frustrated (or seemingly hostile) manner toward the patient, thus completing the loop.

Clinical Approach

Diagnostic Criteria

Patients with antisocial personality disorder show a pervasive disregard for and violation of the rights of others starting by age 15. These individuals often appear to have **no conscience and no remorse about their activities.** They repeatedly perform illegal acts, lie frequently, and are impulsive and irritable. They often engage in physical fights and have an almost **reckless disregard for the safety of others.** They are consistently irresponsible as well. Although **the diagnosis is not made until the patient is older than age 18,** there must be evidence of a conduct disorder in childhood with an onset before the age of 15. The antisocial behavior cannot occur exclusively during the course of another psychiatric illness.

Differential Diagnosis

Patients with antisocial personality disorder must be differentiated from people who perform antisocial acts. The difference is that patients with the personality disorder lack empathy for others, have little to no remorse, and exhibit reckless, impulsive, and antisocial behavior in many areas of life. Not only do they usually run afoul of the law, but they also lack stable relationships with others, and all areas of their lives are permeated by difficulties involving recklessness, impulsiveness, and irresponsibility. It can be difficult to differentiate patients with active substance abuse disorders from those with antisocial personality disorders because many individuals with antisocial personality disorder abuse substances, although many substance abusers commit antisocial acts to facilitate their addiction. However, when the antisocial behavior occurs secondary to a substance abuse disorder, antisocial personality should not be diagnosed. For example, if a person robs a convenience store to support a heroin habit, but this kind of behavior does not occur when he does not need money for drugs, a diagnosis of antisocial personality disorder should not be made.

Interviewing Tips

Patients with antisocial personality disorder can often appear colorful and seductive, or manipulative and demanding. In all instances, a firm, no-nonsense approach with frequent limit setting is necessary. Clinicians should be careful, however, not to allow themselves to become punitive because of their anger over the patient's antisocial behavior and lack of remorse.

Treatment

The treatment of antisocial personality disorder is **difficult** at best and is generally focused on reducing impulsive or aggressive behaviors and antisocial acts rather than on a "cure." **Selective serotonin reuptake inhibitors (SSRIs), mood stabilizers, and propranolol** have shown promise in reducing aggressive symptoms. **Socially based interventions,** such as a group therapy with individuals with the same diagnosis, are considered helpful because patients reduce the amount of rationalization and evasion shown by others in the group because they recognize the patterns. **Psychodynamic psychotherapy has been singularly unhelpful** in these patients.

Comprehension Questions

[25.1] Which of the following diagnostic tests can be used to help confirm a clinical impression of antisocial personality disorder?

A. Urine toxicology screening
B. Dexamethasone suppression test
C. Lumbar puncture
D. Electroencephalogram (EEG)
E. Wechsler intelligence test

[25.2] In which of the following clusters does the diagnosis of antisocial personality disorder belong?

A. Cluster A
B. Cluster B
C. Cluster C
D. Cluster D
E. Cluster E

[25.3] A 39-year-old man with antisocial personality disorder, incarcerated for life after murdering a man, has a multitude of somatic complaints over the course of several years. Yearly physical examinations never show anything physically wrong with him, yet he complains of a variety of aches and pains, neurologic symptoms, and gastrointestinal distress. He does not enjoy the time he spends in the jail's infirmary. Which of the following is the most likely explanation for this patient's complaints?

A. He is malingering.
B. He has developed a psychotic disorder.
C. He has developed a somatization disorder.
D. He has an undiagnosed physical illness.
E. He has an undiagnosed anxiety disorder.

Answers

[25.1] **D.** Patients with antisocial personality disorder often have abnormal EEG results and show soft neurologic signs suggestive of minimal brain damage that occurred in childhood.

[25.2] **B.** Antisocial personality disorder belongs to cluster B, the "bad" cluster.

[25.3] **C.** Development of a somatization disorder becomes more common in patients with antisocial personality disorder as they grow older.

CLINICAL PEARLS

- ❖ Patients with antisocial personality disorder show a reckless disregard for, and violation of the rights of others starting in childhood or adolescence. The disorder itself cannot be diagnosed until the patient is 18 years old, although evidence of conduct disorder must be seen before the age of 15.
- ❖ Physicians should adopt a firm, no-nonsense, yet nonpunitive approach with these patients.
- ❖ Substance abuse disorders are often comorbid in patients with antisocial personality disorders. However, if the antisocial behavior occurs *only* in context of behavior designed to procure drugs and never when the patient is sober, the personality disorder should not be diagnosed.
- ❖ Patients with antisocial personality disorder evidence it in *all* facets of their lives, not just, for example, when robbing a store for personal gain. In the previously discussed case, an episode of antisocial behavior should be noted but not the personality disorder itself.
- ❖ Defense mechanisms commonly used in patients with antisocial personality disorder are projective identification and acting out.

REFERENCES

Ebert M, Loosen P, Nurcombe B, eds. Current diagnosis and treatment in psychiatry. New York: McGraw-Hill, 2000:474–475.

Kaplan H, Sadock B. Synopsis of psychiatry, 9th ed. Baltimore: Lippincott Williams & Wilkins, 2004:744–745.

CASE 26

A 15-year-old girl is brought to your office by her family after a recent hospitalization for a suicide attempt. She made this attempt shortly after a party she attended the previous weekend. At this party, she reportedly argued with her best friend and left very angry. Her history at admission shows a several month history of irritability, worsening performance in school, poor sleep, anhedonia, anergia, and isolation from her family and friends. Her discharge summary has an admitting diagnosis of major depression for which she was started on fluoxetine (Prozac). She sees you 2 weeks after her 3 day hospitalization and is quite cheery, energetic, and happy. She reports no problems and dismisses her earlier suicide attempt as a childish act to get attention. She reports that the staff at the hospital were absolutely wonderful and helped her solve all her problems. She says that she was so impressed with them, that she has decided to go into psychiatry herself so she can help others. Later, while meeting with the parents, they report that at home she is sleeping well and appears in a good mood. But, they are concerned because they also report that she is worried about whether there were cameras in the doctor's office that were recording her. She also reports that she believes she is being stalked by several of the boys at her school.

- **What is the most likely diagnosis?**
- **What is the best therapy for this condition?**
- **Should this patient be hospitalized?**

ANSWERS TO CASE 26: Schizoaffective Disorder

Summary: This is a 15-year-old girl who has a diagnosis of and evidence of major depression with a suicide attempt. She is treated for this and seems to respond well. The parents however note that she has some evidence of paranoia that is still present after the mood symptoms have resolved.

- **Most likely diagnosis:** Schizoaffective disorder (Table 26–1).
- **Best therapy:** An antipsychotic agent (such as haloperidol or risperidone) should be tried initially. If it is ineffective alone, antidepressants (a selective serotonin reuptake inhibitor [SSRI] is generally tried first) should also be administered.
- **Is hospitalization needed:** No. The patient is currently not a danger to herself or others and appears to be able to care for herself. This disorder as presented here should be treated in an outpatient setting unless the suicidal ideation returns and/or worsens.

Analysis

Objectives

1. Recognize schizoaffective disorder in a patient and diagnose it accurately.
2. Know that the disease has two subtypes: depressive and bipolar.
3. Know the recommended pharmacologic treatment for this disorder.
4. Know the indications for hospitalization of a patient with this disorder.

Considerations

This patient has a several month history of what sounds like mood (depressive) symptoms which seem to have remitted with fluoxetine. However, there is evidence of paranoid delusion (believing there are cameras in the doctor's

Table 26–1
DIAGNOSTIC CRITERIA FOR SCHIZOAFFECTIVE DISORDER

1. Patients must exhibit psychotic symptoms consonant with the acute phase of schizophrenia.
2. Psychotic symptoms are accompanied by prominent mood symptoms (mania or depression) during part of the illness.
3. At other points in the illness, the psychotic symptoms are unopposed; that is, no mood symptoms are present. Periods of illness in which there are only psychotic symptoms, and no mood symptoms, must last for at least 2 weeks.
4. The disorder cannot be caused by a substance or by a general medical condition.

office recording her) that persists without mood symptoms. The **psychotic episodes occur during the mood episodes,** but the mood symptoms do not always occur during the psychotic episodes, which is the key to the diagnosis. Although the patient was not asked about manic symptoms, the presence of such symptoms is a crucial element in the patient's history because it changes the subtype of schizoaffective disorder from depressive type to bipolar type and in turn affects the pharmacologic treatment choices. Without these symptoms the patient's disorder would be characterized as depressive type. (For example, a mood stabilizer such as valproic acid might be used in a patient with the bipolar type of schizoaffective disorder.)

APPROACH TO SCHIZOAFFECTIVE DISORDER

Definitions

Anergia: Lack of energy

Anhedonia: Lack of interest in one's usual pleasure-seeking activities, such as hobbies

Tangential speech (tangentiality): A disorder of thought process in which one's thoughts "take off on a tangent" from the initial question or line of thought and do not return to the original line of thinking

Clinical Approach

Differential Diagnosis

The key to developing a differential diagnosis for schizoaffective disorder is to carefully examine the longitudinal functioning of patients by reviewing their histories (provided by the patients and ideally by significant others). Periods of psychosis, and psychosis and mood symptoms (mania and/or depression), must be carefully teased out over a time period of years if possible. Conditions causing substance-induced mood disorder, which can be difficult to differentiate from schizoaffective disorder, include cocaine or amphetamine intoxication (manic symptoms), cocaine withdrawal (depressive symptoms), and the effects of a host of prescribed medications including steroids and antiparkinsonian medications. The symptoms of schizophrenia can appear similar, but the mood symptoms sometimes present in that disorder are generally transient and are brief in relation to the total length of the illness. Patients with bipolar disorder, mania, generally have had mood symptoms (euphoria, irritability) predating development of the psychoses, as have patients with major depression with psychotic features (a depressed mood predating the onset of psychosis).

Treatment

Patients with schizoaffective disorder generally respond to antipsychotic agents and often require long-term therapy. Although haloperidol (Haldol) and typical antipsychotics were once the treatments of choice (indeed, the only options available), newer atypical (second-generation) antipsychotics are now used far more frequently because of their more benign side-effect profile. These medications are not known to cause tardive dyskinesia, most extrapyramidal symptoms, or neuroleptic malignant syndrome. They are likely well tolerated because they also produce fewer anticholinergic side effects. Both typical and atypical antipsychotic medications have approximately the same duration of action, making once or twice per day dosing feasible in both cases.

Mood stabilizers such as lithium, carbamazepine, and valproic acid should be administered to patients with schizoaffective disorder who exhibit manic symptoms. It is sometimes helpful to combine an antidepressant and an antipsychotic for patients with schizoaffective disorder with a depressed mood. However, such patients should be treated with an antidepressant in addition to their antipsychotic only if the antipsychotic alone does not ameliorate the mood symptoms. Other treatment modalities can include hospitalization, particularly when patients are psychotic and unable to care for themselves. Psychosocial rehabilitation, such as is used in the treatment of schizophrenia, is often indicated as well because these patients can suffer from the same social isolation, apathy, and disturbed interpersonal relationships that schizophrenics do, although usually not with the same degree of severity.

Comprehension Questions

[26.1] Schizoaffective disorder, depressed type, is diagnosed in a 32-year-old woman. She is first treated with an antipsychotic, and 3 weeks later her auditory hallucinations have improved. She reports, however, that she still feels "very low" and has no energy or interest in the activities she used to enjoy. Which of the following should the psychiatrist do next?

A. Inform the patient that these symptoms are the negative symptoms common to the disorder.
B. Refer the patient for supportive psychotherapy.
C. Treat the patient with fluoxetine (an SSRI).
D. Increase the dose of the antipsychotic.
E. Add a mood stabilizer to the regimen.

[26.2] A 28-year-old man is brought to a psychiatrist complaining that he has been hearing voices for the past several weeks. He says that he also heard these voices 3 years ago. He notes that his mood is "depressed" and rates it 3 on a scale of 1 to 10 (with 10 being the best he has ever felt). He does not recall if his mood was depressed the last time he had psychotic symptoms. Which of the following actions should the physician take next?

A. Obtain more detailed information about the time course of the psychotic symptoms and the mood symptoms.
B. Treat the patient with an antipsychotic agent.
C. Treat the patient with an antidepressive medication.
D. Request a urine toxicology screening.
E. Refer the patient to supportive psychotherapy.

[26.3] A 40-year-old man with schizoaffective disorder has been hospitalized in an inpatient psychiatry unit for the third time in the last 5 years. During each episode, he becomes noncompliant in taking his medications, develops manic symptoms and auditory hallucinations, and then becomes violent. In the inpatient unit, he physically threatens other patients and staff and is generally agitated. He is put in isolation to help quiet him. The patient is prescribed a mood stabilizer and an antipsychotic medication. Which of the following medications might also help relieve this patient's acute agitation?

A. Buspirone
B. Fluoxetine
C. Chloral hydrate
D. Lorazepam
E. Benztropine

Answers

[26.1] **C.** Although data are not clear as to the efficacy of administering antidepressants to patients with schizoaffective disorder (and depressive symptoms), the continued presence of depressive symptoms makes this treatment worth trying.

[26.2] **A.** The time course of the mood symptoms and psychotic symptoms determines the treatment of the patient because the diagnosis can be schizoaffective disorder versus major depression. Although the patient should undergo a urine toxicology screening, this should not be done until a complete history is obtained so that further targeting of laboratory testing can be accomplished.

[26.3] **D.** Benzodiazepines such as lorazepam and clonazepam have been shown to be effective adjunctive treatments for acute mania both in patients with schizoaffective disorder and in patients with bipolar disorder.

CLINICAL PEARLS

- ❖ Unlike patients with schizophrenia, patients with schizoaffective disorder have mood symptoms that occur during significant portions of their illness.
- ❖ Once a very clear longitudinal history of symptoms and functioning is obtained, it is often possible to diagnose either a bipolar illness or schizophrenia in a patient with schizoaffective disorder.
- ❖ Patients with schizoaffective disorder and manic mood symptoms should be treated with a mood stabilizer and an antipsychotic. Patients with schizoaffective disorder and depressive mood symptoms should be treated with an antipsychotic alone; if this is not effective, an antidepressant should also be used.

REFERENCES

Ebert M, Loosen P, Nurcombe B, eds. Current diagnosis and treatment in psychiatry. New York: McGraw-Hill, 2000:279–281.

Goldman HH. Review of general psychiatry, 5th ed. New York: McGraw-Hill, 2000:253–256.

❖ CASE 27

A 24-year-old woman comes to her outpatient physician with a chief complaint of "smelling bad smells." She reports that several times a week for the past month she suddenly smelled burning rubber. She also noticed a smell of "rotting flesh." During these episodes, she notices that no one else in the vicinity complains about the odors, which are very acrid and pungent. Her friends did not notice anything unusual, except that they saw the patient "staring off into space," sometimes for several minutes at a time and often at the times when she noticed the bad smells. The patient herself is unaware of these periods of lost time, and she has no other complaints. Her medical history is remarkable only for a car accident the prior year in which she lost consciousness, but she reports no headaches. She denies drug use and drinks alcohol only rarely, on special occasions. No one in her family has ever experienced anything like these episodes.

- **What is the likely diagnosis for this patient?**

- **What further diagnostic workup would establish the diagnosis?**

- **On what *Diagnostic and Statistical Manual of Mental Disorders, 4th edition (DSM-IV)* axis are medical problems coded?**

ANSWERS TO CASE 27: Psychosis Caused by a General Medical Condition

Summary: A 24-year-old woman has olfactory hallucinations several times a week for the past month. She smells burning rubber and rotting flesh. Her friends report seeing her "staring off in space," although she herself is unaware of this behavior. The patient has no other psychiatric symptoms. She has a history of a concussion resulting from a car accident 1 year previously.

- **Most likely diagnosis:** Psychosis secondary to a general medical condition (Table 27–1). The medical condition here is most likely a partial complex seizure disorder.
- **Diagnostic test:** An electroencephalogram (EEG) or imaging of the brain using computed tomography (CT) or magnetic resonance imaging (MRI).
- **On what axis are medical problems coded:** Psychosis secondary to a general medical condition is coded on axis I, but the seizure disorder itself is coded on axis III.

Analysis

Objectives

1. Understand the diagnostic criteria for psychosis secondary to a general medical condition.
2. Be aware of some of the common medical conditions that cause psychosis.
3. Understand the rules for coding medical conditions on the *DSM-IV* axes.

Table 27–1
DIAGNOSTIC CRITERIA FOR PSYCHOTIC DISORDER CAUSED BY A GENERAL MEDICAL CONDITION

A. Prominent hallucinations or delusions
B. Evidence that the disturbance is the direct physiologic consequence of a general medical condition as provided by the patient's history, a physical examination, or laboratory studies
C. Not accounted for by another major mental illness and does not occur exclusively during delirium

Considerations

Patients with new-onset psychotic symptoms, particularly **olfactory, and gustatory symptoms,** should have medical conditions ruled out first. One year after experiencing head trauma in which she lost consciousness and suffered a concussion, this patient presents with new-onset olfactory hallucinations. In addition, according to her friends, she has spells of "zoning out," which might point to the **occurrence of a seizure.** The facts that the patient has no other psychotic symptoms, is aware that no one else smells what she smells, and otherwise feels and behaves normally all point away from a major psychotic disorder such as schizophrenia. As a general rule, olfactory and tactile hallucinations are more common with medical conditions rather than psychosis.

APPROACH TO PSYCHOTIC DISORDER CAUSED BY A GENERAL MEDICAL CONDITION

Definitions

Formication: A hallucinated sensation that insects or snakes are crawling over the skin. It is a common side effect of extensive use of cocaine or amphetamines.

Psychosis: Loss of mental functioning and loss of the ability to distinguish fantasy from reality. It can be manifested by delusions, hallucinations, confusion, or impaired memory.

Clinical Approach

This condition is defined by the presence of psychiatric symptoms caused by a nonpsychiatric medical condition. There is objective evidence (obtained from a physical examination or laboratory findings) or a history of cerebral injury/damage/dysfunction. Patients can present with a variety of psychiatric symptoms, including catatonia, personality changes, hallucinations, depression, mania, schizophrenic-like symptoms, and asthenia. The differential diagnosis is extensive and includes neurologic causes, infections, immune disorders, endocrinopathies, metabolic derangements, nutritional deficiencies, and toxic exposures.

Differential Diagnosis

All medical conditions including delirium should be considered. Seizure disorders and brain tumors, especially those arising in the temporal lobe, are likely to produce psychotic symptoms. Hence a complete history and a thorough physical examination are critical. A history of head trauma, increased intracerebral pressure causing nausea and vomiting, increasing headaches, or neurologic symptoms is important. Substance abuse should also be considered.

A CT scan or MRI of the brain is often used as an adjunct to assess for cerebral disorders. A primary psychotic disorder should then be diagnosed if no medical cause is identified. If the full criteria for a definitive diagnosis are not met, psychotic disorder not otherwise specified can be used. A primary mood disorder with psychotic features must also be considered when mood symptoms and psychoses coexist. If the psychotic symptoms are the direct effect of a substance, substance-induced psychotic disorder should be diagnosed. Heavy use of cocaine and amphetamines is a common cause for complaints of formication.

Treatment

If possible, the treatment of a psychosis caused by a general medical condition should be directed toward treating the underlying cause of the medical condition. For example, vitamin deficiencies can be diagnosed and remedied, eliminating the cause of the medical condition and thus the secondary psychosis. In addition, antipsychotics can be used in the immediate treatment of psychosis or in situations in which the general medical condition is not amenable to treatment (e.g., dementias). Either typical antipsychotics (haloperidol, etc.) or atypical antipsychotics (risperidone, etc.) can be used, although the side effects and risks of the former often make them unsuitable in the first-line treatment of psychosis. However, their use can be necessary in recalcitrant cases unresponsive to the newer antipsychotics.

Comprehension Questions

[27.1] The general medical condition causing the psychosis in psychotic disorder caused by a general medical condition is coded on which axis?

A. Axis I
B. Axis II
C. Axis III
D. Axis IV
E. Axis V

[27.2] Which of the following psychotic symptoms indicates that the cause is most likely related to a medical illness?

A. Auditory hallucinations
B. Impairment in reality testing
C. Tactile hallucinations
D. Thought disorder
E. Visual hallucinations

[27.3] A 25-year-old male sustained head trauma as a result of his car hitting a tree. After all other causes have been eliminated, it is determined that he has developed psychotic hallucinations because of the head trauma. Which of the following medications is most likely to be helpful in treating this patient's psychosis?

A. Lithium
B. Valproic acid
C. Risperidone
D. Valium
E. Sertraline

Answers

[27.1] **C.** Medical conditions are always coded on axis III.

[27.2] **C.** Auditory and visual hallucinations are common in all episodes of psychosis regardless of the cause. Tactile hallucinations (along with olfactory and gustatory hallucinations) can be more common in psychoses caused by a medical illness.

[27.3] **C.** Psychoses caused by general medical conditions usually respond to antipsychotic medications.

CLINICAL PEARLS

❖ The psychotic disorder is diagnosed on axis I, and the medical condition causing the psychotic symptoms is listed on axis III.

❖ To diagnose psychosis caused by a general medical condition, other psychiatric conditions should be ruled out.

REFERENCES

Ebert M, Loosen P, Nurcombe B, eds. Current diagnosis and treatment in psychiatry. New York: McGraw-Hill, 2000:287–288.

Yudofsky S, Hales RE, eds. Essentials of neuropsychiatry and clinical neurosciences. Arlington, VA: American Psychiatric Press, Inc., 2004:506–509.

❖ CASE 28

A 7-year-old girl is brought to her pediatrician on the suggestion of her second-grade teacher. The patient has been back in school for 3 weeks following a summer break. According to the teacher, the patient has found it very difficult to complete her classroom tasks since returning to school. The child is seldom disruptive but cannot finish assignments in the allotted time although her classmates do so without difficulty. She is also known to make careless mistakes in her work. Although she is still passing her classes, her grades dropped, and she seems to daydream a great deal in class as well. The teacher reports that it takes several repetitions of the instructions for the patient to complete a task (e.g., in an art class). The patient enjoys physical education and does well in that class.

Although her parents have noticed some of the same behaviors at home, they have not been particularly concerned because they have found ways to work around them. If they monitor the child and her work directly, she can complete her homework, but they must continually check her work for careless mistakes. She does seem to know the right answer when it is pointed out. The parents also report that the patient does not get ready for school in the mornings without moment-by-moment monitoring. Her bedroom is in shambles, and she loses things all the time. The parents describe their daughter as a happy child who enjoys playing with her siblings and friends. They note that she does not like school, except for the physical education classes.

- **What is the most likely diagnosis?**
- **What are the recommended treatments for this disorder?**

ANSWERS TO CASE 28: Attention-Deficit/ Hyperactivity Disorder

Summary: A 7-year-old girl has been referred to a psychiatrist by her teacher because she displays inattention, distractibility, and poor concentration and because her poor academic performance resulted in falling grades. Her parents describe a difficulty in following directions, disorganization, and forgetfulness. She does not have any symptoms of depression, psychosis, or developmental problems.

 **Most likely diagnosis:** Attention-deficit/hyperactivity disorder (ADHD), inattentive type.

◆ **Recommended treatments:** Use of a psychostimulant or atomoxetine along with behavioral parent training and classroom behavior modification programs.

Analysis

Objective

1. Discern a diagnosis of attention-deficit disorder based on the symptoms presented.
2. Understand the differences between the subtypes of attention-deficit disorder.
3. Understand the best treatment choices for this condition.

Considerations

This patient's history is fairly typical of attention-deficit disorder, inattentive type (versus the hyperactive type). She shows numerous traits consistent with this disorder, including inattention, making careless mistakes, difficulty paying attention, difficulty following instructions, difficulty organizing tasks, and forgetfulness (Table 28–1). This disorder is seen more commonly in girls than in boys. She does not have significant hyperactive symptoms, as do patients with the hyperactive and the combined types; specifically, she does not display behaviors such as squirming, leaving her seat, running or climbing, talking excessively, or constantly being "on the go."

Most practice guidelines suggest that the patient be treated with a stimulant, either methylphenidate or an amphetamine preparation. If one is not effective, then the other should be tried. It is important to remember that most treatment guidelines currently available were developed before the release of atomoxetine in 2003. Studies have shown that atomoxetine

Table 28–1
DIAGNOSTIC CRITERIA FOR ATTENTION-DEFICIT/HYPERACTIVITY DISORDER

1. The patient exhibits six or more symptoms of inattention or hyperactivity/impulsivity.
2. There is evidence that these symptoms were present before the age of 7 years.
3. The impairment is present in more than one setting (school, work, or home).
4. There is clinically significant impairment.

Inattention symptoms include:

- Making careless mistakes
- Having difficulty focusing one's attention
- Often seeming not to listen
- Often failing to follow directions
- Having difficulty in organizing tasks
- Avoiding tasks requiring sustained mental effort
- Often losing things
- Often becoming distracted by other stimuli
- Being forgetful

Hyperactivity symptoms include:

- Fidgeting or squirming
- Often leaving one's seat
- Running or climbing excessively and inappropriately
- Difficulty playing quietly
- Often being "on the go"
- Talking excessively

Impulsivity symptoms include:

- Often blurting out on answer before a question is completed
- Difficulty waiting for one's turn
- Often interrupting others

(a selective norepinephrine reuptake inhibitor) is an effective treatment for ADHD and, in revised treatment guidelines, can be placed with the stimulants as a first-line treatment.

If the patient does not respond to stimulants or atomoxetine, then other alternatives include the use of buproprion, imipramine, nortriptyline, and pemoline. Low-dose clonidine is often used in ADHD patients to help with sleep disturbance or agitated behavior after they are on a stable dose of stimulant or other ADHD medication.

Therapy alone is seldom effective. Usually, once medication has controlled symptoms, behavioral parent training to teach them how to adapt their parenting style to the child's special needs is helpful along with classroom behavioral modification approaches.

APPROACH TO ATTENTION-DEFICIT/HYPERACTIVITY DISORDER

Definitions

Distractibility: Inability to focus attention for age-appropriate periods of time

Hyperactivity: Excessive activity significantly above the level expected for the setting and the individual's developmental stage

Impulsivity: Taking action without appropriate thought and consideration, which often leads to a dangerous situation

Clinical Approach

Attention-deficit/hyperactivity disorder is defined as a **persistent pattern of inattention and/or hyperactivity** that is more frequent or severe than expected for a given level of development. Symptoms must be present for **at least 6 months,** begin before age 7, and be observed in more than one setting (e.g., home and school). It is important to remember that sometimes in homes that do not have a lot of structure, the parents can initially not realize that the patient's attention span is poor or that the child is unusually hyperactive or impulsive. In such cases, it is critical to contact other observers besides the school (day cares, after school programs, baby-sitters) to confirm the pervasiveness of the ADHD symptoms. The incidence is 3% to 5% of prepubertal children, and boys are affected with the hyperactive-impulsive type more often than girls. The inattentive type is characterized by failure to pay attention to details, failure to focus attention when performing tasks, failure to follow through with instructions, impaired ability to organize tasks, misplacing items, becoming easily distracted by external stimuli, and forgetfulness during the performance of daily activities. Hyperactivity is manifested by increased fidgeting of the hands and feet, inability to stay seated in a classroom setting, being unduly noisy during playtime activities, and a persistent pattern of increased motor activity not significantly modified by social context. Impulsivity is characterized by the blurting out of answers, difficulty waiting in line or for one's turn, interrupting, and talking excessively without an appropriate response to a given social situation.

Although the exact etiology of ADHD is not yet clear, the body of evidence suggests the dopaminergic and noradrenergic tracts are involved. Dopaminergic tracts of the mesolimbic and cortical areas serve as modulators of persistence, distractibility, motivation, and motor control, whereas the noradrenergic locus coeruleus modulates the child's reaction to novelty or challenging situations. Current research is still trying to refine the exact nature of the interaction of dopamine and norepinephrine in children with ADHD.

Differential Diagnosis

The presence of oppositional defiant disorder (ODD) or conduct disorder in a child or youth with ADHD is relatively common. It is important to remember that medication can do only three things: (1) help the child sit still—if the child wants to sit still, (2) help the child to focus his or her attention—if the child wants to pay attention, and (3) help the child to think before he or she acts—but will not affect whether the child makes a good decision or not. Failing to recognize the presence of ODD or conduct disorder in a child with ADHD results in many physicians trying to medicate away purposeful disruptive behavior.

Patients with ADHD often have learning disabilities, and a thorough evaluation of this problem should be conducted for every child suspected of having this disorder. Patients with bipolar disorder, early onset, can have symptoms of restlessness and distractibility, but their symptoms also have an affective component. **Lead intoxication** can lead to hyperactivity, and the presence of this disorder should be ruled out by determining the lead level in the blood at the initial evaluation.

Treatment

Approximately 70% to 80% of all children with ADHD will respond to stimulant medications, either methylphenidate or amphetamine preparations. Adverse effects typically include decreased appetite (sometimes with subsequent slowed growth rate), initial insomnia, irritability, dysphoria, and headache. Occasionally, the stimulants are associated with the development of **tics** or worsening of tics in those with tic disorders. Stimulants have, as a group, a very rapid onset of action, and typically, their therapeutic effects wear off by the end of the day.

Atomoxetine is a potent selective inhibitor of the presynaptic norepinephrine transporter and is an effective alternative to the stimulants in controlling ADHD symptoms. It is not a stimulant or a controlled substance. It tends to have a more gradual onset of action over a period of two to three weeks and once working seems to have a 24-hour length of action. Many patients sleep well with the medication and occasionally complain of sedation. The patient's appetite needs to be followed. Atomoxetine is not likely to cause tics, but this is still being studied.

Pemoline also has stimulant action, but its association with a **rare hepatotoxic reaction** has resulted in recommendations that a baseline alanine aminotransferase (ALT) be obtained and that it be remonitored every two weeks while the patient is on the medication. The medication should be stopped if there are significant increases above normal or if the patient fails to clinically benefit from adequate dosing after 3 weeks.

Bupropion, imipramine, and nortriptyline all have studies indicating efficacy in the treatment of ADHD. In the case of imipramine and nortriptyline, blood levels and electrocardiograms (EKGs) should be followed because of QT prolongation. Bupropion is contraindicated in individuals with seizure disorder.

Behavioral parent training and classroom behavior modification approaches are often effective approaches, whereas the efficacy of other types of psychotherapy remain to be convincingly demonstrated.

Comprehension Questions

[28.1] A 9-year-old boy is referred to a psychiatrist for the same kinds of school problems discussed in the previously mentioned case. In addition, he appears hyperactive and fidgety at school, which disrupts the class. His parents have noticed no difficulties at home, but his soccer coach has noticed attention problems during practice, and his Sunday school teacher has trouble teaching him because of distractibility. Which of the following is the most likely diagnosis for this patient?

A. ADHD, combined type
B. ADHD, predominantly hyperactive type
C. ADHD, predominantly inattentive type
D. Specific learning disability
E. No diagnosis, because the ADHD symptoms must be reported in the home.

[28.2] Which of the following is the best initial course of action in the treatment of children with ADHD?

A. Stimulant medication or atomoxetine
B. Pemoline
C. Clonidine
D. Bupropion, imipramine, or nortriptyline

[28.3] Which subtype of ADHD is more common in girls than in boys?

A. ADHD, combined type
B. ADHD, predominantly hyperactive type
C. ADHD, predominantly inattentive type
D. Specific learning disability

Answers

[28.1] **A.** Attention-deficit disorder, combined type. The diagnostic criteria for ADHD require that the symptoms be present in more than one setting, usually at home and at school. However, this child seems to have evidence of symptoms observed at school, church, and soccer.

[28.2] **A.** Stimulant medication or atomoxetine and behavioral parent training with classroom behavior modification.

[28.3] **C.** Girls seem to be less likely to demonstrate hyperactivity symptoms than boys. As a result, the condition is more likely to go undiagnosed because their symptoms produce fewer disruptions in the classroom.

CLINICAL PEARLS

- ❖ There are three primary subtypes of ADHD (inattentive type, hyperactive-impulsive type, and combined type), all of which have different presentations.
- ❖ Use of a stimulant medication or atomoxetine is probably the best medication for these children. Pemoline is effective in ADHD, but its association with a rare hepatotoxic reaction has resulted in recommendations that a baseline ALT be obtained and that it be remonitored every two weeks while the patient is on the medication.

REFERENCES

Kratochvil CJ, Heiligenstein JH, Dittmann R, et al. Atomoxetine and methylphenidate treatment in children with ADHD: a prospective, randomized, open-label trial. J Am Acad Child Adolesc Psychiatry 2002;41(7):776–784.

McCracken JT. Attention-deficit disorders. In: Sadock BJ, Sadock VA. eds., Comprehensive textbook of psychiatry, 7th ed. Philadelphia: Lippincott Williams & Wilkins, 2000:2679–2687.

Pliszka SR, Greenhill LL, Crismon ML, et al. Texas consensus conference panel on medication treatment of childhood attention-deficit/hyperactivity disorder. J Am Acad Child Adolesc Psychiatry 2000;39(7):908–919.

CASE 29

A 19-year-old woman is referred to a psychiatrist after her roommates become concerned about her behavior. The patient tells the psychiatrist that for the past 2 years, since beginning college, she has been making herself vomit by sticking her fingers down her throat. This behavior occurs regularly, as many as three or four times a week, and worsens when she is stressed out at school. The patient says that she regularly gorges herself with food and is worried that she will become overweight if she does not vomit it up. She describes her gorging episodes as "eating whatever I can find" in large quantities and mentions one incident in which she ordered three large pizzas and ate them all by herself. The patient states that she feels out of control when she is gorging herself but is unable to stop. She is ashamed of this behavior and goes to great lengths to hide how much she eats. She agreed to see a psychiatrist after her roommates found out about the self-induced vomiting.

A physical examination shows a young woman, 5 ft 6 in tall and weighing 135 lb. Her vital signs are blood pressure 110/65 mm Hg, respirations 12/min, temperature 98.2°F (36.8°C), and pulse rate 72/min. The results of the rest of her physical examination are within normal limits.

- **What is the most likely diagnosis for this patient?**

- **What treatment modalities should the psychiatrist recommend?**

- **What areas of the physical and laboratory evaluation should receive special attention?**

ANSWERS TO CASE 29: Bulimia Nervosa

Summary: A 19-year-old woman has been binging on large quantities of food, above and beyond what most people would eat under similar circumstances. She is embarrassed about the binging and worries that it will make her obese. She then engages in purging behavior, as often as three or four times a week. This behavior accelerates when she is under stress, and the patient feels she has no control over it. The results of her physical examination are normal, and she is of normal weight.

- **Most likely diagnosis:** Bulimia nervosa.
- **Best treatment modalities:** Nutritional rehabilitation, cognitive-behavioral psychotherapy, and treatment with an antidepressant (selective serotonin reuptake inhibitor [SSRI]).
- **Physical examination and laboratory tests:** Parotid glands, mouth, teeth for caries, abdominal examination for esophageal or gastric injury, dehydration from laxative use, ipecac-associated hypotension, tachycardia, arrhythmias. Serum electrolytes, magnesium and amylase levels.

Analysis

Objectives

1. Diagnose bulimia in a patient (Table 29–1).
2. Understand the most effective treatment regimens that should be recommended
3. Be aware of the laboratory tests that most commonly show abnormalities in patients with this disorder.

Considerations

This patient has all the cardinal signs of bulimia. She binges on food, and during these binges she eats more than a normal person would under the same circumstances. She is extremely ashamed of this behavior and goes to great lengths to hide it. She feels her behavior is out of control and purges

Table 29–1
DIAGNOSTIC CRITERIA FOR BULIMIA NERVOSA

- Recurrent episodes (at least twice a week for 3 months) of binge eating and inappropriate compensatory behavior such as purging, fasting, or excessive exercise.
- Self-evaluation is largely (and unduly) based on body shape and weight.
- The behavior does not occur only during an episode of anorexia nervosa.

(in this case vomits) so that she will not gain weight because of her excessive intake of food. These patients use inappropriate ways of controlling weight including fasting, excessive exercise, and misuse of laxatives, diuretics or enemas along with the often seen vomiting. It is a common finding that binging episodes increase during times of stress, and **patients with bulimia are usually normal or near normal in weight.** Frequent exposure to gastric juices from vomiting can result in severe dental erosion. The parotid gland can enlarge, and the patient can have elevated serum amylase levels. The self-induced vomiting can cause acute gastric dilatation and esophageal tears. Severe abdominal pain in these patients requires nasogastric suction tubes, X-ray studies, and possible surgical consultation. Electrolyte abnormalities, especially low magnesium and potassium, are common. Laboratory abnormalities found in individuals with bulimia nervosa demonstrate hypochloremic-hypokalemic alkalosis resulting from repetitive emesis. If they use ipecac to cause vomiting, they can have ipecac intoxication with pericardial pain, dyspnea, and generalized muscle weakness associated with hypotension, tachycardia, and electrocardiogram (EKG) abnormalities. Ipecac intoxication can cause a toxic cardiomyopathy that can lead to death.

According to American Psychiatric Association practice guidelines, individuals with bulimia nervosa should have a three-pronged plan of treatment. (1) There should be a plan developed for nutritional rehabilitation in which the patient is having regular, nutritionally balanced meals to replace the pattern of fasting then binging with vomiting often seen in this population. This should be supplemented with nutritional counseling. (2) Cognitive-behavioral psychotherapy on an individual basis to deal with the underlying cognitive patterns that drive bulimia combined with group therapy (often based on an addiction-model 12-step program) would be the best way for dealing with the immediate issues. If the patient moves back in with her parents, this should be supplemented with family therapy. (3) Treatment with an antidepressant, usually an SSRI, can produce a decrease in vomiting and binging behavior, but it is important to realize that without psychotherapy, purging behaviors can return.

APPROACH TO BULIMIA NERVOSA

Definitions

Binge eating: Eating an amount of food definitely larger than most people would eat during a similar period of time and experiencing a sense of lack of control

Nonpurging type: Type of bulimia where fasting and excessive exercise is utilized without frequent purging

Purging: Self-induced vomiting or misuse of laxatives, diuretics, or enemas for the purpose of preventing weight gain

Clinical Approach

Differential Diagnosis

Bulimia nervosa is estimated to occur in 1% of adolescent and young adult females, but eating-disorder-like behavior (brief times of purging) can affect up to 5% to 10% of young women. Its onset is usually later in adolescence than that of anorexia nervosa, and it can even start in adulthood. Like individuals with anorexia, bulimic patients tend to be high achievers, have a family history of depression, and respond to social pressures to be thin. In contrast to patients with anorexia, those with bulimia often exhibit coexisting alcohol dependence and emotional labiality but more readily seek help. Binge eating and purging are the hallmarks of the disease.

One of the main disorders in the differential diagnoses is anorexia nervosa, binge-eating/purging type. Although binging and purging behavior can be seen in anorexia as well as in bulimia, **anorexia is distinguished by the *requirement* of being underweight and amenorrheic. Bulimic patients can be underweight, of normal weight, or even overweight.** Despite their purging, the sheer amount of high-caloric food eaten can more than compensate for the amount purged.

Another concern is individuals who present with **purging behavior** who do not necessarily meet the criteria for bulimia nervosa. It is not uncommon for adolescents and young adults (especially women) to engage in purging behavior in order to lose weight. This behavior is usually learned from peers and is distinguished from bulimia by being **short-lived, infrequent, and unassociated with physical sequelae.**

Binging behavior can be seen with central nervous system tumors, Kluver-Bucy syndrome, and Klein-Levin syndrome.

Clinical Course

Typical onset is in females during adolescence or early adulthood with the peak onset at ages 18 to 19. It has a mortality rate of up to 3%. After 5 to 10 years of treatment, approximately 50% of bulimic patients will be recovered, 30% will be partially recovered and 20% will meet full criteria for active bulimia. One third of recovered bulimic patients will have a relapse within 4 years of recovery.

Treatment

Cognitive-behavioral psychotherapy to resolve cognitive distortions is the most effective type of psychotherapeutic intervention. Those living at home should have concomitant family therapy. Group therapy is effective because bulimic patients often feel ashamed of their symptoms and have problems dealing with interpersonal problems. Groups show them that they are not alone and give them opportunities to practice interpersonal problem solving skills. Generally, studies of the effects of medication alone show that they are not as effective as when given in combination with psychotherapy. In cases of effective treatment, a reduction of the purging rate by more than 50% over the first 4 weeks of treatment is often seen.

Comprehension Questions

[29.1] In individuals with bulimia nervosa, which of the following behaviors is considered purging?

A. Eating large amounts of food
B. Excessive exercise
C. Fasting
D. Misuse of laxatives

Questions [29.2] through [29.4] pertain to the following vignette: A 34-year-old woman presents with a 10-year history of episodes in which she eats large quantities of food, such as eight hamburgers and three quarts of ice cream, at a single sitting. Because of her intense feelings of guilt, she then repeatedly induces vomiting. This cycle repeats itself several times a week. She is extremely ashamed of her behavior but says, "I can't stop doing it."

[29.2] On examination, which of the following physical findings is most likely to be seen?

A. Dental caries
B. Lanugo
C. Muscle wasting
D. Obesity
E. Body weight at less than the 10th percentile of normal

[29.3] Which of the following laboratory abnormalities would most likely be found?

A. Hypermagnesemia
B. Hypoamylasemia
C. Hypochloremic-hypokalemic alkalosis
D. Elevated thyroid indices
E. Hypercholesterolemia

[29.4] An effective treatment program would consist of which of the following?:

A. Nutritional rehabilitation
B. Cognitive behavioral psychotherapy supplemented by group psychotherapy
C. Careful use of SSRIs
D. All of the above

Answers

[29.1] **D.** Purging includes self-induced vomiting or misuse of laxatives, diuretics, or enemas for the purpose of preventing weight gain. Other behaviors utilized by patients with bulimia to prevent weight gain include fasting and excessive exercise.

[29.2] **A.** The most likely diagnosis for this woman is bulimia nervosa. Physical findings can include dental caries, a round face caused by enlarged parotid glands, or calluses on the fingers resulting from recurrent self-induced vomiting. Lanugo and muscle wasting result from the severe weight loss characteristic of anorexia nervosa.

[29.3] **C.** Laboratory abnormalities found in individuals with bulimia nervosa demonstrate hypochloremic-hypokalemic alkalosis resulting from repetitive emesis. Hyperamylasemia and hypomagnesemia are also not uncommonly seen in such patients. Various electrolyte imbalances can occur as a result of frequent laxative abuse. Thyroid abnormalities are not common in individuals with bulimia nervosa.

[29.4] **D.** An effective treatment program would involve all of the treatment modalities described in this question.

CLINICAL PEARLS

❖ A diagnosis of bulimia nervosa requires both recurrent binging and purging or other compensatory behaviors to prevent weight gain. This behavior cannot occur exclusively during an episode of anorexia nervosa.

❖ Individuals with bulimia can be underweight, of normal weight, or overweight.

❖ Physical findings include dental caries, enlarged parotid or salivary glands, and esophageal tears.

❖ Abnormalities revealed in laboratory studies can include hypochloremic-hypokalemic alkalosis, hyperamylasemia, hypomagnesemia, and various electrolyte imbalances.

❖ Selective serotonin reuptake inhibitors are helpful in reducing both binging and purging behavior, but should not be the sole treatment offered.

REFERENCES

American Psychiatric Association. Practice guideline for the treatment of patients with eating disorders (revisions). Am J Psychiatry 2000;157(suppl 1):1–39.

Fairburn CG, Agras WS, Walsh BT, Wilson GT, Stice E. Prediction of outcome in bulimia nervosa by early change in treatment. Am J Psychiatry 2004; 161(12):2322–2324.

Halmi KA. Eating disorders. In: Sadock BJ, Sadock VA, eds. Kaplan and Sadock's comprehensive textbook of psychiatry, 7th ed. Philadelphia: Lippincott, Williams & Wilkins, 2000:1663–1676.

❖ CASE 30

A 35-year-old man is brought to see a psychiatrist by his friend because "ever since the disaster that killed his wife, he has been out of it." The patient states that 1 week previously the town in which he lived was hit by a tornado. His house was destroyed, and his wife of 2 years was killed. The patient states that he feels as if "I'm living in a fog—this just can't be real." He says that he feels disconnected from everything and everyone—he knows they are trying to help him, but he just feels numb. He claims that when he closes his eyes, all he sees is an image of his wife being buried under rubble, and he hears the loud roar of the tornado. The patient says that since that time he has isolated himself from others as much as possible so that he does not have to talk about what happened. He has not slept well for several days, and when he hears a loud noise, he thinks the tornado is coming back, which makes him very anxious and jumpy. He has been unable to work and has not called any of his insurance companies to tell them about the disaster. The patient states that he has never been to a psychiatrist before and came today only because his friend insisted.

◆ **What is the most likely diagnosis for this patient?**

◆ **What should be the next step in his treatment?**

ANSWERS TO CASE 30: Acute Stress Disorder

Summary: A 35-year-old man presents to a psychiatrist 1 week after living through a tornado that killed his wife. Since that time he has been "in a daze," and he describes feelings of numbness and derealization. He sees recurrent intrusive images of the event and tries to avoid thinking about it. He does not sleep well and becomes anxious when he hears a loud noise. His ability to function has been impaired (he is not able to work or call his insurance companies).

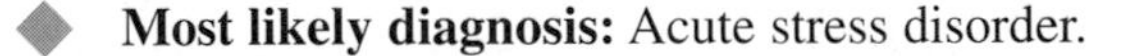

- **Most likely diagnosis:** Acute stress disorder.
- **Next step in treatment:** The major initial approach is support, especially facilitating and strengthening family and community support. Prior spiritual or religious affiliation, which can lend meaning to the event and loss, can be very supportive to the individual. Educating the patient and family about expected symptoms and a variety of coping techniques (such as relaxation training) can be very helpful. The use of sedatives or hypnotics in the short term can also be useful.

Analysis

Objectives

1. Recognize acute stress disorder in a patient.
2. Understand the recommended treatment approaches for patients with this disorder.

Considerations

This patient suffered an acute traumatic episode 1 week prior to his appearance at the psychiatrist's office. The response to the trauma has lasted more than 2 days but less than 4 weeks. The patient experiences several dissociative symptoms (feeling in a daze, derealization, numbing). He relives the event over and over in his mind (seeing his wife killed and hearing the tornado). The patient avoids talking about the trauma to avoid arousing recollections of it. He has symptoms of anxiety (insomnia, anxiety when hearing loud noises) that prevent him from functioning well (not working, failing to call his insurance company to report the loss).

APPROACH TO ACUTE STRESS DISORDER

Definitions

Derealization: A perception that the environment is somehow different or strange, although the individual cannot account for the changes.

Dissociative amnesia: Memory loss of some component of an event, which in the case of acute stress disorder, is usually traumatic.

Clinical Approach

Acute stress disorder (ASD) is a syndrome that develops shortly after an individual is exposed to a traumatic event. It is characterized by intense fear and feelings of helplessness, as well as a number of dissociative symptoms. The traumatic events are usually frightening enough to cause strong reactions in anyone; examples are war (as a combatant, civilian survivor, or refugee), torture, political violence, terrorism, natural or accidental disasters, and sexual or physical assault. The fear response is activated via the hypothalamic-pituitary-adrenal axis and locus ceruleus/norepinephrine system, resulting in a cascade of further physiologic events. Acute stress disorder is defined as occurring within the first 4 weeks after a traumatic event because research indicates that in many individuals this syndrome can resolve without progressing to posttraumatic stress disorder (PTSD).

Diagnostic Criteria

Acute stress disorder has the same criteria as the *Diagnostic and Statistical Manual of Mental Disorders, text revision (DSM-IV-TR)* criteria for PTSD, with the addition of one symptom cluster and a different time frame. **Acute stress disorder occurs within 4 weeks of the traumatic event and lasts for a minimum of 2 days.** The patient must also have **at least three of the following dissociative symptoms** as a response to the traumatic event:

1. A feeling of numbing, detachment, or lack of emotional responsiveness
2. Decreased awareness of surroundings
3. Derealization
4. Dissociative amnesia

Differential Diagnosis

An individual involved in an accident or assault is likely to have suffered a head injury, which can produce a postconcussion clinical picture resembling the dissociative symptoms of ASD. A patient can have an independent substance abuse or dependence problem or drinks and uses street drugs to "self-treat" the symptoms of ASD, complicating the diagnosis of either or both disorders. Cocaine intoxication can resemble the hypervigilance and hyperarousal of ASD. Other anxiety disorders such as panic disorder also can resemble ASD; the occurrence of a traumatic event and the reliving of it, along with avoidance symptoms, differentiate the disorders. Dissociative disorders can resemble ASD because of the dissociative symptoms associated with the latter. In order to make the correct diagnosis, the clinician must ask about the other symptom clusters present in ASD; patients with dissociative disorders do not have the trauma history or display the avoidance behavior of patients with ASD. Malingering should be in the differential diagnosis for patients pursuing financial gain as compensation for a traumatic event; this is especially true considering recent publicity about the disorder. Experienced clinicians should be able to detect genuine symptoms of hyperarousal and reexperiencing of an event in a patient with ASD.

Treatment

Treatment of a patient with ASD consists of supportive intervention; there is a wide range of possibilities based on the type of trauma, the patient's culture, and the presence or absence of a social network. The clinician should attempt to mobilize all active social supports, including family, religious groups, and the community, to assist the individual. Education about the symptoms and coping skills can be very helpful. Research on critical incident stress debriefing (CISD), in which the individual is encouraged to talk about and process thoughts about the event, is inconclusive regarding its effectiveness. When insomnia and marked hypervigilance are problematic, hypnotics and anxiolytics can be used on a short-term basis. There is some emerging research that suggests that beta-blockers, such as propranolol, started directly following the traumatic event, are effective in preventing the development of PTSD.

Comprehension Questions

[30.1] A 28-year-old male assembly-line worker comes in for treatment after developing symptoms a few days after a serious factory accident in which he was briefly knocked unconscious by a machine. He was medically cleared directly following the event but later developed nightmares about the accident. He says he has been very anxious, fears returning to work, and is thinking about seeking disability pay. The differential diagnosis should include all except which of the following?

A. Head injury with postconcussive syndrome
B. Malingering
C. Posttraumatic stress disorder
D. Acute stress disorder

[30.2] Treatment of ASD should focus primarily on which of the following?

A. Pharmacologic treatments, such as selective serotonin reuptake inhibitors
B. Debriefing the individual about the event
C. Biofeedback
D. Mobilizing social supports

[30.3] Acute stress disorder is diagnosed in a 32-year-old woman who witnessed her fiancee being shot to death in a robbery attempt. She has difficulty sleeping and feels that she is not emotionally attached to anything around her. She also has repetitive flashbacks of the event and avoids going near the location where the incident occurred. Which of the following medications might be helpful to this patient over the short term?

A. Zolpidem
B. Risperidone
C. Paroxetine
D. Buspirone

Answers

[30.1] **C.** This man cannot have PTSD because the symptoms appeared only a few days after the accident. He can indeed have ASD, and he can be exhibiting symptoms of a head injury; he can also be malingering, that is, fabricating symptoms for the purpose of financial gain. If the symptoms exceed 9 weeks, PTSD must be considered.

[30.2] **D.** Pharmacologic treatments and biofeedback are primarily interventions for PTSD; the results of research are currently unclear regarding the benefits of debriefing. Mobilizing social supports is the most effective intervention in treating patients with ASD.

[30.3] **A.** The use of a hypnotic for insomnia is likely to be helpful to this patient in the short term.

CLINICAL PEARLS

- ❖ Acute stress disorder occurs within 4 weeks of a traumatic event and lasts at least 2 days for a maximum of 4 weeks.
- ❖ When symptoms of ASD persist beyond 4 weeks, PTSD must be considered.
- ❖ Diagnostic criteria for ASD include a response to the traumatic event characterized by fear, helplessness, and dissociative symptoms (detachment, decreased awareness of surroundings, derealization, dissociative amnesia).
- ❖ Individuals with ASD feel detached, feel "unreal," and can have dissociative amnesia.
- ❖ Mobilizing social supports is the first intervention in treating patients with ASD; most symptoms resolve without pharmacologic treatment.
- ❖ There are many resilience and risk factors in the development of PTSD or ASD, but most individuals develop symptoms given a traumatic stressor of sufficient magnitude.

REFERENCES

Galea S, Ahern J, Resnick H, et al. Psychological sequelae of the September 11, 2001, terrorist attacks in New York City. N Engl J Med 2002;346:982–986.

Harvey AG, Bryant RA. Memory for acute stress disorder symptoms: a two-year prospective study. J Nerv Ment Dis 2000;1888:602–604.

❖ CASE 31

A 54-year-old man comes to the emergency department with a chief complaint of "I'm having a hard time kicking the habit." The patient states that for the past 2 days, he has experienced a depressed mood, muscle aches, diarrhea, insomnia, sweating, and a fever. Three days ago he ceased using his drug of choice, which he used heavily for more than 4 years. On a physical examination, the patient is noted to have a watery nose and eyes, a fever of 100°F (37.8°C), and dilated pupils.

◆ **What is the most likely diagnosis for this patient?**

◆ **What drug can be used to alleviate the patient's symptoms?**

ANSWERS TO CASE 31: Opioid Withdrawal

Summary: A 54-year-old man discontinued use of his drug of choice 3 days previously. Since then, he has experienced dysphoric mood, diarrhea, muscle aches, sweating, and a fever. A physical examination shows pupillary dilation, lacrimation, rhinorrhea, and a fever of 100°F (37.8°C).

- **Most likely diagnosis:** Opioid withdrawal
- **Medication to help alleviate symptoms:** Methadone or any other opioid; clonidine

Analysis

Objectives

1. Recognize opioid withdrawal in a patient.
2. Understand the use of methadone in ameliorating opioid withdrawal symptoms.

Considerations

Shortly after he ceased using his drug of choice after years of heavy use, this patient began to experience classic signs and symptoms of opioid withdrawal. Whereas opiate intoxication causes apathy, psychomotor retardation, constricted pupils, and drowsiness, opiate withdrawal results in nausea and vomiting, muscle aches, lacrimation or rhinorrhea, diarrhea, fever, and dilated pupils. These symptoms can develop within hours or days of the last opiate dose depending on the half-life of the agent and the body's dependence status. In general, agents with a short half-life tend to induce a rapid, severe withdrawal effect, whereas opiates with a long half-life tend to be associated with a less severe, more gradual withdrawal course. The introduction of clonidine to treat the autonomic hyperactivity in the acute phase, followed by administration of a long-acting opiate such as methadone for maintenance, is effective.

APPROACH TO OPIOID WITHDRAWAL

Definitions

Autonomic hyperactivity: Symptoms of autonomic hyperactivity include tachypnea, hyperreflexia, tachycardia, hypertension, sweating, and hyperthermia.

Endogenous opioids: A class of natural peptides that bind to all types of human opioid receptors (mu, delta, and kappa); endorphins are included in this class.

Fasciculation: Muscular twitching of contiguous groups of muscle fibers.

Lacrimation: Secretion of tears from the eyes.

Methadone: An opioid with pharmacokinetic properties (including a long half-life, reliable absorption and availability, administered by oral ingestion, and nonspecific binding to tissues) that make it a helpful substitute for more dangerous and addicting opioids such as heroin.

Opioids: A class of drugs that includes naturally occurring compounds derived from opium, as well as other synthetic drugs that act as similar receptors.

Rhinorrhea: Runny nose

Clinical Approach

Opioid withdrawal is just one of many recognized substance withdrawal syndromes. All these syndromes have in common the development of a substance-specific pattern of symptoms following cessation of use of the drug in question. The drug use is generally heavy and prolonged, and a **physiologic dependence** develops; thus a withdrawal syndrome occurs on its cessation. The symptoms of opioid withdrawal specifically include **sensitivity to touch and light, goose flesh, autonomic hyperactivity, gastrointestinal distress, joint and muscle aches, yawning, salivation, lacrimation, urination, diarrhea, and a depressed or anxious mood.** Although very uncomfortable, opiate withdrawal is rarely **life-threatening unless complicated by a severe preexisting physical condition.** An intense craving for the drug is present. For the diagnosis, these symptoms must cause significant distress or impairment in functioning. They cannot be caused by either a medical condition or another mental disorder.

Differential Diagnosis

The differential diagnosis for opioid withdrawal is generally straightforward because patients undergoing withdrawal are conscious, are usually able to give their history, and know when the last dose of their drug of choice was taken. Other withdrawal syndromes are not manifested in the same way. For example, patients undergoing alcohol and/or benzodiazepine withdrawal present with anxiety, restlessness, irritability, and insomnia, as well as hyperreflexia and tremor. As withdrawal progresses, tachycardia, hypertension, diaphoresis, hyperthermia, and muscle fasciculations are seen. In severe cases, seizures, delirium, and death can occur. Withdrawal from cocaine includes a "crash," including hypersomnia, hyperphagia, and depressed mood. Withdrawal from nicotine produces anxiety, depression, irritability, headaches, poor concentration, sleep disturbance, and increased blood pressure and heart rate. Opioid withdrawal generally does not cause tremors, confusion, delirium, or seizures. Patients are seldom lethargic or tired. If any of these symptoms are present, the concurrent or separate use of other drugs of abuse should be considered.

Treatment

A rule of thumb regarding opioid withdrawal symptoms is that the shorter the duration of action of the drug ingested, the more acute and intense the withdrawal symptoms. The longer the duration of action of the drug being used, the more prolonged, but mild, the symptoms are. An exception to this rule occurs when an opioid antagonist is given to a person who is dependent on a long-acting opioid. In this case, the withdrawal symptoms can be severe. **Clonidine** has been used to **decrease the autonomic symptoms of opioid withdrawal, such as hypertension, tachycardia, sweating, lacrimation, and rhinorrhea.** It does not, however, remove the subjective sensations or cravings for the drug. Blood pressure levels must be monitored carefully if clonidine is used. It is thought that its mechanism of action in the treatment of opioid withdrawal involves the noradrenergic neurons of the locus ceruleus. Of course, methadone can be used in a daily oral dose to ameliorate opioid withdrawal syndromes, although technically, the patient has not withdrawn from drugs in the opioid class.

Comprehension Questions

[31.1] A 25-year-old man comes to the hospital with classic symptoms of opioid withdrawal. He is adamantly opposed to the use of methadone to relieve his symptoms, saying he "wants to kick this thing once and for all." Which of the following medications can be used to help ameliorate his symptoms while he goes through withdrawal?

A. Sertraline
B. Haloperidol
C. Desipramine
D. Lorazepam
E. Clonidine

[31.2] A 42-year-old woman is determined to "kick her heroin habit" at home without the use of methadone or any other prescription drug. Of the following over-the-counter medications, which is most likely to be of benefit to this patient as she goes through opioid withdrawal?

A. Acetaminophen
B. Ibuprofen
C. Benadryl (diphenhydramine)
D. Pseudoephedrine
E. Dextromethorphan

[31.3] A 32-year-old man with a heroin addiction has recently started treatment with methadone as he tries to quit his heroin habit. Three days after starting the methadone regimen, he has not developed any major symptoms and has not taken any heroin. However, he is experiencing some craving, diarrhea, and mild sweating. Which of the following is the most appropriate course of action?

A. Increase the dose of methadone.
B. Decrease the dose of methadone.
C. Keep the dose of methadone the same and assure the patient that the symptoms will subside.
D. Write a prescription for clonidine to be taken along with the methadone.
E. Put the patient on a 1-week methadone taper program and refer him to Narcotics Anonymous.

Answers

[31.1] **E.** Clonidine can be used to help ease the withdrawal symptoms of opioid withdrawal. It is not an opioid and does not have any addictive properties. Withdrawal from the opioid, however, is not as painless as it otherwise would be if an opioid such as methadone were used. Blood pressure levels should be monitored when clonidine is used. Selective serotonin reuptake inhibitor antidepressants, such as sertraline, are not used in treating acute withdrawal, although the tricyclic antidepressant, desipramine was tried for the reduction of craving in cocaine withdrawal. Lorazepam, a benzodiazepine, is commonly used in the treatment of alcohol withdrawal. Haloperidol, an antipsychotic, has no use in treating withdrawal.

[31.2] **B.** Ibuprofen can help relieve the muscle cramps that are common to opioid withdrawal.

[31.3] **A.** Clinical signs of withdrawal appearing very early in the treatment of heroin addiction with methadone are an indication that the dose is not sufficient to ameliorate all the withdrawal symptoms. Because the patient is at great risk of returning to the use of heroin at this point in the process, a dose adjustment upward to prevent craving is appropriate.

CLINICAL PEARLS

- ❖ A mnemonic that is helpful in remembering the signs and symptoms of opioid withdrawal is **SLUD**—**s**alivation, **l**acrimation, **u**rination, and **d**efecation.
- ❖ Opioid withdrawal is extremely uncomfortable for the patient but generally is not life-threatening.
- ❖ Clonidine and methadone (a long-acting opioid) are the two most common treatments for the relief of opioid withdrawal symptoms.
- ❖ Loperamide (for loose stools) and promethazine (for nausea and vomiting) are useful adjunctive treatments for the symptoms of opioid withdrawal, as is ibuprofen for muscle and joint aches.
- ❖ The presence of dilated pupils and anxiety are often the first signs of opioid withdrawal that can easily be seen in the physician's office.
- ❖ Methadone maintenance programs swap one addiction for another, but the social and physical advantages gained make it one of the best choices for treatment of opiate addiction. Other substances of abuse should always be sought in the presence of heroin addiction.

REFERENCES

Ebert M, Loosen P, Nurcombe B, eds. Current diagnosis and treatment in psychiatry. New York: McGraw-Hill, 2000:247.

Goldman HH. Review of general psychiatry, 5th ed. New York: McGraw-Hill, 2000:220.

❖ CASE 32

A 42-year-old woman presents to a primary care physician with a chief complaint of back pain for the past 6 months that began after she was knocked down by a man attempting to elude the police. She states that she has extreme pain on the right side of her lower back, near L4 and L5. The pain does not radiate, and nothing makes it better or worse. She says that since the injury she has been unable to function and spends most of her days lying in bed or sitting up, immobile, in a chair. Immediately after the accident, she was taken to an emergency department where a workup revealed back strain but no fractures. Since then, the patient has repeatedly sought help from a variety of specialists, but the ongoing pain has been neither adequately explained nor relieved. She denies other medical problems, although she mentions a past history of domestic violence that resulted in several visits to the emergency department for treatment of bruises and lacerations.

On mental status examination, the patient is alert and oriented to person, place, and time. She is cooperative and maintains good eye contact. She holds herself absolutely still, sitting rigidly in her chair and grimacing when she has to move even the smallest amount. Her mood is depressed, and her affect is congruent. Her thought processes are logical, and her thought content is negative for suicidal or homicidal ideation, delusions, or hallucinations.

◆ **What is the most likely diagnosis for this patient?**

◆ **What is the best approach for this patient?**

ANSWERS TO CASE 32: Pain Disorder

Summary: A 42-year-old woman has unremitting back pain for 6 months since she was knocked down. The pain is right-sided, located near L4 and L5. There are no exacerbating or alleviating factors, and the pain does not radiate. The patient is nonfunctional since the event. No fractures were found at the time of the accident—a diagnosis of back strain was made. Further workups over the past 6 months show no anatomic or physiologic reason for continued pain. The patient has a history of domestic violence and on multiple occasions was treated in the emergency department for bruises and lacerations. The results of her mental status examination are noncontributory to the diagnosis.

- **Most likely diagnosis:** Pain disorder.
- **Best approach:** Validate the patient's experience of pain. Explain the role of psychological factors as a cause and consequence of pain. Consider antidepressants and referral to a pain clinic.

Analysis

Objectives

1. Recognize pain disorder in a patient.
2. Understand the chronicity, approach, and treatment options for patients with pain disorder.

Considerations

This patient has **chronic back pain (for 6 months or longer)** that is unaccounted for by a general medical condition. As a result, she is distressed and unable to function. There are no data suggesting that the condition was produced intentionally or is being feigned. It is possible (based on her history of domestic violence) that the accident **triggered memories of the psychological trauma** she previously experienced and thus has a role in the severity of her current pain. The patient does not exhibit signs or symptoms of any other disease that might better account for the pain. Table 32–1 lists the diagnostic criteria for pain disorder.

APPROACH TO PAIN DISORDER

Definitions

Biofeedback: A relaxation technique by which patients are trained to induce physiologic changes (most frequently the induction of alpha waves on an electroencephalogram [EEG] or vasodilatation of peripheral capillaries) that result in a relaxation response.

Dyspareunia: Painful sexual intercourse.

Table 32–1
DIAGNOSTIC CRITERIA FOR PAIN DISORDER*

1. Pain at one or more sites that is severe enough for a clinical evaluation; it is the patient's primary complaint.
2. The pain is very distressing to the patient and/or causes significant functional impairment.
3. The clinician judges that psychological factors play an important part in the initiation, worsening, or severity of the pain.
4. The pain cannot be explained by another axis I condition such as major depression or a psychotic disorder, nor can it be solely the pain of dyspareunia.

*The disorder is considered acute if it lasts for less than 6 months, chronic if longer.

Pain disorder: One of several somatoform disorders listed in the *Diagnostic and Statistical Manual of Mental Disorders, text revision (DSM-IV-TR)* that is distinguished by a primary complaint of pain that is not explained by physical factors; psychological factors are significant in the clinical picture. Pain is a very common complaint in medicine and occurs more often in older patients (fourth and fifth decade of life) and in those who are likely to have job-related physical injuries. A number of psychodynamic factors can be involved, including inability to express emotions verbally, an unconscious need to obtain attention by suffering physical pain, or an unconscious need for punishment. Individuals also learn this form of help-seeking in a family that models and reinforces the behavior.

Clinical Approach

Differential Diagnosis

Pain is a very common complaint in medicine and occurs more often in older patients (fourth and fifth decade of life) and in those who are likely to have job-related physical injuries. It is important that the patient undergo an evaluation for all medical or surgical illnesses that could cause the pain. Patients with depression can sometimes present with a primary complaint of pain; however, on evaluation, the depressive symptoms predominate. Patients with hypochondriasis can complain of pain symptoms, but the main clinical feature is a conviction that they have a serious medical illness. Patients with factitious disorder *intentionally* produce an injury or illness in order to assume the sick role. Patients who are malingering can consciously present false reports of pain in order to achieve secondary gain (such as financial compensation, evading the police by being hospitalized). Patients with pain disorders often use substances to relieve distress, which can mask the pain disorder or some other medical or surgical illness.

Treatment

In treating a patient with pain disorder, the clinician must accept that the **condition is often chronic** and that the goal of pain relief can be unrealistic; providing **gradual rehabilitation is a more reasonable approach.** Although the physician must validate the existence of the patient's pain, education about the contributing effect of psychological factors is important. The use of antidepressants can be an effective pharmacologic approach; **both tricyclics and selective serotonin reuptake inhibitors (SSRIs) have been shown to be helpful.** These agents work by decreasing comorbid depression or by exerting an independent analgesic effect. **Analgesic medications are generally not helpful,** and the patient has usually tried this approach before seeking treatment. Narcotic analgesics should be avoided given their abuse and withdrawal potential. Biofeedback is helpful in certain pain disorders, specifically headaches and muscle tension. Hypnosis and nerve stimulation are also used. Psychodynamic psychotherapy focused on the impact of the disorder on the patient's life can be helpful. For treatment-resistant individuals, comprehensive pain clinics (either inpatient or outpatient) should be considered.

Comprehension Questions

[32.1] A 63-year-old woman returns to her family physician with continuing headaches for 9 months. She describes the pain as "constant . . . always with me," around her entire scalp. She does not appreciate much variation throughout the day, and she cannot name any aggravating or alleviating factors. Although she occasionally feels lightheaded when in severe pain, she denies photophobia, visual changes, nausea, or vomiting. She is especially upset about the headaches as she retired in the past year and has been unable to visit her infant granddaughter. Complete neurologic exams, computerized tomography, magnetic resonance imaging, laboratory studies, and lumbar punctures have been unremarkable. Which of the following is her most likely diagnosis?

A. Factitious disorder
B. Hypochondriasis
C. Malingering
D. Pain disorder
E. Somatization disorder

[32.2] Which of the following would be the most useful approach for the patient in question [32.1]?

A. Confrontation regarding the psychological nature of her pain
B. Reassurance that there is no evidence of pain
C. Referral to a mental health professional
D. Validation of her experience of pain

[32.3] The patient in questions [32.1] and [32.2] feels that her headaches are now "unbearable." Which of the following treatments would be the most appropriate?

A. Acetaminophen
B. Biofeedback
C. Lorazepam
D. Nonsteroidal anti-inflammatory
E. Oxycodone

Answers

[32.1] **D.** This patient presents with criteria for pain disorder. She has chronic, unremitting headaches that are the focus of her complaints. They have interfered with her ability to travel, and the onset seems to coincide with her retirement and new grandchild. Her condition is not intentionally produced as in factitious disorder or malingering, nor is there any appreciable secondary gain (avoidance of work, financial compensation, etc.). The concern is not on having a serious medical illness as in hypochondriasis or multiple physical complaints as in somatization.

[32.2] **D.** One of the most important aspects is to validate the patient's experience of pain. An empathic response will serve to strengthen the therapeutic alliance. Conversely, implying that the symptoms are "not real" or denying that "there is anything wrong" will only cause the patient further distress and can actually worsen the pain. Although referral to a mental health professional can be indicated and helpful given the psychological factors present in pain disorder, this subject should first be gently broached with the patient in order to avoid the appearance of not taking the pain seriously.

[32.3] **B.** Biofeedback and relaxation techniques have demonstrated efficacy in patients with pain disorder, particularly with headaches. Analgesics are often not helpful in these patients. Potentially addicting medications such as benzodiazepines and opiates should especially be avoided in these individuals given the chronic nature of this illness.

CLINICAL PEARLS

- ❖ Patients with pain disorder actually feel pain; it does not help to tell them that "it's all in your head."
- ❖ Pain disorder tends to be a chronic condition; patience, acceptance, and regular visits can promote amelioration of the intensity and frequency of complaints. The patient's therapeutic relationship with the clinician is very important in the management of this condition.

REFERENCES

Kaplan H, Sadock B. Synopsis of psychiatry, 9th ed. Baltimore: Lippincott Williams & Wilkins, 2003:655–658.

Massie MJ, ed. Pain: what psychiatrists need to know. Review Psychiatry Series, Vol 19, no 2. 2000;89.

❖ CASE 33

A 42-year-old man comes to see a psychiatrist stating that his life is "crashing down around his ears." He explains that since his girlfriend of 2 months left him, he has been "inconsolable." He says that he is having trouble sleeping at night because he is mourning her loss. When asked to describe his girlfriend, the patient states, "She was the love of my life, just beautiful, beautiful." He is unable to provide any further details about her. He says that they had five dates, but that he simply knew that she was the one for him. He claims that he was often in the "depths of despair" in his life, but that he also felt "on top of the world." He denies any psychiatric history or any medical problems.

On a mental status examination, the patient is dressed in a bright, tropical-pattern shirt and khaki pants. He leans over repeatedly to touch the interviewer on the arm as he speaks, and he is cooperative during the interview. He sometimes sobs for a short period of time when talking directly about his girlfriend but smiles broadly during the interview when asking the interviewer questions about herself. His speech is of normal rate, although at times somewhat loud. The patient describes his mood as "horribly depressed." His affect is euthymic the majority of the time, and full-range. His thought processes and thought content are all within normal limits.

◆ **What is the most likely diagnosis?**

◆ **What is the best initial treatment for this patient?**

ANSWERS TO CASE 33: Histrionic Personality Disorder

Summary: A 42-year-old man comes to a psychiatrist with complaints of a depressed mood and difficulty sleeping. His says that his girlfriend recently left him. Although he is obviously upset about the loss of the relationship, he cannot describe her in any specific detail, and they had not been going out together for long. The patient's speech and manner appear somewhat theatrical and overblown. His affect appears euthymic and full-range, and he appears to be trying to directly engage the (female) interviewer by touching her and asking her direct personal questions. In this manner, he appears to be trying to draw attention to himself by being somewhat seductive. He is shown to have normal thought processes and thought content on a mental status examination.

- **Most likely diagnosis:** Histrionic personality disorder.
- **Best initial treatment:** Supportive psychotherapy while he grieves the loss of his girlfriend. Setting a strict limit on his seductive behavior needs to be implemented as well.

Analysis

Objectives

1. Recognize histrionic personality disorder in a patient.
2. Know the treatment recommendations for patients with this disorder who come in while experiencing some kind of psychologic crisis.

Considerations

This patient provides a somewhat classic presentation of histrionic personality disorder. Newer epidemiological evidence suggests that histrionic personality disorder is equally common in men as in women, affecting approximately 1.8% of Americans. Clues to making the diagnosis include his **theatrical and overblown speech and his seductive manner.** Other clues include the fact that although he describes himself as being deeply depressed about the loss of his girlfriend, he is unable to describe her other than superficially, and his affect appears euthymic. His case is not unusual because patients with this disorder come to a psychiatrist with a depressed mood but rarely with the thought that their difficulties in functioning in daily life and work are secondary to their own maladaptive behaviors.

APPROACH TO HISTRIONIC PERSONALITY DISORDER

Definitions

Dissociation: A defense mechanism by which an individual deals with emotional conflict or stressors with a breakdown in the usually integrated functions of consciousness, memory, perception of self or the environment, or sensory/motor behavior. For example, a woman who has just been told that her child was killed in an automobile accident suddenly feels as if she is not herself but rather is hearing the events unfold as if they are being told to "someone else."

Limit setting: An activity by which a physician clearly tells a patient what is, and what is not, appropriate behavior in a given circumstance. For example, a physician can set limits on how many times a patient can telephone the physician in a week.

Repression: A defense mechanism by which individuals deal with emotional conflict or stressors by expelling disturbing wishes, thoughts, or experiences from their conscious awareness. For example, a patient is told that she has breast cancer and clearly hears what she has been told because she can repeat the information back to the physician. However, when she returns home later, she tells her husband that the visit went well but that she cannot remember what she and the physician spoke about during the appointment.

Supportive psychotherapy: Therapy designed to help patients support their existing defense mechanisms so that their functioning in the real world improves. Unlike insight-oriented psychotherapy, its goal is to maintain, not improve, a patient's intrapsychic functioning.

Clinical Approach

Patients with **histrionic personality disorder** show a **pervasive pattern of excessive emotionality and attention seeking.** They are uncomfortable in settings where they are not the center of attention. Their emotions are rapidly shifting and shallow, and they often interact with others in **a seductive manner.** Their speech is impressionistic and lacks detail. They are **dramatic and theatrical and exaggerate their emotional expressions.** They often consider relationships to be much more intimate than they really are. They are suggestible to the thoughts of others as well, often adopting other's views without thinking them through.

Differential Diagnosis

Patients with borderline personality disorder can often appear similar to those with histrionic personality disorder, although the former make suicide attempts more often and experience more frequent (brief) episodes of psychosis. Patients who are manic can often be overly dramatic, attention seeking, and seductive, but symptoms of insomnia, euphoria, and psychosis are present as well.

Interviewing Tips and Treatment

The clinician should provide emotional support for and show interest in these patients **but should not allow a personal or sexual relationship to form. Tactful confrontation about seductive behavior** can help. Expressing admiration of the patient, without showing inappropriate behavior, can help in forming a therapeutic working alliance. The treatment of histrionic personality disorder is often best attempted in a group therapy setting, where such patients, particularly if there are other patients with the same diagnosis in the group, better tolerate confrontations to avoid being rejected by other group members. Most psychotherapies require insight, which these individuals lack. Dynamic psychotherapy would likely lead to tumultuous results at best.

Comprehension Questions

[33.1] A 35-year-old woman with histrionic personality disorder has seen her psychotherapist once a week for the past year. During a session, the therapist tells the patient that he is going to be on vacation the following 2 weeks. When he returns from the vacation, the patient tells him that she felt he abandoned her and says, "You didn't even bother to tell me that you would be away." This lapse in memory can best be described as which defense mechanism common to patients with histrionic personality disorder?

A. Sublimation
B. Splitting
C. Undoing
D. Repression
E. Displacement

[33.2] To which cluster does histrionic personality disorder belong?

A. Cluster A
B. Cluster B
C. Cluster C
D. Cluster D
E Cluster E

[33.3] A 20-year-old woman comes to see a psychiatrist at the insistence of her mother, who states that her daughter just "isn't herself." The patient has dressed in brightly colored clothes and worn large amounts of makeup for the past 3 weeks. She acts overtly seductive toward her colleagues at work, is more distractible, and is easily irritated. She also sleeps less, claiming that she "no longer needs it." Which of the following diagnoses best fits this patient's presentation?

A. Histrionic personality disorder
B. Borderline personality disorder
C. Bipolar disorder, mania
D. Narcissistic personality disorder
E. Delusional disorder

Answers

[33.1] **D.** Repression is a common defense mechanism in patients with histrionic personality disorder.

[33.2] **B.** Histrionic personality disorder belongs in cluster B, the "bad" cluster (see Case 6).

[33.3] **C.** This patient has a new onset of behavior that is unlike her usual personality. It includes dressing in loud clothing and wearing lots of makeup, as well as being seductive. She is distractible, is irritable, and needs less sleep than usual. All these symptoms point to a manic episode (assuming neither a medical condition nor a substance can account for the sudden change in functioning).

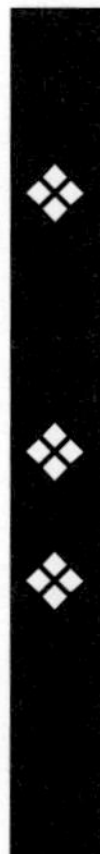

CLINICAL PEARLS

❖ Patients with histrionic personality disorder often appear very dramatic and overemotional. They do not seem to have much depth in either their emotions or their relationships with others. They are uncomfortable when they are not the center of attention.

❖ Patients with histrionic personality disorder use the defense mechanisms of dissociation and repression most commonly.

❖ In interacting with these patients, the physician should use a low-key, friendly approach but should watch interpersonal boundaries. He or she should not become caught up in personal or sexual relationships with such patients, who can be quite seductive.

❖ Patients with histrionic personality disorder can be differentiated from those with mania because the latter often develop dramatic, seductive symptoms as new-onset behavior, not as a pervasive pattern. Patients with mania commonly also have vegetative symptoms, such as a decreased need for sleep, and psychotic symptoms as well.

REFERENCES

Ebert M, Loosen P, Nurcombe B, eds. Current diagnosis and treatment in psychiatry. New York: McGraw-Hill, 2000:477–479.

Grant BF, Hasin DS, Stinson FS, et al. Prevalence correlates and disability of personality disorders in the United States: results from the national epidemiologic survey on alcohol and related conditions. J Clin Psychiatry 2004;65(7):948–958

Kaplan H, Sadock B. Synopsis of psychiatry, 8th ed. Baltimore: Lippincott Williams & Wilkins, 1998:220–221.

❖ CASE 34

A 9-year-old girl is brought to her pediatrician by her mother because of frequent complaints of headaches and stomachaches for the past 3 to 4 weeks. The mother tells you that she has also been doing worse in school during this same time period and believes it is a result of the chronic aches. She has already taken her to the optometrist, and her vision is not a problem. On further questioning by the medical student, we find out that the child's father is part of the army reserve and left for a 6-month assignment in Iraq 5 weeks ago. He e-mails her almost daily, but his daughter notes how much she worries about him and whether he is safe or not. When interviewed, the girl also notes that in addition to her worries about her father, she also sometimes cries about it and feels better when she talks to her friends. She occasionally has a bad dream about her father and feels she sleeps more uneasily as a result.

◆ **What is the most likely diagnosis for this patient?**

◆ **What is the treatment of choice for this disorder?**

ANSWERS TO CASE 34: Adjustment Disorder

Summary: A 9-year-old girl presents to her pediatrician with a number of short-term (3–4 weeks) somatic complaints. In addition, she also has some mild symptoms related to mood as well as anxiety as a result of her father's army commitment. She is able to maintain general functioning, but there does seem to be some decline. She shows evidence of good strengths in that she can express these feelings to others and feels better as a result.

- **Most likely diagnosis:** Adjustment disorder with mixed anxiety and depressed mood
- **Treatment of choice:** Psychotherapy (supportive)

Analysis

Objectives

1. Recognize adjustment disorder in a patient.
2. Understand the best treatment recommendation for patients with this disorder.

Considerations

A few weeks after her father was sent overseas to fulfill an armed-service obligation, his daughter begins to have some difficulties noted by her mother. These seem to show up first in terms of somatic complaints. This is a common presentation for anxious or depressed feelings in children. These should be worked up to reassure both the parents and the patients that there is nothing physically seriously wrong. When further investigated, we find that she has additional, more classically psychiatric symptoms in the areas of mood and worries. She is functioning adequately, but there does seem to be a mild decline. The symptoms have been short in duration (less than 6 months) and occurred within 4 months of the stressor (father going overseas). Her prognosis is good, given her supportive environment and responsiveness to talking about her feelings. (See the diagnostic criteria in Table 34–1.) Supportive therapy would be indicated in this situation as well as an evaluation of the mother to see how she is managing.

APPROACH TO ADJUSTMENT DISORDER

Definitions

Clinically significant symptoms: Distress in excess of what might be expected in response to the particular stressor in question. To be considered clinically significant, these symptoms must include a marked impact on functioning in a variety of settings.

Table 34–1
DIAGNOSTIC CRITERIA FOR ADJUSTMENT DISORDER WITH MIXED ANXIETY AND DEPRESSED MOOD

1. Development of an emotional response to a specific stressor within 3 months of the onset of that stressor.
2. Clinically significant symptoms developed as a response to the stressor.
3. The symptoms do not persist longer than 6 months after the stressor is resolved.
4. Five different subtypes of adjustment disorder are recognized, each characterized by a specific set of moods and/or behavior:
   - With depressed mood
   - With anxiety
   - With mixed anxiety and depressed mood
   - With disturbance of conduct
   - With mixed disturbance of emotions and conduct

Conduct: When used clinically, this term relates to the psychopathology associated with a conduct disorder. The hallmark of this disorder includes violation of the rights of others.

Supportive psychotherapy: A type of therapy in which individuals are taught how to confront issues such as phobias and stressors.

Clinical Approach

Differential Diagnosis

The largest concern in the differential diagnosis for patients with adjustment disorder is major depression. The difference between the two is a matter of degree. Patients with major depression can see its onset following the onset of a stressor, although even after the stressor is removed, the major depression continues. Also, in major depression, marked difficulties involving sleep, appetite, concentration, and energy level are noted, and suicidal ideation (not just transient) and psychotic symptoms can occur. In children or adolescents, irritable mood is often seen rather than the classic depressed mood seen in adults. Mood disorders arising secondary to the use of a substance or a general medical condition must always be ruled out. Clinicians should exclude any symptom complexes characteristic of other stress-induced disorders as well (such as in acute stress disorder or posttraumatic stress disorder [PTSD]) before diagnosing adjustment disorder. With PTSD, the stressor is usually actual or threatened death or serious injury. Finally, normal grief reactions or bereavement can be difficult to differentiate from adjustment disorders, but if the stressor is within expected and/or culturally acceptable ranges, adjustment disorder should generally not be diagnosed.

Treatment

The treatment of choice for adjustment disorder is psychotherapy. Group psychotherapy can often be helpful, especially if the group members all have similar stressors, for example, patients with breast cancer or individuals who have experienced a similar trauma. Individual therapy gives patients an opportunity to work through the meaning of the stressor in their lives and the impact it has on their emotional well-being. Medications are not, in general, indicated, although short-term medications to induce sleep can be helpful if sleep disturbance is part of the symptom presentation. Finally, in the case of extremely acute stressors, for example, a specific traumatic event such as a car accident or an incidence of violence, supportive techniques such as relaxation training, reassurance, and environmental modification (e.g., changing the locks on an apartment door, or moving, if a patient has been the victim of an in-home rape) can be helpful.

Comprehension Questions

[34.1] Adjustment disorder is diagnosed in a 45-year-old woman who was fired from a job she held for 20 years. She undergoes supportive psychotherapy. Nine months later, she is seen by her physician, but none of her symptoms have resolved. During this time, she found another job that is similar to her first position in duties and salary. Which of the following is the most likely diagnosis?

A. Adjustment disorder
B. Posttraumatic stress disorder
C. Major depressive disorder
D. Bipolar disorder
E. Schizoaffective disorder

[34.2] Which of the following treatments would likely be most helpful for a patient with adjustment disorder?

A. Supportive psychotherapy
B. Family therapy
C. A selective serotonin reuptake inhibitor antidepressant
D. Psychoanalysis
E. Behavioral modification therapy

[34.3] In a child who comes in with a diagnosis of major depression, which of the following is the most likely symptom that you might see instead of depressed mood?

A. Irritability
B. Suicidal thoughts
C. Delusions
D. Mania
E. Inattention

Answers

[34.1] **C.** The duration requirement for symptoms occurring *after* the stressor resolved are met.

[34.2] **A.** Symptoms accompanying this disorder most likely will be resolved with a decrease in or elimination of the stressor. Brief supportive psychotherapy is indicated to help the patient deal with the response to the stressor.

[34.3] **A.** In the clinical presentation of children and adolescents, one will often find evidence of irritability or short temper rather than a feeling of sadness or depression. The ability to understand the concept of depression seems to be developmentally mediated.

CLINICAL PEARLS

❖ Adjustment disorder has several different subtypes of symptoms: depressed mood, anxiety, or disturbance of conduct.

❖ Children often feel irritable rather than depressed.

❖ The chronology of the symptoms is very important in making the correct diagnosis.

❖ The most important treatment modality for adjustment disorder involves psychotherapy and not a somatic intervention.

REFERENCES

Ebert M, Loosen P, Nurcombe B, eds. Current diagnosis and treatment in psychiatry. New York: McGraw-Hill, 2000:460–466.

Kaplan H, Sadock B. Synopsis of psychiatry, 9th ed. Baltimore: Lippincott Williams & Wilkins, 2003:1111–1112.

❖ CASE 35

A 41-year-old nurse presents to the emergency department with concerns that she has hypoglycemia from an insulinoma. She reports repeated episodes of headache, sweating, tremor, and palpitations. She denies any past medical problems and only takes nonsteroidal anti-inflammatory medications for menstrual cramps. On physical examination, she is a well-dressed woman who is intelligent, polite, and cooperative. Her vital signs are stable except for slight tachycardia. The examination is remarkable for diaphoresis, tachycardia, and numerous scars on her abdomen, as well as needle marks on her arms. When asked about this, she says that she feels confused because of her hypoglycemia.

The patient is subsequently admitted to the medical service. Laboratory evaluations demonstrate a decreased fasting blood sugar level and an increased insulin level, but a decreased level of plasma C-peptide, which indicates exogenous insulin injection. When she is confronted with this information, she quickly becomes angry, claims the hospital staff is incompetent, and requests that she be discharged against medical advice.

◆ **What is the most likely diagnosis?**

 **How should you best approach this patient?**

ANSWERS TO CASE 35: Factitious Disorder

Summary: A 41-year-old female health care worker presents to the emergency department with symptoms typical of an insulinoma, including headache, diaphoresis, palpitations, and tremors. She denies a medical history, although her physical examination demonstrates prior surgeries and injections. When confronted with this evidence, she becomes hostile and asks to leave the hospital.

- **Most likely diagnosis:** Factitious disorder.
- **Best approach:** In order to engage the patient in psychiatric treatment, attempt to ally with her regarding her compulsion to "be sick."

Analysis

Objectives

1. Recognize factitious disorder (Table 35–1).
2. Differentiate factitious disorder from conversion disorder and malingering.
3. Understand the best approach to patients with factitious disorder.

Considerations

Although this patient initially presents with classic symptoms of hypoglycemia possibly caused by an insulinoma, discrepancies are noted in her story, especially her **denial of a medical history in light of the numerous scars.** Her laboratory evaluations are consistent with the use of insulin, which she undoubtedly injects herself. Specifically, although her insulin levels are increased, her serum C-peptide levels are decreased**. When confronted, she becomes hostile and defensive and asks to leave the hospital. No obvious external incentives** are present. Thus, it appears that her motivation is merely to be sick as primary gain. The fact that the patient consciously created the hypoglycemia rules out the diagnosis of a somatoform or conversion disorder. The absence of a secondary gain differentiates factitious disorder from malingering. It is useful to note that she is an intelligent woman who works in the health care field, a common scenario for this disorder.

Table 35–1
DIAGNOSTIC CRITERIA FOR FACTITIOUS DISORDER

Intentional production or feigning of physical or psychological signs or symptoms.
The motivation is to assume the sick role (primary gain).
External incentives for the behavior (as in malingering) are absent.

APPROACH TO FACTITIOUS DISORDER

Definitions

Pseudologia phantastica: The telling of "tall tales," or lying, commonly seen in factitious disorder

Münchhausen syndrome: Factitious disorder, especially involving repeated episodes, seeking admission at different hospitals, and pseudologia phantastica

Münchhausen syndrome by proxy: Factitious disorders induced in children by parents, who are usually very cooperative after taking them to the hospital

Clinical Approach

Although the true incidence of this disorder is unknown, it seems to be more common in hospital and health care workers. The etiology is unclear and can have to do with poor parent–child relationships during childhood. Affected individuals usually have average to above-average intelligence, poor self-identity, and strong dependency needs. They feign physical symptoms so convincingly that they are hospitalized or operated on.

Differential Diagnosis

The possibility of an authentic underlying medical cause with an unusual presentation should be ruled out. In addition, given the self-inflicted nature of the symptoms, it is essential that the patient be examined for any legitimate complications as well. Examples include adhesions resulting from frequent (unnecessary) abdominal surgeries leading to obstruction, serious infections produced by the injection of urine or feces into the veins, and coma caused by hypoglycemia.

Differentiating factitious disorder from conversion and other somatoform disorders, as well as malingering, can be difficult. Whereas the etiology of the compulsion to fabricate physical or psychiatric illness is likely rooted in unconscious, primitive dynamics, **in factitious disorder the *conscious* motivation is to assume the sick role.** Patients **consciously feign illness in order to be taken care of in a health care setting.** This behavior is in contrast to that seen in conversion and other somatoform disorders, in which both the underlying conflicts and the production of the symptoms are *unconscious.* In malingering, both the motivation (an external incentive) and the fabrication are *conscious.*

Patients with factitious disorder can also meet criteria for borderline personality disorder. Patients with both disorders frequently have histories of childhood mistreatment such as physical, sexual, or emotional abuse.

Treatment

There is no treatment per se for factitious disorders. If there is an underlying psychiatric disorder such as major depression or an anxiety disorder, it should be treated as indicated. Like patients with somatoform disorders, these individuals are extremely resistant to mental health treatment. When discovered, they usually flee the hospital, frequently repeating the same or a similar cycle at another facility. *Managing* this disorder is more appropriate than *treating* it. Liaison with a psychiatric consultation service is helpful in engaging the patient in psychiatric treatment, as is working with the hospital staff to cope with the feelings of anger, betrayal, and mistrust that frequently come to the forefront. It is useful to keep in mind that individuals with factitious disorder are very ill and that, like other "genuine" patients, they require help and caring.

Comprehension Questions

[35.1] Which of the following is most likely the motivation behind the behavior displayed in factitious disorder?

A. Desire to avoid jail
B. Desire to be taken care of
C. Desire to obtain compensation
D. Desire to obtain narcotics

[35.2] Which type of personality disorder is most likely to occur comorbidly with factitious disorder?

A. Antisocial
B. Avoidant
C. Borderline
D. Schizoid

[35.3] Which of the following scenarios is most consistent with factitious disorder?

A. Lying about back pain to receive time off from work
B. Pseudoseizures in the context of a family conflict
C. Placing feces in urine to receive treatment for a urinary tract infection
D. Recurrent fears of having a serious illness

[35.4] Which of the following is the most useful approach for patients with factitious disorder?

A. Confronting their feigning of symptoms
B. Discharging them from the hospital
C. Establishing a therapeutic alliance
D. Referring them to legal authorities

Answers

[35.1] **B.** The primary desire in factitious disorder is to assume the sick role and be taken care of. In contrast, in malingering, the motivation is to achieve a tangible gain (such as avoiding work, school, or a prison sentence) or to obtain narcotics or financial compensation.

[35.2] **C.** Borderline personality disorder is not uncommon in patients with factitious disorder. Individuals with either of these disorders often have similar histories of abuse, molestation, and emotional neglect. Patients with borderline personality disorder also act out their internal psychological conflicts on an interpersonal level, and they display the chaotic, labile affective state seen in factitious disorder.

[35.3] **C.** The hallmark of factitious disorder is intentional feigning of a physical or psychiatric illness in order to assume the sick role. Examples include injecting oneself with insulin to create hypoglycemia, taking anticoagulants to fake a bleeding disorder, and contaminating urine samples with feces to simulate a urinary tract infection. Lying about back pain in order to avoid work is an example of malingering. Pseudoseizures are an example of a conversion disorder. Fear of having a serious disease caused by misinterpretation of bodily sensations is characteristic of hypochondriasis.

[35.4] **C.** Although there is no specific treatment for factitious disorder, the best way to help these patients is to attempt to establish a therapeutic alliance and a working relationship. Although this can be difficult, only then can the patient's compulsion to feign illness be addressed and dealt with in a psychotherapeutic environment. Confrontation is necessary in some circumstances, but if an accusatory or judgmental manner is employed, patients flee care and begin the cycle again at another hospital. Prematurely discharging patients from the hospital or referring them to legal services has the same result, although in cases of factitious disorder by proxy (where a caretaker simulates illness in a child), referral to child protective services is necessary because this behavior is considered a form of child abuse.

CLINICAL PEARLS

- Factitious disorder is characterized by the intentional production of physical or psychiatric signs or symptoms in order to assume the sick role.
- Factitious disorder is more common in women and in those in the health care professions.
- The course of factitious disorder is chronic, with a pattern of lying, self-inflicted injuries, repeated hospitalizations, and premature discharges.
- The best management of factitious disorder involves early identification, avoidance of unnecessary tests and treatments, empathic understanding of the need to be sick, establishment of a therapeutic working relationship, and potential referral to a mental health professional.

REFERENCES

Ebert M, Loosen P, Nurcombe B, eds. Current diagnosis and treatment in psychiatry. New York: McGraw-Hill, 2000:378–383.

Kaplan H, Sadock B. Synopsis of psychiatry, 9th ed. Baltimore: Lippincott Williams & Wilkins, 2003:843–846.

CASE 36

The $2^1/_2$-year-old, first-born son of married parents is brought to a pediatrician's office by his father. Before this visit, the patient visited the pediatrician only for regular well-child checks and for treatment of one episode of otitis media. The father is concerned about the behavioral problems his son has developed. He reports that for the past month, after the patient goes to bed and to sleep, the parents hear him get up in the middle of the night. This behavior occurs perhaps once or twice a week. On these occasions, the child is found standing somewhere in the house, crying and seemingly disoriented with rapid breathing and profuse sweating. When the parents attempt to comfort him or return him to his room, he becomes quite upset, striking out at them and screaming loudly. He continues to scream and fight for several minutes but then stops spontaneously. If he can be awakened, he will continue to act frightened and cannot share any dream content. Once the child is calmed, the parents put him back in his bed, and he sleeps through the rest of the night without incident. In the morning, he wakes up in his usual happy mood and does not remember what occurred the previous evening. The parents are worried that he might be having seizures or developing a severe behavioral problem.

- **What is the most likely diagnosis for this child?**

- **What treatments would you recommend for this child?**

ANSWERS TO CASE 36: Sleep Terror Disorder

Summary: The patient is a 2½-year-old boy with new-onset sleep problems who has no significant other history. He wakes at night, screaming with autonomic hyperarousal, and his parents are unable to soothe him. These episodes last a few minutes, after which he goes back to normal sleep. The child has no memory of the events in the morning.

 **Most likely diagnosis:** Sleep terror disorder.

◆ **Recommended treatments:** Protect the child from injury and do nothing. The disorder is usually time-limited.

Analysis

Objectives

1. Recognize sleep terror disorder in a patient (Table 36–1).
2. Offer treatment suggestions to the parents.

Considerations

This patient's presentation is typical for sleep terror disorder, a disorder that is found in 3% of all children and less than 1% of adults and typically manifests itself as emotional and behavioral disturbances at night. These events usually occur early in the nightly sleep cycle during **delta (slow-wave) sleep. With sleep terror disorder,** the affected **child does not remember the episodes in the morning. Fever, sleep deprivation, and central nervous system depressants may increase frequency of sleep terror episodes. Typically, these children have no psychopathology.** The episodes are usually self-limiting without treatment, and the prognosis is very good. Reassuring the parents is the usual indicated intervention. Nightmares occur during rapid eye movement (REM) sleep and are typically associated with the report of a "bad dream." If the child is awakened, he or she can typically recall the dream, even the next morning.

Table 36–1

DIAGNOSTIC CRITERIA FOR SLEEP TERROR DISORDER

Episodes of apparent abrupt awakening from sleep usually occurring in the early part of the sleep cycle.
Behavioral exhibition of intense emotion, often with extreme autonomic responses seen.
Patient is often unresponsive to efforts to soothe or calm.
Little memory of episode in the morning after a normal awakening.

APPROACH TO SLEEP TERROR DISORDER

Definitions

Delta sleep: Sleep stage characterized by low frequency (0.5 to 2 waves/sec), high voltage (amplitudes greater than 75 microvolts) waves in at least 20% of the waves

Dysomnias: Sleep difficulties associated with the duration and type of sleep

Parasomnias: Sleep disorders associated with problems during the stages of sleep

Rapid eye movement: A sleep stage characterized by fast eye movements and a wakeful pattern of electrical activity in the brain

Sleep cycle: The brain-wave activity associated with varying stages of sleep from light to deep

Somnambulism: Sleepwalking

Clinical Approach

Normal Sleep

The human sleep cycle is divided into several different stages defined by brain wave patterns that can be measured in a sleep study. Parameters measured include an electroencephalogram (EEG), which measures and records electrical activity on the surface of the brain, an electro-oculogram (EOG), which records eye movements during sleep, and an electromyogram (EMG), which records the electrical activity emanating from active muscles in the body (Figure 36–1). The stages of sleep defined by the sleep study include:

Stage 1: The EEG may show theta waves, muscle tone may be relaxing, and eye movements may be slow and rolling; typically the "nodding off" period.

Stage 2: The EEG shows K complexes and sleep spindles, no eye movements, and little muscle activity.

Delta sleep: The EEG shows low frequency, high voltage waves. Delta sleep has been divided into Stages 3 and 4 by some, depending on the number of delta waves seen.

Rapid eye movement: Low, fast voltage on the EEG, no muscle tone (cataplexy), and very rapid eye movements.

The sleep cycle is a dynamic presentation of the stages in a typical night's sleep. Sleep disorders are classified and defined based on their occurrence and manifestation in the context of the sleep cycle. Dyssomnias are disorders characterized by excessive sleepiness or difficulty initiating or maintaining sleep. They include such intrinsic sleep disorders as narcolepsy and obstructive sleep apnea, and such extrinsic sleep disorders such as poor sleep hygiene, allergies, and insufficient sleep. Parasomnias are sleep disorders that occur during sleep or on arousal. They include such disorders as sleep terrors, sleepwalking (somnambulism), rhythmic movement disorder, sleep talking, nightmares, sleep paralysis, bruxism, and enuresis.

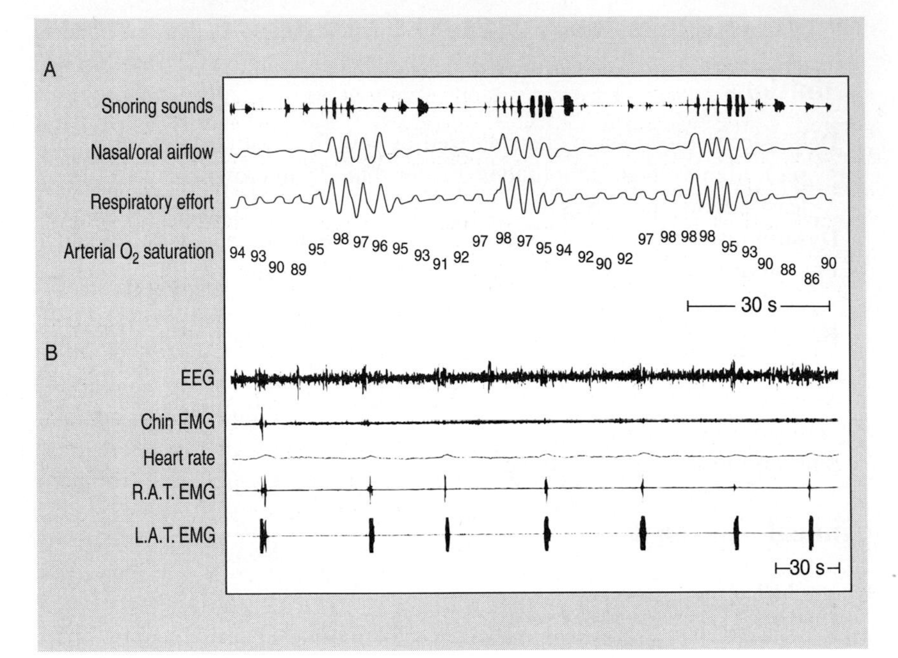

Figure 36–1. The parameters measured during a sleep study.

Differential Diagnosis

Night terrors and somnambulism tend to occur during periods of arousal from delta sleep. As a result, these disorders are more common in children who have more delta sleep and they often occur during the first half of the night when there is more delta sleep occurring. It is not uncommon for both disorders to occur in the same person. Patients with both disorders are difficult to awaken, confused if they are awakened during a parasomnia and typically do not remember the incident. Sleepwalking (somnambulism), is characterized by repeated episodes of rising from bed and walking during the sleep. Often patients have a blank look on their face and seem indifferent to what is around them. They typically are not very reactive and thus do not show the behavior, such as screaming and violent thrashing, seen in sleep terror disorder. Patients who sleepwalk often show amnesia to the event on awakening as well. They are not dreaming but typically show an arousal pattern during delta sleep. The potential for harm to self or others from a sleepwalker (falls, walking into streets, starting a fire) means that families must take steps to protect the child and in serious cases may require pharmacologic intervention.

Individuals with nightmare disorders have dreams of a very frightening nature characterized by limited verbalization and movement. These dreams occur during REM sleep, and the patient can often recall them in detail on awakening. The absence of screaming and thrashing, plus the detailed memory of the dream, differentiates this disorder from sleep terror disorder. Patients with posttraumatic stress disorder may have frightening dreams or dissociative experiences, because this disorder is one of autonomic reactivity and an exaggerated startle response following exposure to a traumatic experience. However, these patients typically remember frightening dreams and/or flashbacks that do not occur exclusively at night. Temporal lobe epilepsy is a type of seizure disorder that includes active, often violent, motor responses, but these typically occur during waking hours.

Perhaps one of the most common disorders of sleep in childhood is **enuresis.** The treatment of enuresis in childhood is best approached by **diagnosing the core problem correctly and advising the parents to be supportive of and not punish the child. Primary enuresis is** defined as **nighttime urination** in a child **with no previous significant period of dryness. Secondary enuresis is nighttime urination following a period of dryness (usually at least several months).** Secondary enuresis is often the result of a physical problem, such as a urinary tract infection, or a psychological stressor, such as regression associated with the arrival of a newborn sibling.

Treatment

The treatment of sleep terror disorder usually consists of reassuring the parents that, with time, the child will outgrow these harmless events. They should be instructed to take measures to maintain the patient's safety during these episodes, as unrestrained thrashing can result in injury.

In somnambulism, special care must be taken to ensure that the patient cannot wander out of windows or out of the house or access dangerous materials. There have been case reports on using drugs such as diazepam or imipramine but no controlled studies.

Primary enuresis can be treated in a number of ways, although the developmental level of the child should also be considered. It often remits spontaneously as the child becomes older. Generally, pharmacologic or extensive behavioral treatment should not be considered prior to **age 7.** The behavioral treatment for enuresis primarily involves the use of **an enuresis alarm, alternatively known as a "bell and pad."** This device consists of a moisture-sensitive sensor attached to the child's underwear and an alarm linked to the sensor close by. When the sensor is activated, the alarm goes off, waking the child as well as the caretaker. The child should then be quickly and directly taken to the bathroom to urinate. This method of enuresis control has a 75% success rate, as well as a low rate of recidivism after the alarm is taken away. Buzzer ulcers sometimes can develop and should be discussed as a potential adverse effect.

Desmopressin (DDAVP) is a synthetic analog of a natural antidiuretic hormone that has been found effective in 18 randomized, controlled trials. A study comparing bell-and-pad method to DDAVP found comparable efficacy: bell-and-pad, 86% and desmopressin, 70%. It was used successfully in both tablet and nasal form to control enuresis in children. Again, it is an effective short-term treatment for enuresis, but there is a high rate of recidivism once the medication is discontinued.

Another common treatment for enuresis involves medication. **Imipramine** was an effective treatment in more than 40 double-blind studies. Given in relatively low doses, it is very effective in controlling nighttime wetting. However, there is a high rate of recidivism after the medication is discontinued. **Electrocardiogram (EKG) monitoring is recommended in doses above 3.5 mg/kg/day, and the dangerousness of imipramine in overdosage should be stressed to parents and children.**

Comprehensive Questions

[36.1] A child with nightmare disorder experiencing a nightmare is in which of the following stages of sleep?

A. Stage 1
B. Stage 2
C. Stage 3
D. Rapid eye movement sleep
E. Light sleep

[36.2] Which of the following is not true related to night terror disorder?

A. The child has intense autonomic arousal.
B. The child typically can relate details of a bad dream.
C. They tend to occur in the first half of the night.
D. They tend to occur during delta sleep.
E. The frequency is higher in children than adults.

[36.3] The best treatment for sleep terror disorder is which of the following?

A. A selective serotonin reuptake inhibitor antidepressant
B. A benzodiazepine sleeping agent
C. Reassuring the parents
D. Gradually changing the sleep/wake cycle
E. Warm milk before bedtime

Answers

[36.1] **D.** Nightmare disorder is a parasomnia usually associated with the REM stage of sleep. Night terrors usually occur during non-REM sleep.

[36.2] **B.** Because night terrors typically do not occur during REM sleep, there is usually no dream to recall.

[36.3] **C.** The best treatment for night terrors and nightmares is to assure the parents that their child will probably grow out of this developmental stage rather quickly. Precautions should be taken to maintain the patient's safety during these episodes because unrestrained thrashing can result in injury.

CLINICAL PEARLS

- Patients with sleep terror disorder need to be protected from injuring themselves during these episodes, but otherwise do not require pharmacologic intervention.
- Sleep terror disorder occurs almost exclusively during delta sleep.
- Enuresis may be effective treated with the bell-and-pad method, desmopressin, and imipramine.

REFERENCES

Gillin JC, Seifritz E, Zoltoski RK, Salin-Pascual RJ. Basic science of sleep. In: Saddock BJ, Saddock VA, eds., Comprehensive textbook of psychiatry, 7th ed. Philadelphia: Lippincott Williams & Wilkins, 2000:199–209.

Mikkelsen EJ. Elimination disorders. In: Sadock BJ, Sadock VA, eds. Kaplan and Sadock's comprehensive textbook of psychiatry, 7th ed. Philadelphia: Lippincott Williams & Wilkins, 2000:2720–2728.

Moore CA, Williams RL, Hirshkowitz M. Sleep disorders. In: Sadock BJ, Sadock VA, eds. Kaplan and Sadock's comprehensive textbook of psychiatry, 7th ed. Philadelphia: Lippincott Williams & Wilkins, 2000:1677–1700.

❖ CASE 37

A 28-year-old woman comes to her primary care physician with a chief complaint of not getting enough sleep and feeling fatigued for the past 2 months. She says that she has a problem falling asleep and often wakes up numerous times during the night as well. She claims that her sleep problems began after she had an argument on the telephone with her boyfriend. She noted that after that she was "all keyed up" and could not go to sleep that night. Subsequently, she faces every evening with dread because she is preoccupied with getting enough sleep. She becomes very frustrated with her inability to sleep, which just makes the problem worse. She has no other signs or symptoms other than the fatigue caused by failure to get her usual 8 hours of sleep each night. She states that her mood is "Okay, except for this sleep thing." She is still seeing her boyfriend, and their relationship has been stable. She has no medical problems, she denies the use of drugs, and she drinks alcohol only very rarely—not at all since she began having problems sleeping. The results of her physical examination are entirely normal.

◆ **What is the most likely diagnosis for this patient?**

◆ **What treatment recommendations should be made to this patient?**

ANSWERS TO CASE 37: Primary Insomnia

Summary: A 28-year-old woman has had sleeping problems for the past 2 months that were precipitated by an argument with her boyfriend. Since that time, she is preoccupied with getting enough sleep and is worried and frustrated. She has problems falling and staying asleep. She reports no other medical or psychiatric problems, and the results of her physical examination are normal. She denies the use of drugs or alcohol.

- **Most likely diagnosis:** Primary insomnia.
- **Recommended treatment:** Suggestions regarding sleep hygiene should be offered. Helpful medications include zolpidem, zaleplon, and benzodiazepines, although these medications should in general not be used for more than 2 weeks because tolerance and withdrawal can result.

Analysis

Objectives

1. Recognize primary insomnia in a patient.
2. Understand the recommended treatment approaches for patients with this disorder.

Considerations

This patient experienced a psychological upset that interfered with her ability to sleep. Subsequently, she developed a vicious cycle of worrying about whether or not she will be able to sleep, which is invariably followed by a poor night's sleep. She has no signs or symptoms of a mood or other psychiatric disorder and no evidence of a physical disease or a substance abuse/dependence problem.

APPROACH TO PRIMARY INSOMNIA

Clinical Approach

Diagnostic Criteria

Primary insomnia is diagnosed when problems sleeping have occurred for at least 1 month and cause significant distress or impairment. These problems include nonrestorative sleep or an inability to initiate or maintain sleep, often presenting as complaints of difficulty falling asleep and multiple awakenings during the night. Patients are often quite preoccupied with getting enough sleep and the fact that they are not doing so, which further increases their frustration and inability to sleep. Psychological and physiologic arousal at night and negative conditioning for sleep are often evident. The sleep disorder cannot be caused by the effects of a substance or general medical condition or occur exclusively during an episode of another psychiatric disorder. Narcolepsy, breathing-related sleep disorder, circadian rhythm sleep disorder, or parasomnias (e.g., sleepwalking, sleep terrors) must first be ruled out, which makes the diagnosis of primary insomnia disorder basically one of exclusion.

Differential Diagnosis

As noted earlier, the diagnosis of primary insomnia is one of exclusion, and so physical factors (sleep apnea, sleep-related epilepsy, sleep-related asthma, sleep-related gastroesophageal reflux disease, etc.) must all be ruled out before such a diagnosis can be made. In addition, mental disorders that cause disturbances in sleep, such as psychosis, major depression, alcoholism, anxiety disorders, and mania should also be excluded. Sleep-related disorders such as narcolepsy and circadian rhythm sleep disorder (in which the individual's sleep–wake pattern is out of synchrony with the desired schedule) must also be ruled out.

Treatment

Primary insomnia can be very difficult to treat. When patients have been negatively conditioned to sleep, deconditioning is necessary. This procedure includes instructing them to use their beds only for sleeping. If they cannot fall asleep after 5 minutes, they should get up and do something else in another room. Relaxation training such as meditation and biofeedback can be helpful. Pharmacotherapy can be useful in the short term and includes the use of benzodiazepines, zolpidem, or zaleplon. These drugs should not be used consecutively for more than 2 weeks because tolerance and withdrawal can occur. Neither melatonin nor L-tryptophan have demonstrated clear efficacy in research trials. Nonspecific sleep hygiene techniques can also work (Table 37–1). Telling patients that their health will not be endangered if they get fewer than 6 hours of sleep per night for a short time can reduce frustration and anxiety about their sleeplessness, which often is contributing to their insomnia.

Table 37–1
SLEEP HYGIENE MEASURES

1. Eat at regular times during the day and not late at night
2. Take a long, very hot bath near bedtime
3. Drink a glass of warm milk near bedtime
4. Avoid daytime naps
5. Get up at the same time every day
6. Go to sleep at the same time every night
7. Do not use substances that impair sleep, such as caffeine, alcohol, nicotine, or stimulants
8. Begin a physical fitness program
9. Avoid evening stimulation—listen to the radio or read a book instead

Comprehension Questions

[37.1] A 33-year-old married physician presents to your primary care practice with complaints of "depression." On interview, he denies pervasive feelings of sadness or anhedonia, and he has not had any change in appetite or weight, or any problems concentrating. He has felt tired much of the time for the past 6 weeks, with ongoing, multiple awakenings during the night. On further questioning, he reveals that these difficulties began when he was involved in a malpractice suit after the death of a patient. He was "up obsessing about it" prior to the trial when his sleep disturbance began. Although the suit was dropped, he continues to wake up frequently, worrying about not being able to fall back asleep. He denies medical problems, alcohol, or drug use. Which of the following is the most likely diagnosis for this patient?

A. Breathing-related sleep disorder
B. Circadian rhythm sleep disorder
C. Major depressive disorder
D. Primary insomnia

[37.2] You offer the patient in question [37.1] a short course of lorazepam, but he declines. Which of the following should you next recommend to help his sleep?

A. Eat a late evening meal
B. Exercise prior to bedtime
C. Sleep later on the weekends
D. Take a hot bath in the evening
E. Take naps during the day

[37.3] A patient comes to her physician stating that for the last 6 months, since she started a new job, she has difficulty getting up in time for work. She notes that she is not tired around bedtime, and so she stays up for several hours playing computer games. When she finally does go to sleep, she has time to sleep for only 4 to 5 hours before she has to get up to go to work. She then finds herself groggy in the morning and fatigued throughout the day. This problem is interfering with her work at her job and thus is causing her distress. Prior to starting her new office job, the patient worked evening hours as a bartender and did not have a problem with sleeping. She takes no medications and uses no substances that could explain her sleep problems. The results of her physical examination are normal. Which of the following is the most likely diagnosis for this patient?

A. Breathing-related sleep disorder
B. Circadian rhythm sleep disorder
C. Primary hypersomnia
D. Primary insomnia

Answers

[37.1] **D.** The patient likely suffers from primary insomnia. There is no evidence of sleep apnea or a disconnect between the environment and the circadian rhythm of the patient. Despite the insomnia and fatigue, there is no pervasive depressed mood, anhedonia, or other neurovegetative symptoms suggestive of a major depression.

[37.2] **D.** Taking a hot bath near bedtime is an effective technique for inducing sleep in some patients. The other options listed do not help and are actually likely to *worsen* insomnia.

[37.3] **B.** This patient is suffering from a delayed-sleep-phase type of circadian rhythm sleep disorder. Circadian rhythm sleep disorder is characterized by a recurrent pattern of sleep disruption leading to excessive sleepiness and/or insomnia because of the mismatch between the sleep–wake schedule required in a person's environment (in this case, the demands of the patient's new job) and her circadian sleep–wake pattern. The sleep disorder must cause distress and must not be caused by a substance, a physical condition, or another mental disorder.

CLINICAL PEARLS

- Primary insomnia is characterized by trouble falling asleep and multiple awakenings throughout the night. Individuals with this disorder are often preoccupied with getting enough sleep and become more and more frustrated every night, which further inhibits their ability to sleep.
- Primary insomnia is a diagnosis of exclusion because interfering physical and mental disorders must all be ruled out before the diagnosis can be made.
- Primary insomnia can be treated in the short term (to break the cycle of insomnia and worrying about it) with benzodiazepines or other hypnotics. Melatonin and L-tryptophan do not have proven benefit.
- Deconditioning, relaxation training, and sleep hygiene training can be useful in helping patients with primary insomnia sleep.

REFERENCES

Ebert M, Loosen P, Nurcombe B, eds. Current diagnosis and treatment in psychiatry. New York: McGraw-Hill, 2000:437–440.

Kaplan H, Sadock, B. Synopsis of psychiatry, 9th ed. Baltimore: Lippincott Williams & Wilkins, 2003:763–767.

❖ CASE 38

A 28-year-old woman presents to her primary care physician with a chief complaint of a headache that "will not go away." The patient states that she had a headache every day for the past month and that she obtained relief only by lying down in a darkened room. The pain radiates through her head to the back. Tylenol with codeine helps somewhat but does not completely alleviate the pain. The patient notes that she had these headaches for "at least a decade," along with frequent chest pains, back pains, and abdominal pains. She reports vomiting and diarrhea, most commonly occurring with the abdominal pain but sometimes in isolation. She notes that she vomited throughout her one and only pregnancy at age 24. The patient states that along with the headaches and abdominal pains she sometimes experiences numbness and tingling in her upper arms. She has been to see neurologists, obstetricians, and other primary care physicians, but no one has found the cause of any of her problems. The patient underwent one prior surgery, for a ruptured appendix at age 18. She has one 4-year-old child. She has been unable to work for the past 5 years because of her symptoms and claims that they have "destroyed her life." A mental status examination is notable for the patient's depressed mood and affect.

◆ **What is the most likely diagnosis for this patient?**

◆ **What is the best treatment?**

◆ **What is the most likely prognosis?**

ANSWERS TO CASE 38: Somatization Disorder

Summary: A 28-year-old woman presents with a chief complaint of a headache every day for the past month. Lying down in a dark room and taking Tylenol with codeine help somewhat. The pain radiates through her head to the back. Her headaches have occurred for 10 years, along with chest pain, back pain, and abdominal pain. Associated symptoms include numbness and tingling in the upper arms, vomiting, diarrhea, and "continual" vomiting throughout her pregnancy 4 years ago. No physical abnormalities have been found. The patient is disabled by her symptoms, and they are distressing to her. A mental status examination reveals a depressed mood and a dysphoric affect.

 **Most likely diagnosis:** Somatization disorder (Diagnostic criteria in Table 38–1).

◆ **Best treatment:** Identify one physician as the primary caregiver and schedule regular, brief, usually monthly visits. Psychotherapy is useful if it is acceptable to the patient.

◆ **Prognosis:** Patients with somatization disorder generally have a chronic disease that is often debilitating. Rarely does a patient with this disease go for longer than 1 year without medical attention.

Analysis

Objectives

1. Recognize somatization disorder in a patient.
2. Understand the treatment recommendations for this disorder.
3. Be aware of the prognosis for this disorder.

Table 38–1

DIAGNOSTIC CRITERIA FOR SOMATIZATION DISORDER

1. The patient has a history of many physical symptoms that began before age 30, have persisted over several years, and cause considerable distress and impairment in function.
2. The patient's symptoms have met the following criteria over the course of the illness:
   a. Four pain symptoms (involving four different sites or body systems)
   b. Two gastrointestinal symptoms (nausea, vomiting, abdominal pain)
   c. One sexual or reproductive symptom
   d. One pseudoneurologic symptom, such as localized weakness or sensory loss
3. The symptoms cannot be explained by a medical condition or a substance.
4. If there is a known medical condition, the complaints and decreased functioning cannot be explained by this condition.
5. The patient does not intentionally produce the symptoms.

Considerations

This patient has a long history, **beginning before the age of 30,** of numerous physical complaints that cannot be accounted for by any physical illness. She complains of **pain symptoms** (headaches and abdominal, back, and chest pains), **gastrointestinal symptoms** (vomiting and diarrhea), sexual symptoms (vomiting throughout pregnancy), and **pseudoneurologic symptoms** (pain and tingling in her upper arms). She is significantly impaired by these complaints. There is no evidence that the symptoms are feigned or intentionally produced. A brief physical examination should be performed to address each new complaint. Laboratory and diagnostic procedures should generally be avoided unless there are clear, objective signs that they are needed. If the patient can be convinced that psychological factors might be contributing to her problems, a referral for psychotherapy can be made, which can be helpful in decreasing health care expenditures.

APPROACH TO SOMATIZATION DISORDER

Definitions

Somatization disorder: A syndrome in which the individual has **multiple physical symptoms** that cannot be explained on the basis of a medical evaluation. It is a **chronic condition** that usually begins before the age of 30 and consists of complaints involving **multiple organ systems:** pseudoneurologic, pain, gastrointestinal, and sexual symptoms. The patient is distressed and repeatedly seeks medical attention. The condition causes marked impairment in functioning in the social and occupational areas.

Clinical Approach

Differential Diagnosis

Some medical illnesses are characterized by diverse symptoms such as those present in somatization disorder—multiple sclerosis, acquired immunodeficiency syndrome (AIDS), lupus erythematosus, porphyria, hyperthyroidism, hyperparathyroidism, and myasthenia gravis. The clinician must rule out these disorders in making an evaluation.

Many patients with depression have somatic symptoms, including gastrointestinal and neurologic complaints, however, these symptoms are found from the patient's history to **have begun *after* the mood symptoms.** Patients with psychotic disorders can have somatic delusions that are expressed as physical symptoms, but other symptoms such as hallucinations, bizarre delusions, or negative symptoms are present as well. Patients can misinterpret the sympathetic hyperarousal of anxiety as various physical symptoms, although these symptoms usually consistently involve one body area (e.g., a stomachache) rather than being spread throughout the body and its systems as in somatization disorder. Other somatoform disorders must be ruled out as well: Hypochondriasis is distinguished by the patient's having a conviction that he or she has a particular illness, and pain disorder by the prominence of the pain symptoms. In conversion disorder, the patient's complaints are limited to neurologic symptoms.

Comorbidity with other axis I disorders is very common in somatization disorder as well, particularly with depressive disorders, and can further cloud or complicate the diagnosis.

Treatment

The **course of somatization disorder is often chronic, and the prognosis is guarded to poor;** patients with this disorder often "doctor-shop." The most important intervention is establishment of an ongoing treatment relationship with one physician, usually a primary care doctor. Regular, brief visits should be scheduled for the patient to discuss concerns. The physician should avoid excessive diagnostic testing and consider the patient's symptoms expressions of emotions. If affected patients are willing to engage in psychotherapy, they can gradually learn to live with their symptoms more adaptively and learn to be aware of, and express their emotions directly instead of developing physical symptoms.

Comprehension Questions

[38.1] In order to fulfill the criteria for somatization disorder, symptoms must be present in which of the following areas?

A. Gastrointestinal
B. Cardiac
C. Urinary
D. Musculoskeletal
E. Respiratory

[38.2] A 35-year-old woman with somatization disorder comes to see a new doctor. Prior to seeing this physician, she obtained complete evaluations from at least four clinics. The most important part of the treatment plan for this patient is which of the following?

A. A trial of analgesics
B. Intensive psychodynamic psychotherapy
C. Antidepressant medication
D. Establishing a schedule for regular visits

[38.3] For a diagnosis of somatization disorder, which of the following criteria must be met?

A. Symptoms began prior to age 30.
B. Symptoms last less than 6 months.
C. Patient is without significant impairment.
D. Symptoms are intentionally feigned or produced.

Answers

[38.1] **A.** Gastrointestinal symptoms(2) are required in the diagnosis of somatization disorder.

[38.2] **D.** Analgesics are generally not helpful in treating these patients, and they probably cannot be relied on to take psychotropic medications. Patients with somatization disorder have difficulty recognizing affects and so are not candidates for dynamic therapy, especially early in their treatment. The most important treatment intervention is establishing a relationship with one clinician and scheduling brief, regular visits.

[38.3] **A.** The symptoms must have occurred prior to age 30 and be present for several years.

CLINICAL PEARLS

- For somatization disorder the prognosis is generally poor. The clinician should set very modest goals, establishing an ongoing therapeutic relationship and the scheduling of regular appointments as the foundation of treatment.
- Even when a diagnosis of somatization disorder is established, the patient can still develop a medical illness over time. The clinician must keep an open mind and at the same time try to avoid unnecessary tests.

REFERENCES

Kirmayer LJ, Robbins JM, Dworkind M, Yaffe MJ. Somatization and the recognition of depression and anxiety in primary care. Am J Psychiatry 1993;150:734–739.

Phillips KA, ed. Somatoform and factitious disorders. Review of Psychiatry series vol 20, 2001;pp 95–99.

❖ CASE 39

A psychiatrist is called in to interview a 23-year-old woman 2 days after she delivered a healthy 7-lb boy by cesarean section. One day after the birth, she told the nurses that her baby was "the devil" and that to rid the world of evil she would have to kill him. The patient tells the psychiatrist the same story and claims that she hears the voice of God telling her that she must kill her baby.

On a mental status examination, the patient is alert and oriented to person, place, and time. Her hair is not combed and she has poor eye contact. She seems anxious and distracted. Her speech is within normal limits. She states that her mood is "upset" by the news that she must kill her child, and she notes she feels agitated, is not sleeping well, and wonders what she has done to be punished by God like this. Her affect is congruent with her mood and full-range. She denies suicidal ideation.

The patient's husband states that previously, she never had thoughts or ideas that were considered strange. He claims that the both of them were anxiously (and happily) awaiting the birth of the baby, who was planned for and wanted. The patient does not use drugs or alcohol and has no medical problems.

◆ **What is the most likely diagnosis?**

◆ **What are the next steps?**

ANSWERS TO CASE 39: Mood Disorder Not Otherwise Specified

Summary: A 23-year-old woman experiences auditory hallucinations in which God tells her to kill her baby, and the delusion that the baby is evil and must be killed in order to save the world coupled with a sudden-onset depression with extreme mood lability. These mood and psychotic symptoms appeared suddenly 24 hours after the delivery of the baby, and the patient did not have them before. Her husband reports that she was not depressed prior to the delivery either. The patient does not have a history of drug use/abuse or of medical problems.

- **Most likely diagnosis:** Mood Disorder Not Otherwise Specified. This patient can be developing a major depression, single episode, postpartum onset, severe with mood-congruent psychotic features.

- **Next steps:** The mother should be allowed to see her child, but only under close observation at all times. Under no circumstances should she be discharged home with the infant. The patient may require hospitalization in a psychiatric inpatient unit if the psychoses and depression do not remit immediately. She should be treated with an antipsychotic agent and an antidepressant.

Analysis

Objectives

1. Understand the diagnostic criteria for postpartum depression and the range of postpartum psychiatric disorders.
2. Recognize the danger in this situation for both parent and infant and take appropriate steps to keep both safe.
3. Know the recommended pharmacologic treatment for this disorder.

Considerations

This patient presents with sudden-onset psychotic symptoms (hallucinations and delusions) and depression after the birth of her child. She has no previous history of a psychiatric disorder. The symptoms lasted for more than 1 day and less than 1 month; because of the brief duration the patient cannot be diagnosed as having a major depression with psychotic features at this time. However, the possibility that she is having an incipient major depression with psychotic features needs to be at the forefront of your considerations.

APPROACH TO POSTPARTUM DEPRESSION

Definition

Delusion: A fixed, false belief that is held to be true by a patient. It is a symptom of psychosis.

Postpartum blues: Transient mood changes occurring shortly after delivery characterized by mood labiality, depressed or irritable mood, interpersonal hypersensitivity and tearfulness that usually resolves within 7 to 14 days after delivery.

Clinical Approach

Diagnostic Criteria

Postpartum blues are observed commonly and can be considered normative in the first few days after delivery with an incidence of 49% to 75%. Obstetricians should alert pregnant women to the possibility of developing postpartum blues to make sure that patients know it is not uncommon but should be reported so the physician can monitor for the development of more severe psychiatric disorders. Otherwise, the new mother can fear that something is wrong with her for not feeling joy at the birth of a new child and can conceal feelings of depression or thoughts of psychosis.

The criteria for diagnosing nonpsychotic postpartum depression are no different from those used for diagnosing major depression at other periods in a patient's life. Because the mother is often having her sleep disrupted by the infant, it can be difficult get a clear history of sleep disturbance. However, these women often cannot sleep or nap even when their baby is sleeping and not needing attention. The postpartum year is the time of greatest risk for first-onset depression in women, with up to 65% of all women experiencing their first episode of major depression in that time interval.

Postpartum psychosis occurs in 1–2 women per 1,000 deliveries. These episodes are often associated with confusion and extreme mood lability along with the psychosis.

Treatment

Use of the tricyclic antidepressants (TCAs) and selective serotonin reuptake inhibitors (SSRIs) are commonly used to treat the depressive component of this disorder and in those with psychotic symptoms should be treated with a neuroleptic. Because two-thirds of mothers breast-feed their infants, considerations of the transfer of medication into the breast milk and then the infant must be kept in mind. Although there is no evidence to suggest that exposure to antidepressants is harmful, similarly, there is no evidence to say that it is safe either. Because of their potential for anticholinergic effects and cardiotoxicity, TCAs are typically used as second-line drugs to SSRIs in this population. Doxepin has been reported to accumulate in breast milk at elevated levels. Of the SSRIs, sertraline and paroxetine are the least detectable in nursing infants.

A limited number of studies suggest that placing a patient with a history of postpartum depression on an antidepressant before delivery can help prevent recurrences.

Hormone therapy to prevent postpartum depression is currently being investigated but cannot be clinically recommended at this time.

Patients can also benefit from trained lay person support and group and individual psychotherapy.

Care must always be taken to assure that the mother does not present a danger to the infant especially in the case of postpartum psychosis.

Comprehension Questions

[39.1] A 28-year-old woman delivered her first child 2 months previously and is noted to have significant postpartum depression. She is reluctant to take antidepressant medications and asks about the use of hormonal therapy. Which of the following is the most accurate statement about hormonal therapy?

A. It is strictly investigational.
B. It can be used in small doses with success.
C. It must be used in large doses and is associated with side effects.
D. It must be used with deep venous thrombosis prophylaxis.

[39.2] Which of the following statements regarding postpartum mood disturbances is most accurate?

A. The second year after birth is a high-risk period for first-onset depression in women.
B. Postpartum mood disturbances are relatively rare, occurring in 1% of births.
C. The incidence of postpartum psychosis is more common than that of postpartum depression.
D. Criteria for postpartum-onset major depression are no different from at other times.
E. The mother's sleep patterns don't seem to play a role.

Answers

[39.1] **A.** Hormonal therapy is strictly in the investigational stages.

[39.2] **D.** The criteria for postpartum depression are the same for other individuals. The baby blues are quite common, occurring in up to 65% of delivering mothers.

CLINICAL PEARLS

- Baby blues are a common phenomenon.
- Treating a patient with antidepressants for several weeks to a month before delivery can prevent recurrence of postpartum depression in patients with a history of this disorder.

REFERENCES

Abreu AC, Stuart S. Pharmacologic and hormonal treatments for postpartum depression. Psychiatric Annals 2005;35(7):569–576.

Flynn HA. Epidemiology and phenomenology of postpartum mood disorders. Psychiatric Annals 2005;35(7):544-551.

Kopelman R, Stuart S. Psychological treatments for postpartum depression. Psychiatric Annals 2005;35(7):556–566.

❖ CASE 40

A 19-year-old man comes to a psychiatrist with a chief complaint of "I think I am going crazy." He states that for the past year, at irregular intervals, he had episodes of seeing flashes of color and halos around lights. In the past year, he experienced such events approximately 10 times. The last time was the day before his appointment with the psychiatrist, while he was commuting to his job but stuck in traffic. Each episode lasts only a few minutes, but the patient finds them extremely frightening. He states that he knows that "normal people" do not have such experiences. He claims he never had episodes like these before, except when he became intoxicated on "mushrooms" with his friends while he was in high school. He has not used such drugs since he was 18 years old. The patient has no medical problems, and the results of a recent complete physical examination by his primary care physician were normal.

◆ **What is the most likely diagnosis?**

 **What medical disorders should be considered in the differential diagnosis?**

ANSWERS TO CASE 40: Hallucinogen Persisting Perception Disorder

Summary: In the past year, a 19-year-old man experienced approximately 10 episodes of visual hallucinations, including flashes of color and halos around lights. Each episode lasts only a few minutes, and the patient has insight into the pathologic nature of the symptoms. The patient admits to the use of "mushrooms" with his friends while in high school, although he has not used these drugs since he was 18 years old. He has no medical problems, and the results of a recent physical examination were normal.

- **Most likely diagnosis:** Hallucinogen persisting perception disorder (see diagnostic criteria, Table 40–1).
- **Most common medical disorders in the differential diagnosis:** Migraines, seizures, and visual system abnormalities.

Analysis

Objectives

1. Recognize hallucinogen persisting perception disorder in a patient.
2. Understand the medical problems that must be ruled out in patients presenting with symptoms of this disorder.

Considerations

This patient, a previous user of hallucinogens, has been experiencing episodes of visual hallucinations lasting several minutes in duration, which appear frequently and were triggered at least once by sensory deprivation (monotonous driving). He knows that the symptoms are not normal and thus has insight into his perceptual disturbances. Episodes that linger only for a few seconds are

Table 40–1
DIAGNOSTIC CRITERIA FOR HALLUCINOGEN PERSISTING PERCEPTION DISORDER (FLASHBACKS)

- The reexperiencing of perceptual disturbances following cessation of the use of a hallucinogen.
- The symptoms cause significant distress or impairment in functioning.
- The symptoms are not caused by a general medical condition or another mental disorder.

typically called flashbacks. These longer episodes are more properly considered hallucinogen persisting perception disorder. Prolonged visual disturbances have been described up to 40 years after lysergic acid diethylamide (LSD) usage. Approximately half of the patients with this disorder have a complete remission of episodes within 5 years. This disorder can arise from a single dose of hallucinogen.

APPROACH TO HALLUCINOGEN PERSISTING PERCEPTION DISORDER

Definitions

Flashbacks: Visual symptoms that occur sporadically after hallucinogen use and last only for a second or two.

Macropsia: A scale misperception in which surroundings seem very large.

Micropsia: A scale misperception in which surroundings seem very small.

Clinical Approach

Differential Diagnosis

It is essential to rule out other mental disorders that cause hallucinations, such as schizophrenia or posttraumatic stress disorder (PTSD). Whereas in schizophrenia and other primary psychotic illnesses the hallucinations are more commonly auditory in nature, in hallucinogen persisting perception disorder, they are almost always visual. Examples include geometric shapes, perceptions of movement in the peripheral fields, color flashes, trails left by moving objects, and halos. Patients can report that the entire visual field is reticulated, grainy, or filled with vibrating dots to the point that they believe they can see air (aeropsia). Although patients can become extremely anxious about these experiences, the associated symptoms seen in psychotic disorders are not present, such as loose associations, delusions, disorganized behavior, and a flat affect. Another distinguishing feature is that patients with these episodes retain their insight, even in severe cases. Their reality testing remains intact. In PTSD, the perceptual disturbances revolve around a traumatic experience. Although hallucinogen abuse is not uncommon in patients with schizophrenia or PTSD, it is a *necessary* criterion for hallucinogen persisting perception disorder.

After hallucinogen use, episodes of hallucinogen persisting perception disorder can be triggered by use of amphetamines, cocaine, pseudoephedrine, methamphetamine, and exposure or even second-hand exposure to marijuana smoke.

If a patient presents with psychotic symptoms with impaired reality testing after ingesting a hallucinogen, then hallucinogen induced psychotic disorder should be considered.

In the differential diagnosis, it is also important to consider medical illnesses that can cause visual changes similar to those described. These include migraine headaches, seizures, and visual problems. A detailed history (especially prior hallucinogen use) and a physical examination usually illuminate the correct diagnosis. In individuals with hallucinogen persisting perception disorder, it is common to find consistent triggers for the flashbacks, such as emotional stress, sensory deprivation (such as driving a car as in the above case), or use of alcohol or marijuana.

Treatment

Although the symptoms of this disorder are usually transient, **treatment with a long-lasting benzodiazepine such as clonazepam or an anticonvulsant such as valproic acid or carbamazepine can be beneficial in reducing symptoms.** Antipsychotics should be avoided as they can actually worsen the psychotic symptoms within 72 hours of administration. As mentioned earlier, minimizing emotional stress and abstaining from alcohol and drugs are helpful in reducing the triggering of the flashbacks.

Comprehension Questions

[40.1] Which of the following characteristics most distinguishes hallucinogen persisting perception disorder from schizophrenia?

A. Impairment in functioning
B. Presence of hallucinations
C. Retention of insight
D. Significant distress

[40.2] Which of the following modalities is most often affected in hallucinogen persisting perception disorder?

A. Auditory
B. Olfactory
C. Tactile
D. Visual

[40.3] Which of the following situations is most likely to trigger a flashback?

A. Alcohol use
B. A brightly lit room
C. Loud music
D. A relaxed state

[40.4] A 21-year-old woman presents to the emergency department with a complaint of "seeing trails" around objects. In relating further history, she reluctantly admits to recent use of LSD but has not used it for several weeks. She denies having any medical problems, and the results of her physical and laboratory examinations (including urine toxicology screenings) are normal. She appears quite upset and finds her symptoms extremely bothersome. What is the least appropriate pharmacologic treatment?

A. Clonazepam
B. Valproic acid
C. Risperidone
D. Carbamazepine

Answers

[40.1] **C.** Both hallucinogen persisting perception disorder and schizophrenia can be manifested by hallucinations, although with flashbacks, they tend to be visual, and with schizophrenia, they tend to be auditory. In both disorders, there is an associated impairment in functioning as well as significant distress. Patients with hallucinogen persisting perception disorder retain their insight, whereas patients with schizophrenia (and other primary psychotic disorders) have impaired reality testing.

[40.2] **D.** Flashbacks are visual phenomena, whereas hallucinations in schizophrenia and other primary psychotic illnesses are more commonly auditory. Olfactory hallucinations are common in temporal lobe epilepsy, whereas tactile hallucinations are consistent with drug-induced states such as in formication (the feeling of insects crawling on the skin seen in cocaine withdrawal).

[40.3] **A.** Alcohol and marijuana use commonly triggers flashbacks. Other triggers include emotional stress and sensory deprivation (such as sitting in a quiet, darkened room).

[40.4] **C.** Antianxiety medications can be helpful in treating the distress associated with the flashbacks. Antidepressants are appropriate if there is a comorbid depressive illness. Antipsychotics are not indicated in the treatment of flashbacks, as they can paradoxically worsen the symptoms. Mood stabilizers many be beneficial.

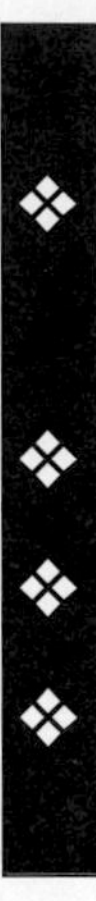

CLINICAL PEARLS

❖ In hallucinogen persisting perception disorder, the flashbacks are usually visual and include geometric objects, perceptions of movement, flashes of color, trails of moving objects, halos, and micropsia/macropsia.

❖ Medical disorders causing visual changes, such as migraines, epilepsy, and visual pathway disturbances should be ruled out.

❖ Triggers for flashbacks include emotional stress, sensory deprivation, and the use of alcohol and marijuana.

❖ Treatment with benzodiazepines can be useful in reducing anxiety, but antipsychotics can worsen the symptoms.

REFERENCES

Abraham HD. Hallucinogen-related disorders. In: Sadock BJ, Sadock VA, eds. Kaplan and Sadock's comprehensive textbook of psychiatry, 7th ed. Philadelphia: Lippincott Williams & Wilkins, 2000:1015–1025.

❖ CASE 41

A 45-year-old man was admitted to a cardiac intensive care unit after suffering a heart attack. Twenty-four hours after admission, the consultation psychiatrist is called in to make an evaluation because the patient is trying to sign himself out against medical advice. When the psychiatrist enters the patient's hospital room, she finds him getting dressed and yelling at the top of his lungs, "I won't be treated in this manner! How dare you!" The patient does agree to sit down and speak with the psychiatrist, however. He tells the psychiatrist that staff members are simply rude and do not treat him "in the manner to which he is accustomed." He says that he is a small business owner, but that he is on the way up and "as soon as people realize my full potential, I will be a millionaire." He cannot understand why the staff will not bring food up from an outside cafeteria for him because the food in the hospital is so bad. He asks the psychiatrist whether, after the interview, she will get some food for him, and he becomes angry when she declines. He then eyes her new, expensive watch enviously. On a mental status examination, the psychiatrist finds no disorders of thought process or content, and the patient is found to be oriented to person, place, and time.

◆ **What is the most likely diagnosis?**

◆ **What would be the most successful approach in dealing with this patient?**

ANSWERS TO CASE 41: Narcissistic Personality Disorder

Summary: A 45-year-old man is admitted to the hospital after a heart attack. Twenty-four hours later, he tries to leave the hospital against medical advice because he is angry about the way the staff has treated him. He has a grandiose sense of self-importance and feels entitled. He is interpersonally exploitative with the psychiatrist who interviews him and is obviously envious of a watch that he thinks is expensive. He shows no other abnormalities on a mental status examination.

- **Most likely diagnosis:** Narcissistic personality disorder.
- **Most successful approach:** If the psychiatrist and/or the treatment team can show validation for the patient's experience, feelings, and concerns, he will most likely calm down and agree to stay in the hospital for treatment.

Analysis

Objectives

1. Know the diagnostic criteria for narcissistic personality disorder.
2. Know some strategies to employ when working with patients with this disorder.

Considerations

This patient has suffered a "narcissistic injury" at the hands of the staff in that they refuse to cater to his need for admiration and special treatment. This injury has been inflicted on top of the injury of realizing that his body is not immortal. The patient has responded by becoming arrogant, hostile, and demanding, and has tried to sign himself out against medical advice. He continues to demand attention when speaking with the psychiatrist by telling her how important he is and how he feels entitled to special treatment. He even tries to manipulate her and is angry when she does not comply. He is envious of her success as evidenced by her watch. Patients like these respond best to a show of honest admiration from another individual—it can be difficult to react in this manner because these patients often engender strong negative countertransference feelings.

APPROACH TO NARCISSISTIC PERSONALITY DISORDER

Definitions

Denial: A defense mechanism in which an individual deals with emotional conflict or stress by refusing to acknowledge some painful aspect of external reality or subjective experience that is apparent to others. For example, a patient hospitalized after a severe heart attack tells a physician he feels "as fit as a fiddle" and jumps out of bed and starts performing jumping jacks. When there is gross impairment in reality testing, the denial can be termed psychotic.

Devaluation: A defense mechanism in which an individual deals with emotional conflict or stress by attributing exaggerated negative qualities to themselves or to others. This behavior can alternate with idealization. For example, a patient states that her therapist is "the worst doctor in the world."

Grandiosity: An exaggerated concept of one's importance, power, or fame.

Idealization: A defense mechanism in which an individual deals with emotional conflict or stress by attributing exaggerated positive qualities to themselves or to others. This behavior can alternate with devaluation. For example, a patient states that her therapist is "the most empathic person on the planet."

Clinical Approach

Diagnostic Criteria

Patients with this disorder exhibit a pervasive pattern **of grandiosity, a need for admiration, and a lack of empathy for others.** They often exaggerate their accomplishments and are jealous of the achievements or possessions of others. They believe they are special or are deserving of special treatment. They have **fantasies about obtaining unlimited power and success.** They take advantage of others and can appear haughty or arrogant. They handle criticism poorly and can become enraged quickly.

Differential Diagnosis

Patients with narcissistic personality disorder can often be difficult to differentiate from those with other cluster B disorders. Individuals with borderline personality disorder generally live more chaotic lives, have multiple failed relationships, and make suicidal gestures. Patients with antisocial personality disorder are often in trouble with the legal system because they have committed one or more impulsive, irresponsible, and often violent acts. Patients with histrionic personality disorder can appear to be dramatic but do not claim to be entitled to special behavior and do not appear as arrogant or haughty.

Interviewing Tips and Treatment

Patients with this disorder try to appear perfect and invincible in order to protect their fragile self-esteem. When this is lost, they are especially prone to develop depression. They often denigrate their physicians in a defensive effort to maintain a sense of mastery. The clinician should be tactful and admiring if at all possible. **Treatment of these individuals is difficult because they rarely desire to change and seldom seek help.** Group therapy is helpful only if the therapist can make the inevitable confrontation by group members somehow palatable to the patient. Psychotherapy with these individuals is challenging, and the patient often terminates treatment when confrontation is attempted. Psychopharmacology can be employed to treat symptoms associated with narcissistic personality disorder (e.g., lithium for the affective lability, selective serotonin reuptake inhibitors [SSRIs] for depressive symptoms).

Comprehension Questions

[41.1] A 22-year-old, single graduate student with narcissistic personality disorder is admitted to a hospital after a car accident in which his right femur is fractured. A medical student has been assigned to follow the patient, but when she enters the room and introduces herself as a medical student, the patient states, "Oh, I wouldn't let a medical student touch me—I need someone with much more experience than you." Which of the following statements by the medical student is most likely to lead to a successful interview with this patient?

A. I know this will be boring for you, but it's just one of the things that you will have to put up with in the hospital.
B. I know you must be scared to be in the hospital, but you will be safe here.
C. I'm told that you are a very articulate person, and so I'm hoping you'll teach me what I need to know.
D. I understand that you think you deserve only the best, but *I* have been assigned to you.
E. Please don't make this difficult, I have to interview you as part of my job.

[41.2] To which cluster of personality disorders does the patient in question [41.1] belong?

A. Cluster A
B. Cluster B
C. Cluster C
D. Cluster D

[41.3] The patient in questions [41.1] and [41.2] would be most likely to become depressed after which of the following life occurrences?

A. Aging
B. Graduation
C. Job promotion
D. Marriage

[41.4] A 36-year-old man with narcissistic personality disorder sees his therapist two times a week and has done so for the past 2 years. The therapist and the patient have a good working alliance. During one therapy session, the therapist comes to the session 4 minutes late. He apologizes to the patient, stating that he had an emergency involving another patient. During the session, the patient notes that the therapist "isn't as sharp as some of the therapists I hear on the talk shows." Which of the following defense mechanisms is the patient using?

A. Denial
B. Devaluation
C. Isolation of affect
D. Rationalization
E. Splitting

Answers

[41.1] **C.** Appealing to the patient's narcissism by being admiring most often deescalates the patient as well as improves the therapeutic alliance in these cases.

[41.2] **B.** Cluster B is the "bad" cluster (see Case 6) and includes narcissistic, antisocial, borderline, and histrionic personality disorders. Cluster A includes paranoid, schizoid, and schizotypal personality disorders. Cluster C includes avoidant, dependent, and obsessive-compulsive personality disorders.

[41.3] **A.** Patients with narcissistic personality disorder do not handle aging well because beauty, strength, and youth are often highly valued. Any blow to their fragile (but covert) self-esteem can raise their feelings of envy, anger, and subsequently lead to depression.

[41.4] **B.** The patient defends against his feelings of hurt and anger toward the therapist by using devaluation. Devaluation, along with idealization and denial are considered primitive (lower-functioning) defense mechanisms used by patients with personality disorders such as narcissistic and borderline.

CLINICAL PEARLS

- ❖ Patients with narcissistic personality disorder show a pervasive sense of grandiosity and entitlement in their thoughts and behavior. They are very seldom capable of true empathy with others and often manipulate them for personal gain.
- ❖ Clinicians should try to maintain an admiring stance with these patients. Tact is important as well, as these individuals handle criticism poorly.
- ❖ Defense mechanisms in patients with narcissistic personality disorder include denial, devaluation, and idealization.

REFERENCES

Ebert M, Loosen P, Nurcombe B, eds. Current diagnosis and treatment in psychiatry. New York: McGraw-Hill, 2000:479–480.

Kaplan H, Sadock B. Synopsis of psychiatry, 9th ed. Baltimore: Lippincott Williams & Wilkins, 2003:811–812.

❖ CASE 42

A 7-year-old boy in second grade is brought to a pediatrician by his parents for an evaluation of his eyes. They state that he blinks them repeatedly, and that this behavior seems to be worsening. They first noticed it a year or more ago, but it became very obvious in the past several weeks. They note that their son cannot control the blinking, and that it appears worse at some times of the day compared to others. The boy's teacher reports that other children tease him because of his rapid eye blinking. The pediatrician observes that in addition to blinking, the child seems to clear his throat frequently, although his nose and throat appear normal on physical examination. The parents report that this behavior occurs several times daily as well. The patient is doing well at school, although he sometimes has trouble completing his homework. The patient's father has a history of attention-deficit/hyperactivity disorder (ADHD).

◆ **What is the most likely diagnosis?**

◆ **What is the best therapy for this condition?**

ANSWERS TO CASE 42: Tourette Disorder

Summary: A 7-year-old boy presents to a pediatrician with a year-long history of uncontrollable blinking, which has worsened over the past several weeks. The blinking is worse at some times than at others, and the boy is teased at school because of it. The child also clears his throat repeatedly, although nothing physically wrong can be found. He is doing well at school although he sometimes has trouble completing his homework. The patient has a paternal history of ADHD.

- **Most likely diagnosis:** Tourette disorder.
- **Best treatment:** The first line of somatic treatment involves the use of a dopamine-2 receptor antagonist such as haloperidol or pimozide. If side effects prohibit their use, clonidine, a selective alpha-2-adrenergic receptor agonist can also be of use.

Analysis

Objectives

1. Recognize Tourette disorder in a patient (see Table 42–1 for diagnostic criteria).
2. Describe the basic evaluation and treatment of this disorder.

Considerations

A 7-year-old boy shows signs of a motor tic in the form of eye blinking. This behavior has been present to some degree for more than a year and has recently worsened. The tics affect how other children at school interact with him. He also exhibits a vocal tic in the form of throat clearing, which has been present for a long period of time. This combination of multiple motor and vocal tics occurring for **at least 1 year** is consistent with Tourette disorder.

Table 42–1
DIAGNOSTIC CRITERIA FOR TOURETTE DISORDER

1. Presence of both motor and vocal tics during the course of the illness but not necessarily at the same time.
2. Tics occurring almost every day for a period of at **least a year,** and during this year there is never a tic-free period lasting more than three consecutive months.
3. The disturbance must cause marked distress or impairment in functioning.
4. Onset must be before 18 years of age.
5. The disorder must not be due to a substance or a general medical condition.

There is a genetic predisposition to this disease, probably via autosomal dominant inheritance. There are also relationships among Tourette disorder, obsessive-compulsive disorder (OCD), and attention-deficit disorder. Haloperidol is the most commonly prescribed agent for treating this problem. It is important to note that symptoms such as these in a child could also be related to an environmental allergen, and this should be thoroughly worked up before diagnosing Tourette disorder and beginning treatment.

APPROACH TO TOURETTE DISORDER

Definitions

Athetoid movements: Slow, irregular, writhing movements.

Choreiform movements: Dancing, random, irregular, nonrepetitive movements.

Coprolalia: Vocal tic involving the involuntary vocalization of obscenities.

Dystonic movements: Slower than choreiform movements, these are twisting motions interspersed with prolonged states of muscular tension.

Hemiballistic movements: Intermittent, coarse, large-amplitude, unilateral movements of the limbs.

Myoclonic movements: Brief, shocklike muscle contractions.

Tic: A sudden, rapid, recurrent, nonrhythmic, stereotyped motor movement or vocalization.

Clinical Approach

The lifetime prevalence of Tourette disorder is approximately 4 to 5 per 10,000 in the general population, and it tends to be more common in boys. The motor component (eye blinking, shoulder shrugging, neck jerking) usually emerges by 7 years of age, and the vocal component (grunting, sniffing, snorting, using obscene words) by 11 years of age. Epidemiologic studies involving twins indicate a strong genetic etiology, probably via autosomal dominant inheritance. There is a strong relationship between Tourette disorder, OCD, and ADHD. The dopamine system can be involved in the tic disorders; thus, dopamine antagonists such as haloperidol suppress the tics.

Differential Diagnosis

Tic disorders must be differentiated from general medical conditions that can cause abnormal movements. Involuntary movements such as myoclonus, athetosis, dystonias, and hemiballismus can be seen in such diseases as Sydenham chorea, Huntington chorea, Wilson disease, and stroke. The long-term use of a typical antipsychotic such as haloperidol can cause tardive dyskinesia, another involuntary movement disorder. The presence of a family history of these disorders, findings on a physical examination, or a history of long-term use of antipsychotic medication can help rule out these conditions.

Tics must be differentiated from compulsions seen in OCD. Compulsions are typically fairly complex behaviors performed to ward off the anxiety of an obsession or according to a rigid set of behavioral rules. Certain vocal and motor tics such as barking, coprolalia, or echolalia must be distinguished from the psychotic behavior seen in schizophrenia. However, in the latter case patients have other findings congruent with psychosis, such as hallucinations or delusions. Transient tic disorders last at least 4 weeks but for no longer than 1 year. Patients with a chronic motor or vocal tic disorder can have it for more than 1 year, but there is an absence of multiple motor tics and/or motor and vocal tics occurring simultaneously.

Treatment

The treatment of Tourette disorder involves **both somatic therapies and psychotherapies.** In children, tics are often worsened or triggered by anxiety-producing events. Children and families can be taught to reduce the manifested anxiety at home, which in turn can help to reduce the triggers for tics. A child can be taught **relaxation techniques** that can help in the reduction of this anxiety.

In addition to anxiety reduction and trigger reduction, there are medications that are helpful in controlling tics associated with Tourette disorder. First-line medications currently used include **clonidine and guanfacine.** Approximately two thirds of children with tics respond to reasonable doses of these agents. In addition to these two classes of medications, some antipsychotic medications can be effective in the treatment of tic disorders. The most commonly used medication in this category is **haloperidol.** Most patients have a favorable response to antipsychotics, but their long-term side effect profiles are causes for concern. Other methods of symptom reduction should be tried prior to using this potentially risky agent.

Comprehension Questions

[42.1] Which of the following disorders has a higher likelihood of developing in a patient with Tourette disorder?

A. Obsessive-compulsive disorder
B. Sleep terror disorder
C. Primary insomnia
D. Developmental disability
E. Sydenham chorea

[42.2] Which of the following pathologies would be most important to rule out before starting treatment of Tourette disorder in a child presenting as described earlier?

A. Streptococcus infection
B. Environmental allergies
C. Autism
D. Marijuana abuse
E. Rett disorder

[42.3] Which of the following medications sometimes used to treat Tourette disorder has the least likelihood of causing tardive dyskinesia?

A. Pimozide
B. Clonidine
C. Risperdal (risperidone)
D. Haloperidol
E. Clozaril (clozapine)

[42.4] A patient with ADHD is treated with methylphenidate during the school year. After several months of treatment, his teachers and parents note that he has developed both motor and vocal tics. What should be the first line of treatment for these symptoms?

A. Begin treatment with haloperidol
B. Discontinue the use of methylphenidate
C. Refer the child for family therapy
D. Reduce the dose of methylphenidate
E. Administer an anticonvulsant

Answers

[42.1] **A.** Obsessive-compulsive disorder has been associated with Tourette disorder, along with ADHD and other learning disorders.

[42.2] **B.** Environmental allergies can have a presentation most resembling this presentation of Tourette disorder. Although the other pathologies mentioned are important, they are not usually considered as part of the differential diagnoses for Tourette disorder so probably warrant less consideration in the active work up of this particular patient.

[42.3] **B.** Clonidine is an alpha-2 agonist that does not cause tardive dyskinesia as a side effect. It is moderately effective in the treatment of vocal and motor tics, although not as effective as some antipsychotics.

[42.3] **D.** The development of tics as a side effect of stimulant medication is relatively common. These tics diminish in severity or cease when the dose is reduced, or the medication is discontinued. Because stimulants are quite effective in treating ADHD, a reduction in the dose of the stimulant or management of its side effects should be tried before the medication is discontinued.

CLINICAL PEARLS

- A diagnosis of Tourette disorder requires both vocal and motor tics and a duration of 1 year.
- Vocal tics can consist not only of words but also throat clearing, grunting, and squeaking.
- Motor tics can involve complicated movements such as brushing hair or repetitive and intricate hand or arm movements.

REFERENCE

Kaplan H, Sadock B. Synopsis of psychiatry, 9th ed. Baltimore: Lippincott Williams & Wilkins, 2003:1421–1422.

CASE 43

A 12-year-old boy attends a summer camp for children with attention-deficit/hyperactivity disorder (ADHD) every summer. He always looks forward to this 3-week experience in the summer, and this year is no different. His parents drop him off at camp without incident as usual, and he moves into his cabin and renews his friendships from years past very quickly. Over the next several days, he comes to the camp infirmary several times daily complaining of feeling scared, short of breath, worried, and tearful. He sometimes feels so scared and short of breath, he thinks he is going to die. He has not experienced these feelings in the past with any regularity. His daily routine has changed considerably over the past several days given the camp environment, living in a cabin with several other boys, and the increased amount of exercise, including team sports, swimming, horseback riding, and campfires.

- **What is the most likely diagnosis?**
- **What is the best diagnostic test?**
- **What is the best treatment for this disorder?**

ANSWERS TO CASE 43: Anxiety Disorder Caused by Asthma

Summary: A 12-year-old boy comes to the camp infirmary with a primary complaint of anxiety symptoms, including worry, feeling frightened, short of breath, tearful, and worried that he is going to die. These symptoms seem to be related to beginning camp and are interfering with his ability to participate fully in the camp's activities. On physical examination by the camp physician, she hears wheezing when auscultating his lungs. She then checks his tidal volume and finds it significantly reduced. She chooses to give him an asthma inhaler and checks his tidal volume several minutes later when he feels much better, and it is normal.

- **Most likely diagnosis:** Anxiety disorder secondary to a general medical condition (asthma).
- **Diagnostic tests:** Complete blood count (CBC) with differential, physical examination, peak flow respiratory testing.
- **Best treatment:** His anxiety symptoms are related to his newly induced asthma. Treating the asthma is the best way to reduce the anxiety symptoms.

Analysis

Objectives

1. Recognize anxiety disorder secondary to a general medical condition (see Table 43–1 for diagnostic criteria).
2. Use laboratory tests appropriately to finalize the diagnosis of this disorder in a patient.
3. Understand the treatment of patients with this disorder.

Table 43–1

DIAGNOSTIC CRITERIA FOR ANXIETY DISORDER SECONDARY TO A MEDICAL CONDITION

1. Anxiety, panic attacks, or obsessions or compulsions are the primary symptoms in the clinical picture.
2. The patient's history, a physical examination, or laboratory findings strongly suggest that the symptoms are a direct physiologic consequence of a general medical condition.
3. The symptoms are not better explained by another mental disorder.
4. The symptoms do not occur only during the course of a delirium.
5. The symptoms cause clinically significant distress and/or impairment in functioning.

Considerations

This patient has obvious problems with anxiety but cannot pinpoint any psychological trigger. He attended the camp many times in the past and was looking forward to it this year. The patient began to feel a number of psychological symptoms that are often felt with the shortness of breath experienced with asthma. The anxiety has been present since starting camp, which also could be the trigger for the asthma. Environmental allergens associated with being outdoors in the summer and exercise can be related to asthma exacerbation. A physical examination can reveal wheezing in the lung fields, and the peak flow expiratory levels are likely to be below normal. All these symptoms occurred over the past few weeks, and the patient did not previously consider himself anxious or a worrier, suggesting something other than generalized anxiety disorder (GAD).

APPROACH TO ANXIETY DISORDER SECONDARY TO A MEDICAL CONDITION

Definition

Sjögren syndrome: A chronic disease in which white blood cells attack the moisture-producing glands. The hallmark symptoms are dry eyes and a dry mouth, but it is a systemic disease, affecting many organs and causing fatigue. It is one of the most prevalent autoimmune disorders, striking as many as 4 million Americans annually.

Clinical Approach

Many medical conditions can manifest symptoms that resemble a variety of anxiety disorders, including panic attacks, GAD, and obsessions and compulsions.

Differential Diagnosis

Multiple medical illnesses can cause syndromes in which anxiety is prominent; these include a host of neurologic disorders, systemic conditions, endocrine diseases, immune system disorders, deficiency states, and toxic conditions. **The criteria for GAD are met in up to 60% of patients with Graves disease.** Sjögren syndrome can produce prominent anxiety symptoms. In hypothyroidism, hypoparathyroidism, hypoglycemia, and B_{12} deficiency, anxiety can be the initial or predominant symptom. A pheochromocytoma can cause episodes of anxiety that mimic panic attacks. Patients with cardiomyopathy awaiting a cardiac transplant have a high incidence of panic disorder, probably as a result of increased noradrenergic tone. Parkinson disease and chronic obstructive pulmonary disease (COPD) can also lead to panic attacks. Obsessive-compulsive symptoms have been reported in individuals with Sydenham chorea and multiple sclerosis. The clinician must keep in mind that the patient can have a coexisting but independent medical illness and anxiety disorder; in this case, the patient's previous psychiatric history, course of illness, and current symptoms can be helpful diagnostically.

Other possible diagnoses include axis I disorders such as major depression, schizophrenia, and bipolar disorder, mania, all of which can cause anxiety, and the presence of other symptoms (e.g., depressed mood, hallucinations, excessive spending) can help in differentiating among them.

Treatment

Treatment of an anxiety disorder secondary to a general medical condition includes addressing the causative medical illness. Some anxiety symptoms can linger long after treatment of the condition has been otherwise successful, especially in the case of obsessions and compulsions; in such cases, the symptoms can be treated as if they were primary psychiatric syndromes. As in the case of primary anxiety disorders, selective serotonin reuptake inhibitors (SSRIs), benzodiazepines, and buspirone can all be helpful, depending on the nature of the anxiety. For example, an individual with mainly obsessions and compulsions tends to respond to SSRIs, whereas a person with primarily generalized anxiety symptoms responds to buspirone.

Comprehension Questions

[43.1] A 62-year-old man with a history of diabetes mellitus, chronic COPD, hepatitis C, peripheral neuropathy, and a pacemaker for control of cardiac arrhythmia complains of new-onset episodic anxiety occurring over the past 3 weeks. He has no history of anxiety symptoms. Episodes of intense anxiety tend to occur in the daytime, last for 30 minutes to an hour, and are accompanied by hyperventilation and a sense of "palpitations," as well as some confusion and disorientation. Of the following, which is least likely to be the diagnosis in this case?

A. Panic disorder
B. Episodic hypoglycemia
C. Hypoxia caused by COPD
D. Hypoxia caused by arrhythmia

[43.2] A 45-year-old man with schizophrenia, type II diabetes, and alcohol and cocaine dependence comes to the emergency department 2 hours after drinking half of a fifth of whiskey and smoking cocaine, after which he fell and hit his head. He describes losing consciousness for several minutes. He states that he feels extremely anxious, saying, "I can't calm down." In the emergency department, he is noted to be hyperventilating. Which of the following tests should be performed immediately?

A. Blood glucose level determination
B. Thyrotropin (TSH) level determination
C. Abdominal ultrasound examination
D. Test for human immunodeficiency virus disease

[43.3] Generalized anxiety disorder secondary to a medical condition is diagnosed in a 23-year-old woman after she began having obsessions and compulsions after falling from a horse. Although her head trauma was treated, and she apparently suffered no sequelae, her obsessions and compulsions have continued. If medication is given, which of the following medication side effects will most likely develop?

A. Orthostatic hypotension
B. An increase in the QT interval
C. Anorgasmia
D. Tardive dyskinesia

[43.4] A patient experiencing tachycardia, derealization, paresthesias, and shortness of breath most likely would be diagnosed with?

A. Myocardial infarction
B. Asthma
C. Hyperthyroidism
D. Agoraphobia
E. Panic attacks

Answers

[43.1] **A.** This man has multiple medical problems that can cause anxiety symptoms and no history of anxiety. He can be inadvertently overdosing on insulin or hypoglycemic medications, or his pacemaker is not functioning properly. Although a primary diagnosis of an anxiety disorder is possible, it is the least likely in this case.

[43.2] **A.** This patient is hypoglycemic, or his anxiety is caused by alcohol withdrawal or cocaine intoxication. Because he has history of a head injury, a computed tomography scan of the head should be performed to rule out a hemorrhage. The other laboratory or imaging tests are unnecessary in the short term.

[43.3] **C.** Selective serotonin uptake inhibitors are the treatment of choice for obsessions and compulsions, and the most common side effect of these agents is sexual dysfunction, primarily anorgasmia in women and delayed ejaculation in men.

[43.4] **E.** Tachycardia, derealization, paresthesias, and shortness of breath are the classic presentation for panic attacks. Panic attacks are also associated with agoraphobia but are distinct from that disorder.

CLINICAL PEARLS

- Many medical illnesses produce prominent anxiety symptoms, and a carefully recorded history, a review of symptoms, and a physical examination usually point to the underlying medical problem.
- The presence of a psychiatric history should not preclude careful evaluation for a medical cause of symptoms.

REFERENCES

Cassem EH. Depression and anxiety secondary to medical illness. Psychiatr Clin North Am 1990;13:597–560.

Gorman JM. Anxiety disorders. In: Sadock BK, Sadock VA, eds. Kaplan and Sadock's comprehensive textbook of psychiatry, 7th ed., vol. 1. Philadelphia: Lippincott Williams & Wilkins, 2000:1441–1445.

❖ CASE 44

A 17-year-old girl is brought to see a psychiatrist because her parents have become increasingly alarmed about her weight loss. The patient claims that her parents are "worrying about nothing" and that she has come to the office just to appease them. She states that she feels fine, although her mood is slightly depressed. She denies having problems with sleeping or appetite and with any kind of drug or alcohol abuse. She says that she thinks she looks "fat," but that if she could lose another couple of pounds, she would be "just right." She notes that her only problem is that she stopped having her period 3 months ago; she is not sexually active and therefore cannot be pregnant.

When questioned separately, the parents report that the patient has been steadily losing weight over the past 8 months. They say that she started dieting after one of her friends commented that she "looked a little plump." At that point, they noted that their daughter weighed approximately 120 lb. The patient lost 5 lb and, according to the parents, felt good about the comments made by her friends. Since that time, she has eaten less and less. She now dresses in baggy clothes and does not discuss with her parents how much she weighs. Despite this, she helps her mother cook elaborate meals for party guests when the family entertains. She exercises throughout the day, and her parents say they can often hear her doing jumping jacks and sit-ups in her room in the evening. On a physical examination, the patient is found to be 5 ft 2 in tall; she weighs 70 lb and appears cachetic.

◆ **What is the most likely diagnosis?**

◆ **What are the next therapeutic steps?**

ANSWERS TO CASE 44: Anorexia Nervosa

Summary: A 17-year-old girl appears in a psychiatrist's office grossly underweight. Despite this, she denies having any problems other than being mildly depressed, and she has not come to the office willingly. She views herself as overweight despite obvious appearances to the contrary. Her parents note that she has increasingly restricted her intake of calories and exercises excessively. She has been amenorrheic for the past several months.

- **Most likely diagnosis:** Anorexia nervosa.
- **Next steps:** The patient would benefit from **hospitalization,** but it is unlikely that she will agree. However, because she is 17 years old, her parents can sign her into a hospital without her consent. Her initial treatment should be aimed at restoring her nutritional status, as she is grossly malnourished. Dehydration, starvation, and electrolyte imbalances must be corrected. The patient should be weighed daily, and her daily fluid intake and output should be monitored. Therapy (behavioral management, individual psychotherapy, family education, and therapy) should also be started, but her unstable nutritional status needs to be addressed first.

Analysis

Objectives

1. Recognize anorexia nervosa in a patient.
2. Make recommendations about the hospitalization and initial treatment of a patient with anorexia nervosa.

Considerations

This patient meets all four criteria for anorexia nervosa: First, she has a refusal to maintain her body weight above a minimally normal level for her age. This young woman is in need of immediate hospitalization, as her weight (70 lb) is 64% of the normally expected weight for her height (110 lb). Second, she has disturbance in the way her shape and body weight is perceived and a denial of the seriousness of her current low body weight. Her dieting began after she heard a derogatory comment about her weight, and it has accelerated over the past 8 months. The patient, **despite being quite cachectic, believes herself to be fat** and wants to lose still more weight. Third, her intense fear of gaining weight is consistent with anorexia nervosa. Finally, the **weight loss has caused amenorrhea.** She is not interested in psychiatric treatment and denies that there is anything wrong with her other than a mild depressed mood; this is commonly seen in patients with anorexia. Despite severely restricting her caloric intake, she seems very much interested in food and its preparation. She

exercises excessively as well. Individuals with this disorder are often difficult to treat; they **deny** their behavior and try to mislead their parents or physicians. **She has the restricting type of the disorder. Anorexia nervosa can also present with a pattern in which the patient binge eats and then uses vomiting, laxatives, diuretics, and enemas to lose weight.**

Although not part of the official *Diagnostic and Statistical Manual of Mental Disorders, 4th edition (DSM-IV)* criteria, these patients tend to be perfectionistic high achievers, who are socially withdrawn and have a poor self-concept. The anorexia is often an attempt to gain a sense of control over their lives as they are going through the physical and emotional changes of adolescence.

APPROACH TO ANOREXIA NERVOSA

Definitions

Amenorrhea: Absence of at least three consecutive menstrual cycles.

Anorectic abnormal body weight: Body weight that is less than 85% of normal for the age and produced by conscious weight loss efforts.

Lanugo: Fine body hair present on prepubertal children and commonly seen in patients with anorexia.

Clinical Approach

There is a strong female predominance of individuals with eating disorders. Anorexia nervosa is observed as either a food-restricting or a binge-eating/purging subtype. **A strong distortion of body image is present, and even at an extremely low weight, the patient thinks she is overweight.** Table 44–1 lists the diagnostic criteria. Anorexia nervosa is rare in non-Western societies, and immigrants who move from these societies to the Western cultures (and adopt Western concepts of female thinness as being desirable) have much higher incidences of anorexia.

Table 44–1

DIAGNOSTIC CRITERIA FOR ANOREXIA NERVOSA

1. Refusal to maintain weight at or above the normal weight for one's age and height (85% of expected weight caused either by weight loss or by lack of expected weight gain).
2. Intense fear of gaining weight or becoming fat despite being underweight.
3. Disturbance in the way one's body weight or shape is experienced, undue influence of body weight or shape on self-evaluation, or denial of the severity of the current low body weight.
4. In females who are beyond menarche, amenorrhea may be present.

Differential Diagnosis

Weight loss caused by a general medical condition should be listed first on the differential diagnosis. Many medical conditions cause weight loss and must be ruled out prior to the initiation of treatment for anorexia nervosa. Major depressive disorder can be associated with weight loss caused by a decreased appetite; however, patients with this disorder are not concerned about their body image and readily admit that they have not put any effort into achieving the weight loss. If the decreased food intake is caused by odd or paranoid thoughts, then schizophrenia and obsessive-compulsive disorder must be considered. Patients with body dysmorphic disorder typically fixate on one particular part of their body that they consider imperfect rather than having the more global desire for thinness expressed by patients with anorexia.

Patients with bulimia nervosa have sudden urges to overeat and during one of these binges have a sense of lack of control over the ability to stop, resulting in their consuming large quantities of food followed by purging via laxatives, self-induced vomiting, diuretics, enemas, fasting, or exercise. These behaviors occur at least twice a week for 3 months. The self-concept of these patients is unduly influenced by their body shape, but not to the extent of individuals with anorexia nervosa.

Diagnosing anorexia nervosa can sometimes be quite difficult. **Adolescents can be experienced at hiding the symptoms.** In addition, the onset of the illness is gradual, and severe changes are not noticed. Patients should be weighed regularly in a physician's office, and any significant weight loss should be evaluated with anorexia nervosa in the differential diagnosis. Additionally, the differential diagnosis **for amenorrhea** in a previously menstruating girl should include anorexia. **Abnormalities in blood chemistry studies and electrocardiogram (ECG) changes** can be detected and considered evidence of anorexia when they are discovered. Common lab abnormalities include hypokalemia, hypochloremic metabolic acidosis, low albumin levels (common in starvation), elevated liver enzymes, or leukopenia and a relative lymphocytosis. **This is a disease that by its nature tends to be hidden.** Clues should not be ignored by clinicians and, when found, should be addressed in a respectful but assertive manner.

Treatment

The treatment of anorexia nervosa can be quite complicated and difficult. It is best accomplished in a series of steps. First, it is critical to engage in nutritional rehabilitation. This is often best done in a special inpatient psychiatric unit for eating disorders. This is because the patients are often able to subvert initial outpatient attempts to structure their eating to encourage weight gain, and even inpatient units must be alert for patient noncompliance. Patients are placed in structured regimens to restore weight, normalize eating patterns, achieve normal perceptions of hunger and satiety, and correct the biological and psychological effects of starvation. Given the cognitive impairment that goes along with starvation, **psychotherapy alone is not enough to treat severely malnourished patients with anorexia nervosa.** As their nutritional status improves, psychotherapy becomes a critical component of the treatment. Psychiatric medications generally do not have a prominent role to play in the treatment of anorexia nervosa itself. However, if the patient has other significant symptoms (depression, obsessions, anxiety) then use of medications for treating these symptoms can be indicated. In general, use of psychiatric medications is delayed until metabolic abnormalities are corrected, and the patient's starvation status is significantly improved.

Comprehension Questions

[44.1] Which of the following laboratory tests is most helpful in assessing the severity of starvation in anorexia nervosa?

A. Complete blood count and differential white blood cell count
B. Thyroid function studies
C. Serum potassium level
D. Determination of albumin level
E. Liver function studies

[44.2] Which of the following most closely characterizes adolescent girls with anorexia nervosa?

A. Poor academic performance
B. An obsession with boys and sex
C. Feelings of entitlement
D. Low self-esteem
E. No feelings of helplessness

[44.3] Anorexia nervosa has been diagnosed in a 14-year-old girl, and she has been admitted to an inpatient psychiatric unit for treatment. On admission, she is found to be 5 ft 4 in tall and to weigh 82 lb. Over the next week in the hospital, she is weighed daily. She gains 4 lb the first day but subsequently loses 1 lb, and so at the end of the week she weighs 85 lb. It is discovered that the patient exercises all night long and hides all her food in napkins. What might account for the 4-lb weight gain early in the hospital stay?

A. Early treatment motivation
B. Excessive intake of water before the first weigh-in
C. A decrease in metabolism, resulting in weight gain
D. Scale error
E. Patient binged on the first day but was unable to purge until after her first weigh-in

Answers

[44.1] **D.** A determination of the albumin level can assist in assessing the current extent of starvation in a patient. It is an important index in the treatment of anorexic patients.

[44.2] **D.** In addition to low self-esteem, girls with anorexia are often perfectionists in school and are seen as academic overachievers. They are often socially withdrawn and do not engage in age-appropriate social activities. They feel helpless and as if they have a limited sense of self-control, but they do not display a sense of entitlement.

[44.3] **B.** Patients admitted to psychiatric units for treatment of anorexia must be watched carefully because they go to great lengths to make it appear as if they are being compliant without really gaining any weight. Binging on water, placing heavy objects in their pockets before weighing, and other such maneuvers are often attempted.

CLINICAL PEARLS

❖ Anorexia nervosa is a serious, life-threatening disorder that can require inpatient medical and psychiatric hospitalization.

❖ Patients with anorexia nervosa rarely (at least at the beginning of their treatment) comply with refeeding and other treatment regimens willingly.

❖ Patients with anorexia nervosa can exhibit symptoms such as obsessions, performing rituals, and depression as a part of their clinical presentation.

REFERENCES

American Psychiatric Association. Practice guideline of the treatment of patients with eating disorders (revised). Am J Psychiatry 2000;157(suppl 1):1–39.

Halmi KA. Eating disorders. In: Sadock BJ, Sadock VA, eds. Kaplan and Sadock's comprehensive textbook of psychiatry, 7th ed. Philadelphia: Lippincott Williams & Wilkins, 2000:1663–1676.

❖ CASE 45

An 18-year-old man presents to a psychiatrist insisting, "I have schizophrenia and need to be admitted." For the past several days, he heard voices telling him to kill himself. He says that he is possessed by the devil. The patient denies feeling depressed, but thinks he will hurt himself if he is not admitted to a hospital immediately. However, he denies having any specific suicide plan. He has no prior history of psychiatric treatment or complaints, no medical problems, and is not taking any medication. He drinks one or two beers a week and denies using drugs. At the end of the interview, he again requests hospitalization. He then adds that he is currently on leave from the Navy and is due back on his ship, which is leaving in 2 days.

On a mental status examination, the patient is initially cooperative and forthcoming but becomes increasingly irritated when asked to give more details about his symptoms. His mood and affect are euthymic but full-range. His thought processes are logical, without looseness of association or thought blocking, and his thought content has suicidal ideation but no homicidal ideation. He reports having delusions and auditory hallucinations. His insight seems good considering the severity of his symptoms.

◆ **What is the most likely diagnosis?**

◆ **How would you approach this patient?**

ANSWERS TO CASE 45: Malingering

Summary: An 18-year-old man without a psychiatric or medical history presents with a sudden onset of hallucinations, delusions, and suicidal ideation and asks to be admitted to the hospital. His social history is notable for his upcoming deployment with the Navy. His mental status examination is relatively unremarkable except for his reported symptoms, some irritability when he is questioned, and his high level of insight.

- **Most likely diagnosis:** Malingering.
- **Best approach:** Obtain collateral information (if possible) from family and/or friends, gently confront the inconsistencies in the patient's presentation, explore and validate his feelings regarding his military duty, and refer him for an appropriate follow-up (if possible).

Analysis

Objectives

1. Recognize malingering.
2. Differentiate malingering from factitious and conversion disorders.
3. Understand how to approach a patient suspected of malingering.

Considerations

This man initially presents with symptoms of a psychotic disorder. Although he admits to some criteria consistent with schizophrenia, such as hallucinations and delusions, the time course is too brief. There does not appear to be any substance use or a medical condition causing his symptoms. An important factor seems to be his upcoming military duty. His mental status examination is remarkable for the lack of a flat or inappropriate affect, loose associations, or thought blocking commonly seen in a psychotic disorder. In fact, **he displays a surprisingly high level of insight into his "illness"** considering his lack of a psychiatric history. He insists that his self-diagnosis is correct and that he needs immediate hospitalization. He becomes irritable only when pressed for more details. Although a psychotic disorder should be considered, the patient's reluctance to provide more details, a lack of objective findings on the mental status examination, and his intact insight in the context of required military duty make malingering the most likely diagnosis.

APPROACH TO MALINGERING

Definition

Malingering: The intentional feigning, production, or exaggeration of psychiatric or medical signs/symptoms to obtain external gain (e.g., financial compensation or avoidance of work, a prison sentence, or military service)

Thought blocking: The unpleasant experience of having one's train of thought curtailed absolutely

Clinical Approach

Diagnostic Criteria

Malingering is not a psychiatric or medical diagnosis, but in the *Diagnostic and Statistical Manual of Mental Disorders, text revision (DSM-IV-TR),* it is listed as an additional condition that can be the focus of clinical attention (a V code), which is listed under axis I. Factors consistent with malingering are an unusual history or presentation, a vague or inconsistent history, a history of antisocial behavior, defensiveness in response to questioning, and a lack of findings on a mental status or physical examination and/or in laboratory studies. A necessary component is the *intentional* production of symptoms or signs in order to achieve some *tangible external gain.*

Differential Diagnosis

The primary, most essential differentiation must be made between malingering and an actual psychiatric or medical diagnosis. Collateral information gathered from family or friends can be helpful in further elucidating the diagnosis. Also important in the differential diagnosis for malingering are both factitious and conversion disorders. In factitious disorder, a patient *intentionally* produces a physical or psychiatric illness in order to assume the *sick role*. In conversion disorder, a patient *unconsciously* produces a physical or neurologic symptom as the result of an *intrapsychic conflict.* Table 45–1 illustrates these differences.

Approach to the Malingering Patient

As malingering is not a psychiatric disorder, there is no specific treatment for it. However, there are several factors that can be helpful to both the clinician and the patient. An important issue to keep in mind is the physician's own feelings toward malingering. Accusations, anger, and rejection serve only to inflame the situation, promote further defensiveness, send the patient elsewhere, or perhaps provoke the individual to violence. As in all other psychiatric and medical interventions, maintenance of a therapeutic alliance is

Table 45–1
DIFFERENTIAL DIAGNOSIS FOR MALINGERING

CONDITION	PRODUCTION OF SYMPTOMS OR SIGNS	MOTIVATION
Malingering	Conscious	External gain
Factitious disorder	Conscious	Assumption of the sick role
Conversion disorder	Unconscious	Unconscious conflict

essential. Whereas gentle confrontation can be necessary, empathic exploration and understanding of the feelings and issues contributing to the feigning of illness can lead to increased trust in the clinician and truth telling by the individual. If it is practical or desired, a referral for further supportive therapy can then be made to address the underlying issues.

Comprehension Questions

For the following clinical vignettes (questions [45.1] through [45.4]), choose the one descriptor (A through D) that *best* describes the situation:

A. Conscious production of symptoms because of a desire to assume the sick role
B. Conscious production of symptoms to obtain external gain
C. Unconscious production of symptoms as the result of an unconscious conflict
D. Unconscious production of symptoms based on imitative behavior
E. Referred symptoms caused by transference

[45.1] A 23-year-old pregnant female complains of an inability to feel her legs. She wonders if the fetus is grabbing her spinal cord. Although she does not appear concerned about her condition, on further questioning she admits that her pregnancy was unplanned and that it has been a source of stress for her and her husband. Her neurologic examination is unremarkable except for decreased sensation below her waist. The results of a computed tomography scan and magnetic resonance imaging of her brain and spine are normal.

[45.2] A 45-year-old male complains of lower back pain and weakness in his legs after lifting heavy boxes while at work. He has not been able to go to work for several days, and he requests treatment and a letter excusing him from work. On examination, he is found to have significant lumbar pain without spasms. The strength in his legs is decreased because of a lack of effort. His reflexes are within normal limits.

[45.3] A 38-year-old woman comes in for evaluation of an abscess on her thigh. Her chart documents numerous out- and inpatient hospital visits. She is admitted, her abscess is drained, and she is treated with antibiotics. Culture studies demonstrate microorganisms consistent with fecal matter, and a further physical examination reveals many old scars, presumably self-inflicted.

[45.4] A 50-year-old male is referred to a physician because he has ongoing migraine headaches. His headaches are chronic and bilateral, are worse with loud noises and light, and occur without aura or vomiting. His physical examination is unremarkable except that the patient does not appear be in significant distress. When he is presented with various options for treatment, including nonsteroidal anti-inflammatory medications, he becomes angry, demanding that Tylenol with codeine is the only thing that helps him. When he is told that nonnarcotic medications should be tried first, he accuses the doctor of not believing him and walks out of the room.

Answers

[45.1] **C.** The most likely diagnosis for this woman is conversion disorder. She presents with symptoms of a neurologic disorder without an obvious cause or trauma. She does not appear particularly concerned about her symptoms *(la belle indifference),* and there is no obvious possibility of obtaining external gain. Her motivation does not seem to be assuming the sick role but rather expressing an unconscious conflict involving her unwanted pregnancy.

[45.2] **B.** In this case the most likely diagnosis is malingering. Although this man can indeed have a minor injury, his physical examination is remarkable only in revealing tenderness without spasms. His complaints of weakness and inability to work appear exaggerated given the lack of objective findings. The patient clearly has an obvious external motivation for embellishing his symptoms, namely, avoiding work.

[45.3] **A.** The most likely diagnosis for this woman is factitious disorder. She presents with a self-induced infection, as well as a history of other self-inflicted injuries that have resulted in numerous hospitalizations. Her illnesses are consciously created, without a desire to obtain obvious external gain other than assumption of the patient role.

[45.4] **B.** In this case the most likely diagnosis is malingering. This man presents with only subjective complaints; there are no significant medical findings or apparent suffering. He is angry and defensive, and he appears to be motivated solely by a desire to obtain narcotics rather than appropriate treatment.

CLINICAL PEARLS

- ❖ Consider malingering when there is an inconsistent history or presentation, coupled with the possibility of obtaining an obvious external gain.
- ❖ Patients with factitious disorder also consciously produce symptoms, but their motivation is to assume the patient/sick role.
- ❖ Gentle confrontation can be necessary with malingerers, but an empathic stance often promotes a more effective physician–patient alliance.
- ❖ Referral to a mental health professional can be indicated to help a malingering individual cope with the ongoing stressors promoting the deception.

REFERENCES

Ebert M, Loosen P, Nurcombe B, eds. Current diagnosis and treatment in psychiatry. New York: McGraw-Hill, 2000:383–384.

Kaplan H, Sadock B. Synopsis of psychiatry, 9th ed. Baltimore: Lippincott Williams & Wilkins, 2004:1541–1545.

❖ CASE 46

A $2^1/_2$-year-old boy is brought to a pediatrician by his parents for his regular yearly examination. He is the couple's only child. The parents relate a normal medical history with a single episode of otitis media. They recently placed their son in day care for 2 half-days a week. However, he has not adjusted well, crying and having tantrums during the first hour of school. Then he usually quiets down, but he does not interact with the rest of the children. The teacher cannot seem to make him follow directions and notes that he does not look at her when she is near him and attempting to interact with him.

On further discussion with the parents, the pediatrician finds that the patient has only a limited vocabulary of perhaps 10 words. He does not use these words in any greater length than two words in a row and often uses them inappropriately. He did not speak his first clear word until 6 to 9 months previously. The patient does not interact well with other children but does not seem upset by them. His favorite toys are often used inappropriately—he performs single, repetitive movements with them for what seems like hours on end. The pediatrician picks the child up to help him onto the examination table and notices that he seems quite stiff, pushing himself away from the examiner with his hands. Although his hearing and eyesight appear to be intact, the child does not respond to requests by the pediatrician and does not make eye contact. All other gross neurologic and physical features are within normal limits.

◆ **What is the most likely diagnosis?**

◆ **What is the most likely prognosis for this condition?**

ANSWERS TO CASE 46: Autistic Disorder

Summary: A 2½-year-old child is brought to a pediatrician for his yearly physical examination. His history reveals various behavioral issues, including poor interaction with peers and family, delayed language development, repetitive movements, and difficulty accepting change. The child stiffens physically when touched, does not respond to the examiner, and does not make eye contact.

- **Most likely diagnosis:** Autistic disorder.
- **Prognosis:** The child will likely experience a number of developmental delays, but with intensive treatment at home and at school, he could achieve near-normal or normal development. Language development is the most important indicator of future developmental potential in autistic children.

Analysis

Objectives

1. Recognize autistic disorder based on symptoms.
2. Understand the unique symptomatic aspects of autistic disorder.
3. Understand the importance of early treatment.

Considerations

The patient's presentation and history are typical of a child with autistic disorder. The symptoms of autism often go unrecognized until the child is placed in an environment with other children of a similar age. This lack of recognition of the problem is especially likely to occur in a family with no other children, where it is not possible to compare developmental milestones. The patient displays typical symptoms: difficulty with social reciprocity, poor peer interaction, poor language development, and repetitive and odd play. His language development is poor for his age. A normal 2½-year-old child should have a much larger vocabulary—hundreds of words—and should easily be able to use several words in a sentence. His comprehension of words should be even better than his ability to use them. The presence of autism does not necessarily indicate mental retardation, but a large percentage of autistic individuals have this disorder. The parents have come for help relatively early in the course of the illness. Intensive behavioral and educational interventions will be necessary to help accelerate the child's development.

Definitions

Asperger disorder: A disorder of unknown etiology in which affected individuals display social impairment and restricted interests and behavior (stereotyped behavior) but have normal language and cognitive skills.

Mental retardation: A classification of cognitive functioning involving both a low intelligence quotient (IQ) and an impairment in adaptive functioning

Rett disorder: A childhood developmental disorder of unknown etiology in which the patient develops progressive encephalopathy, loss of speech capacity, gait problems, stereotyped movements, microcephaly, and poor social interaction skills. The child must have shown normal development in early infancy, and only females are affected.

Social reciprocity: The ability to read and to exhibit verbal and nonverbal behaviors as a result of interacting with others.

Stereotyped behaviors: Purposeless, repetitive movements and behaviors such as spinning toys, toe walking, or hand flapping.

Clinical Approach

Boys are more often affected by autistic disorder than girls by a three- to five-fold increased prevalence. Typically, the disorder is noticed by the parents of an affected child before 3 years of age and is characterized by developmental delay, aloofness, and stereotyped behavior. The etiology of autistic disorder is unknown, but a genetic etiology is likely. Family studies show a markedly increased incidence in monozygotic twins and a low risk in dizygotic twins. Elevated serum serotonin levels can be a clue to the neurochemical abnormality. Approximately 40% of children with autistic disorder are mentally retarded; however, some demonstrate unusual or extremely precocious abilities, so-called islets of precocity. One such talent is the ability to perform extraordinary mathematical calculations although the child is cognitively impaired in other ways.

Diagnostic Criteria

Patients demonstrate a qualitative impairment in social interaction skills, manifested by symptoms such as **a marked impairment in nonverbal behaviors, a failure to develop appropriate peer relationships, or a lack of social reciprocity.** There are also qualitative impairments in their ability to communicate, manifested by a delay in learning or a failure to learn spoken language. Patients exhibit **repetitive and stereotyped patterns of behavior,** including inflexible adherence to rules or stereotyped motor mannerisms. They can also be persistently preoccupied with parts of objects.

Differential Diagnosis

Autistic disorder must be differentiated from other pervasive developmental disorders, including Asperger disorder, childhood disintegrative disorder, Rett disorder, and pervasive development disorder not otherwise specified (NOS). This can usually be done on the basis of age of onset (autistic disorder and Rett disorder have an age of onset prior to 36 months), whether or not there was a period of normal development (present in childhood disintegrative and Rett disorders), and whether or not skills were attained and subsequently lost (also typical of childhood disintegrative and Rett disorders). Autistic children often function within the mentally retarded range, however, unlike autistic children, mentally retarded children generally do not exhibit restricted activities and interests or impairments in communication and social skills. Although a child with schizophrenia can exhibit poor social functioning and affective withdrawal, the onset of childhood schizophrenia usually occurs later, there is a family history of schizophrenia, and the child is less impaired in the area of intellectual functioning. Children with obsessive-compulsive disorder (OCD) can display stereotypical behavior or perform rituals, but they have a more normal course of development otherwise. They also do not exhibit an impairment in social interaction or communication.

Treatment

Autism, perhaps more than any other child psychiatric disorder, requires a well-rounded, multisystemic treatment approach: **family education, behavior shaping, speech therapy, occupational therapy, and educational planning.** Care should be taken to coordinate these activities across school and home settings. Parental support and training are essential to a successful outcome. Applied behavioral analysis can be helpful in autistic patients, especially those with limited verbal skills. This treatment involves an intensive behavioral program that works best if started early in the course of the illness. The goals of this treatment are to teach the child a variety of **basic skills,** such as attending to adults, language use, and how to interact with their peers, all of which can increase the child's ability to be more successful in educational as well as social settings.

No specific medications are used in treating the core symptoms of autism, although some recent studies using low dose Risperdal (risperidone) show some promise. Other psychiatric disorders such as attention-deficit/hyperactivity disorder, OCD, behavior disorders, and psychotic disorders can be present in children with autism. These conditions should be targeted and treated if the symptoms meet the diagnostic criteria for that particular illness. Proper recognition and treatment of comorbid psychiatric disorders can have a significant impact on the overall outcome for children with autism.

Comprehension Questions

[46.1] Which of the following factors is most likely associated with a more positive prognosis for autistic disorder?

A. Physical development/performance IQ
B. Family socioeconomic status
C. Language development/verbal IQ
D. Presence of a seizure disorder
E. Sibling order

[46.2] What percentage of children with autistic disorder are mentally retarded?

A. 100%
B. 50% to 75%
C. 25% to 50%
D. 1% to 5%

[46.3] Stereotyped behaviors in autistic individuals are best illustrated by which of the following?

A. Interacting preferentially with other children of a specific race
B. Preference for similar schedules of play everyday
C. Focus of play on only one aspect of a toy
D. Difficulty playing with a toy creatively beyond its most obvious use
E. Spinning or repetitively using a toy in a specific manner for extended periods of time

[46.4] Autism can be distinguished best from Rett disorder by which of the following?

A. Age of onset
B. Early language development
C. Presence of a period of normal development
D. Evidence of mental retardation
E. Sex of the child

Answers

[46.1] **C.** One of the best predictors of the ability to improve the development of autistic children is the extent to which they have, or have begun to develop, language skills. This ability is often measured in verbal IQ testing.

[46.2] **B.** Because 50% to 75% of autistic individuals are mentally retarded, it is important to have an autistic child thoroughly evaluated for mental retardation so that appropriate educational programs can be developed as quickly as possible.

[46.3] **E.** Spinning or repetitively using a toy in a specific manner for extended periods of time is characteristic of stereotyped play. Autistic individuals often play with toys or objects in odd or eccentric ways. A typical example of stereotyped behavior in playing with toys is spinning or moving an object or toy in the same way for long periods of time.

[46.4] **C.** Both syndromes show evidence of presence prior to the age of 36 months; however, in Rett disorder, the child has an early phase of normal development then gradually loses those skills toward further decline.

CLINICAL PEARLS

❖ Language development is the best predictor of future outcome in autistic disorder.

❖ Mental retardation is often but not always associated with autism.

❖ In cases where early autism is suspected, a full medical workup should always be scheduled to rule out hearing or vision difficulties that can result in poor language development.

REFERENCES

Ebert M, Loosen P, Nurcombe B, eds. Current diagnosis and treatment in psychiatry. New York: McGraw-Hill, 2000:546–551.

Kaplan H, Sadock B. Synopsis of psychiatry, 9th ed. Baltimore: Lippincott Williams & Wilkins, 2003:1642–1646.

❖ CASE 47

A 21-year-old woman comes to the student-counseling center with complaints of being depressed and feeling anxious. She states that 2 weeks ago, while in class, she was called on by the teacher and gave the wrong answer. She says that she felt "humiliated" and has not gone back to the classroom since then. She describes a lifelong history of being painfully shy. She admits that she would like to have a boyfriend but that she is afraid to meet anyone because "I'll get dumped." She describes herself as "socially retarded" and avoids going out with anyone new. She has two close friends and does go out to dinner with them weekly, which she enjoys. She denies trouble sleeping or with her appetite, although she does admit to feeling ashamed of her social ineptitude. She is worried that she will be unable to finish college because of her problems.

 **What is the most likely diagnosis?**

◆ **What is the best therapy for this patient?**

ANSWERS TO CASE 47: Avoidant Personality Disorder

Summary: A 21-year-old patient comes to the counseling center after an embarrassing interpersonal interaction in class. She has a long history of avoiding close interpersonal relationships because of her fear of being rejected. She avoids new interpersonal situations because she feels inadequate.

◆ **Most likely diagnosis:** Avoidant personality disorder

◆ **Best therapy:** Psychodynamic or cognitive-behavioral psychotherapy

Analysis

Objectives

1. Recognize avoidant personality disorder in a patient.
2. Understand the treatment that is likely to be helpful to patients with this disorder.

Considerations

This young woman presents a classic picture of avoidant personality disorder. Although she desperately desires friends and intimate relationships, she is **excruciatingly sensitive to rejection** (or the chance of being rejected) and therefore avoids all but a few safe relationships. These patients usually view themselves as socially inept or otherwise unappealing and then assume that other people will have the same opinion of themselves. Rejections, especially in a public setting, are particularly humiliating, and patients can experience depressed and anxious moods as a result. (These moods do not, however, fit the criteria for any other psychiatric diagnosis.)

APPROACH TO AVOIDANT PERSONALITY DISORDER

Definition

Displacement: A defense mechanism in which an individual avoids emotional conflict or stress by transferring a feeling about, or a response to, one object to another (usually a less threatening or dangerous one). For example, after being yelled at by his boss, a man comes home and lets his anger out by yelling at his children.

Projection: A defense mechanism in which individuals attribute feelings they have about themselves or the world to others. For example, a man feels hostility toward his boss, so he attributes hostile motives to his supervisor's actions, even if others would see the actions as benign.

Clinical Approach

Patients with this disorder experience pervasive **social discomfort, feelings of inadequacy, and hypersensitivity to criticism and rejection.** They are often seen as very timid, and they avoid occupational or social activities because they are afraid of rejection. These patients view themselves as socially inept or inferior to others. Prevalence rates range from 0.5% to 1% in the general population.

Differential Diagnosis

Patients with this disorder can often be confused with patients with schizoid personality disorder because both have very few, if any, close friends or relationships. The difference lies in the reason why they lack these relationships. Patients with **avoidant personality disorder desperately wish to have close friendships** but are afraid to initiate them for fear of rejection. Patients with schizoid personality disorders do not really wish for close relationships and are happy without them. Patients with dependent personality disorder can appear similar to those with avoidant personality disorder—the difference is subtle. Patients with dependent personality disorder cling to others in their inner circle because they are afraid to function on their own. Patients with avoidant personality disorder, although appearing timid, are more afraid of rejection itself than of being able to take care of themselves.

Social phobia is an intense, persistent fear of being exposed to unfamiliar people or scrutiny by others because of the belief that one will be humiliated or embarrassed. When exposed to such a situation, the patient can have a situationally bound panic attack. As a result, the patient avoids feared situations even though he or she can recognize that the fear is excessive or unreasonable. In the case described, the patient is not having the anxiety attacks. If she was, the patient could be diagnosed with social phobia on axis I and axis II with avoidant personality. Social phobia often has a significant response to selective serotonin reuptake inhibitors (SSRIs) along with cognitive behavioral psychotherapy.

Treatment

Patients with this disorder are afraid of being rejected or criticized, and **so the clinician must be very tactful, accepting, and encouraging in approaching these patients.** Coercive or confrontational behavior does not work with these individuals, who can agree with the clinician at the time of the confrontation but never return.

Patients with avoidant personality disorder often have dysfunctional beliefs regarding the world. Often, they view people in general as critical and rejecting, thus they are reluctant to place their trust in people and withdraw. The goal of psychotherapy is to help patients critically examine if their assumptions about people are correct. SSRIs or beta-blockers such as betaxolol can help reduce anxiety associated with some social situations. Benzodiazepines, with their high potential for being habit-forming, should be avoided.

Comprehension Questions

[47.1] A 29-year-old man comes to see his physician because he has just been hired at a new job. He states that since he has been hired, and even before his first day on the job, which is to start in 3 days, he has been so anxious he has been unable to sleep. He says that his mood has been good but that he knows he will fail at the new job because "I am such a dope when it comes to working with other people." The patient tells the physician he has previously received a diagnosis of avoidant personality disorder. Which of the following should the physician do to help the patient manage his anxiety regarding the new job?

A. Tell the patient that everything will be all right and that he should just be confident about his abilities.
B. Prescribe cognitive therapy for the patient to help him deal with his negative self-image.
C. Give the patient a beta-blocker to help him control his anxiety.
D. Treat the patient with an antidepressant such as fluoxetine.
E. Tell the patient that he is probably not ready to hold a job if he is this anxious.

[47.2] Avoidant personality disorder belongs to which of the following clusters of personality disorders?

A. Cluster A
B. Cluster B
C. Cluster C
D. Cluster D
E. Cluster E

[47.3] Which of the following answers best characterizes the difference between patients with avoidant personality disorders and those with schizoid personality disorders?

A. Patients with avoidant personality disorders have fewer friends than those with schizoid personality disorders.
B. Patients with avoidant personality disorders have higher self-esteem than those with schizoid personality disorders.
C. Patients with avoidant personality disorders would like to have friends more than patients with schizoid personality disorders.
D. Patients with avoidant personality disorders are better at accepting criticism than patients with schizoid personality disorders.
E. Patients with avoidant personality disorders are less anxious than are patients with schizoid personality disorders.

[47.4] Which of the following defense mechanisms is typically used by patients with avoidant personality disorder?

A. Undoing
B. Splitting
C. Isolation of affect
D. Idealization
E. Displacement

Answers

[47.1] **C.** The use of beta-blockers can be helpful in the management of anxiety in patients with avoidant personality disorder, especially when they are being asked to approach feared situations.

[47.2] **C.** Avoidant personality disorder belongs in the cluster C, the "sad" cluster. There is no such thing as cluster D or E.

[47.3] **C.** Patients with avoidant personality disorders would desperately like to have social relationships, but they are afraid of criticism and/or rejection.

[47.4] **E.** Displacement and projection are the two defense mechanisms most commonly used by patients with avoidant personality disorders.

CLINICAL PEARLS

❖ Patients with avoidant personality disorder have a pervasive hypersensitivity to criticism and rejection. They avoid interpersonal relationships in every setting because they fear criticism and rejection. Their self-esteem is low, and they usually believe that they are inferior or inadequate, especially in the social arena.

❖ Patients with avoidant personality disorder are differentiated from those with schizoid personality disorder by the fact that they desperately would like interpersonal relationships but are afraid of them. Individuals with schizoid personality disorders do not have relationships but do not miss them.

❖ Patients with avoidant personality disorder are differentiated from those with dependent personality disorder by the fact that the former are afraid of rejection and criticism in relationships. Patients with dependent personality disorder are afraid of being left alone to fend for themselves.

❖ Physicians need to be tactful, encouraging, and accepting of these patients, especially regarding their fear of rejection. Confrontation and coercion are not appropriate, as they can drive the patient away.

❖ Defense mechanisms used by patients with avoidant personality disorder include displacement and projection.

REFERENCES

Cloninger CR, Svrakic DM. Personality disorders. In: Sadock BJ, Sadock VA, eds. Kaplan and Sadock's comprehensive textbook of psychiatry, 7th ed. Philadelphia: Lippincott Williams & Wilkins, 2000:1723–1764.

CASE 48

A 10-year-old boy is brought to a pediatrician for his 6-month check up for chronic asthma. In addition, he has complained of chronic headaches for the past 3 months, as well as increasing gastric upsets, which his family believes are caused by multiple food allergies. The patient also has a severe allergy to peanuts, which limits the number of places he can go in public. Thus, he has been home-schooled for a year and is doing well. A review of his history shows that he is a highly articulate, thoughtful child who grossly appears to be at or above the educational level of his peers. The child does not agree to be interviewed separately from his mother, stating, "I don't go anywhere without my mother." The two of them are almost never apart. Two years ago, the mother was hospitalized after a serious bout with lupus. She continues to a struggle with her disease, and despite having a thriving career before her illness; she can do very little now. She is home all the time, dealing with her own recovery and the management of her illness. During her hospitalization, the patient was quite worried about her illness and even now believes that if he is not around to monitor her condition, she might get sick and require hospitalization again—or even worse. The mother has difficulty sleeping and is most comfortable on the living room couch. The patient no longer uses his own room but sleeps in a chair next to his mother to continue to keep an eye on her. He has very few friends and can be separated from his mother only briefly, and only if he is in the company of his brother or father. After a short period, he becomes anxious and upset and must be reunited with his mother.

- **What is the most likely diagnosis?**
- **What is the prognosis for this disorder?**
- **What treatments might be helpful in this disorder?**

ANSWERS TO CASE 48: Separation Anxiety Disorder

Summary: A 10-year-old, late latency/early adolescent boy exhibits extreme anxiety when not in the presence of his mother. As a result, he no longer attends school but seems quite bright and cognitively on target. His anxiety symptoms began after the mother experienced a serious, life-threatening illness. The patient believes that if he is separated from her, something terrible might happen to her. In addition, he reports several somatic complaints that have been difficult to diagnose.

- **Most likely diagnosis:** Separation anxiety disorder (a childhood disorder).
- **Prognosis:** Difficult to treat; the patient is possibly more likely to develop depression and psychotic disorders.
- **Best treatment:** A multisystemic treatment approach is required. Selective serotonin reuptake inhibitors (SSRIs) can be helpful in the management of mood symptoms and anxiety. Relaxation techniques can help, along with a gradual separation program.

Analysis

Objectives

1. Recognize the symptoms of a typical case of separation anxiety disorder.
2. Understand the predisposing factors contributing to the disorder.
3. Understand what other disorders the patient is at a higher risk of developing.

Considerations

The patient has a typical presentation for separation anxiety disorder, which usually begins in the late latency period (11 to 12 years of age; Table 48–1).

Table 48–1
DIAGNOSTIC CRITERIA FOR SEPARATION ANXIETY DISORDER

Developmentally inappropriate anxiety about separation from home or from the caretaker to which an individual is attached.
Duration of the illness must be at least 4 weeks.
Onset of the illness should be prior to 18 years of age.
The disturbance should cause clinically significant impairment in important areas of functioning.

It is often precipitated by the life-threatening disease of a parent—most typically the mother or primary caretaker. Patients become extremely anxious and worried when they are physically separated from the parent. They worry that the parent will die if they are separated and thus are very difficult to console during these periods. Their beliefs can be quite strong and are minimally amenable to reason or reassurance. These patients often report a number of difficult-to-diagnose somatic complaints themselves. They are at risk for comorbid mood disorders, especially major depression, and should be monitored closely. Treatment is difficult but involves managing symptoms with medication (typically a SSRI) and teaching the patient relaxation techniques to control anxiety symptoms. These treatments should occur in conjunction with the development of a gradual plan to incrementally separate the patient from the parent, with a final goal of returning the patient to his or her earlier level of school and social functioning.

APPROACH TO SEPARATION ANXIETY DISORDER

Definitions

Multisystemic treatment: A philosophy of treatment used with children and adolescents. It can involve several specific theories and modalities of treatment, but the essential feature is the involvement of various social systems essential to the life of a child. Examples of the systems involved include school, church, family, and peers.

Somatic symptoms: Vague or diffuse feelings of pain or discomfort for which it is difficult to pinpoint an etiology.

Clinical Approach

Some degree of anxiety about separation from a parent is normal, and clinical judgment must be used to evaluate the severity of the anxiety and its impact on the functioning of the child. In generalized anxiety disorder, the anxiety does not center exclusively around the issue of separation from a parent but is much more diffuse and occurs in many situations. In major depression, which often coexists with separation anxiety disorder and should be diagnosed concurrently if the criteria for the disorder are met, patients typically have vegetative symptoms including insomnia and anorexia. Panic disorders are rarely seen before the age of 18, and in that case, the fear is of having another panic attack, not of separation.

In childhood, this disorder can be very difficult to treat and is resistant to improvement. However, the best prognosis is achieved with a **timely diagnosis and rapid initiation of treatment, usually psychotherapeutic modalities** directed toward the **individual, family, and school.** The role of medications is less clear; they can be helpful in short-term use with children who show extreme anxiety symptoms at specific times. However, **the mainstay**

of treatment continues to be behavioral interventions. Family therapy can be necessary to identify and address anxiety triggers and in helping the child develop skills to lessen anxiety symptoms, for example, relaxation techniques. School consultations can be helpful to aid in rapid, assertive reintroduction of the child into the school setting. A **successful transition to separations should result in generous praise for the child.**

Comprehension Questions

[48.1] A typical SSRI used in the treatment of separation anxiety disorder includes which of the following?

A. Methylphenidate
B. Bupropion
C. Fluoxetine
D. Valproic acid
E. Imipramine

[48.2] Children or adolescents with separation anxiety disorder are at higher risk for which other psychiatric disorder?

A. Malingering
B. Somatization disorder
C. Bipolar disorder
D. Learning disability
E. Major depression

[48.3] When starting an SSRI, such as fluoxetine, in an adolescent patient with separation anxiety disorder, the Food and Drug Administration (FDA) recommends the clinician monitor closely for which of the following?

A. Hypovolemia
B. Hypertension
C. Anorexia
D. Suicidal thoughts
E. Delusions

Answers

[48.1] **C.** This medication is one of several agents in the class collectively called SSRIs. The other medications are not in this class and are not used to treat separation anxiety disorder.

[48.2] **E.** Children and adolescents with separation anxiety disorder often present with or later develop symptoms of major depression. In children, this can include a depressed, sad, or irritable mood over an extended period of time.

[48.3] **D.** The FDA recently placed a "black box" warning for the use of antidepressants in children and adolescents. This warning reminds clinicians of some evidence indicating a possible increased incidence of suicidal thoughts among adolescents using antidepressants—particularly SSRIs.

CLINICAL PEARLS

- ❖ Separation anxiety disorder is often associated with a severe illness of the caretaker, usually the mother.
- ❖ This disorder often coexists with major depression, and this possibility should be evaluated carefully.
- ❖ The earlier separation anxiety disorder is treated, the better the prognosis.

REFERENCES

Ebert M, Loosen P, Nurcombe B, eds. Current diagnosis and treatment in psychiatry. New York: McGraw-Hill, 2000:579–580.

Kaplan H, Sadock B. Synopsis of psychiatry, 9th ed. Baltimore: Lippincott Williams & Wilkins, 2003:1229–1235.

❖ CASE 49

A 45-year-old man is brought to the emergency department after a fight in the bar where he has been employed for the past 3 weeks. The patient says that his name is "Roger Nelson," but he has no identification. He states that he does not know where he lived or worked prior to 3 weeks ago, although he does not seem upset by this. He says that the fight broke out in the bar because one of the customers attempted to steal money from the cash register.

On a mental status examination, the patient is seen to be alert and oriented to person, place, and time. The results of all other aspects of the examination are normal. A physical examination shows a 3-in-long laceration on the patient's right forearm, which requires suturing. There is no head trauma or any other abnormalities. When the police run a description check on the patient, they find that he fits the description of a missing person, Charles Johnson, who disappeared from a town 50 miles away 1 month prior to his emergency department admission. Mrs. Johnson is able to identify Roger Nelson as her husband, Charles. The patient claims not to recognize her, however, Mrs. Johnson explains that in the months prior to his disappearance, her husband was under increasing work pressures and was afraid that he was going to be fired. She says that the day before his sudden disappearance, her husband had a huge fight with his boss. He came home and had a fight with her as well, culminating in her calling him a "loser." She woke up the next morning to find him gone. She states that the patient has no psychiatric history or problems and denies that he uses drugs or alcohol. He has no medical problems.

◆ **What is the most likely diagnosis for this patient?**

◆ **What are the course of and the prognosis for this disorder?**

ANSWERS TO CASE 49: Dissociative Fugue

Summary: A 45-year-old man is brought to the emergency department after a fight in the bar where he is employed. Other than a laceration on his forearm, there are no physical abnormalities. The results of his mental status examination are normal. The patient has been working at the bar for the past 3 weeks but has no memory of his life prior to that. When his wife is located, the patient does not recognize her. The wife reports that the patient has been missing for 1 month, his disappearance apparently precipitated by increasing problems at work and fights with his boss and his wife. The patient has no history of psychiatric problems, drug or alcohol use, or medical problems.

- **Most likely diagnosis:** Dissociative fugue.
- **Course and prognosis:** Dissociative fugue is usually brief in duration, lasting hours to days. Occasionally it lasts for months, and the patient can travel thousands of miles from home. Generally, there is a rapid, spontaneous recovery, and a recurrence after recovery is rare.

Analysis

Objectives

1. Recognize dissociative fugue in a patient (see Table 49–1 for diagnostic criteria).
2. Understand the usual course of illness in this disorder.

Considerations

This man suddenly disappeared after experiencing a series of difficulties and traumatic events in his life. He appears suddenly several weeks later with a different name and a different life and does not recognize his wife. The results of his mental status examination are otherwise normal. There is no history of a dissociative identity disorder, drug use, or a general medical condition that might better account for his behavior. Individuals experiencing **dissociative**

Table 49–1
DIAGNOSTIC CRITERIA FOR DISSOCIATIVE FUGUE

1. Unexpected, sudden departure from home and travel to a new location; the individual is unable to recall his or her past.
2. The individual is not aware of his or her identity and may create a new one.
3. The condition does not occur in an individual with dissociative identity disorder and is not caused by a medical condition or substance.
4. The condition must be distressing or impair social and/or occupational functioning.

fugue suddenly and unexpectedly travel far away from their homes and cannot recall their previous identity or past. The person usually adopts a **new identity** in the course of the fugue. Dissociation is a way in which people defend themselves against overwhelming trauma; most instances of dissociative fugue occur during times of war or other overwhelming disasters but can also be triggered by severe marital, family, or occupational distress. It is a rare disorder.

APPROACH TO DISSOCIATIVE FUGUE

Definitions

Depersonalization: Persistent or recurrent alteration of one's perception of oneself as unreal or strange.

Dissociation: A form of defense against trauma; the individual "splits off" the memory of the traumatic event, emotions, thoughts, or behaviors, which then exist on a "parallel" level of awareness.

Dissociative amnesia: Inability to recall specific information, usually about one's identity, but having an intact memory about general information; usually caused by a traumatic or stressful memory. This disorder does not involve traveling and adopting a new identity.

Dissociative identity disorder: Commonly known as multiple personality disorder, a disorder in which a person invents multiple personalities to help deal with a traumatic event, usually one that has occurred in childhood. Two or more identities or personality states recurrently take control of the person's behavior.

Clinical Approach

Severely traumatic events, such as those occurring during a war, or intense personal crises can precipitate these rare events. Individuals affected by dissociative fugue display more purposeful behavior than those with dissociative amnesia. They travel away from their families, take on new identities, and often new occupations. Alcohol abuse and certain mood and personality disorders can predispose one to this disorder but are not the cause.

Differential Diagnosis

The main purpose of dissociative fugue appears to be escape from a traumatic experience; therefore there is always a history of the occurrence of an overwhelming event in these cases. However, a clinician faced with such patients is unlikely to be aware of this history, as the patients have blocked the events from their memories. The clinician must therefore consider and rule out other diagnoses. In **dissociative amnesia,** individuals lose their memory of the past but **do not leave home or invent a new identity.** In **dissociative identity disorder,** the patient **experiences himself or herself as at least two separate identities** with individual behaviors, emotions, and histories.

Patients with **dementia or delirium have memory problems and can wander far from home,** but their travels are purposeless and disorganized, and they **do not invent new identities.** Patients with complex partial seizures can travel away from home, but they do not invent new identities, and there is usually no history of a traumatic event. Patients with **bipolar disorder** experiencing an episode of mania often travel far from home, but they are often delusional, have hallucinations, and display other symptoms of bipolar illness. Intoxication caused by many different substances can cause amnesia and result in sudden travel; alcohol and hallucinogens, in addition to barbiturates, benzodiazepines, steroids, and phenothiazines, can all produce retrograde amnesia. Another possibility is malingering, that is, falsifying a fugue to obtain some gain, such as to escape creditors or drug dealers.

Treatment

There is no indicated psychopharmacologic treatment for dissociative fugue, although an interview under Amytal Sodium (amobarbital sodium) or a benzodiazepine can render helpful diagnostic information. It is generally treated by first obtaining a complete psychiatric history, perhaps aided by the use of hypnosis, so that the psychological stressors that precipitated the fugue can be discovered. On identification of the precipitating event, psychodynamic psychotherapy is typically helpful in helping the patient deal with the stressor in a more healthy, integrated way to minimize the risk of a dissociative recurrence.

Comprehension Questions

[49.1] A man who appears to be approximately 70 years of age is brought to the emergency department by the police. He was picked up after he tried to order food in a restaurant but had no money to pay the bill. He is oriented to place and time and gives his name as "Bill," but he cannot remember where he lives, his telephone number, or the names of his family members. He does recall that he served in the Pacific during World War II and that he was raised in rural New Hampshire. The results of his physical examination are essentially normal, and his routine laboratory tests reveal mild anemia. Which of the following is the most likely diagnosis?

A. Dissociative amnesia
B. Dissociative fugue
C. Alcohol dependence
D. Dementia

[49.2] Dissociative fugue is distinguished from dissociative amnesia by which of the following?

A. The presence of retrograde amnesia
B. Travel far from home or family
C. A precipitating traumatic event
D. Creation of multiple identities

[49.3] A 38-year-old woman has adopted a new identity in a city 120 miles away from her hometown and has no memory of her prior life. Apparently, this event was precipitated by confrontation of her addiction to gambling and a threat of divorce. Which of the following is most likely to be an associated factor in her illness?

A. History of head trauma
B. Paranoid personality disorder
C. Birth of a baby within 3 months
D. Female gender

Answers

[49.1] **D.** Dementia. This patient has preserved some past memory, which is characteristic of dementia but not of dissociative fugue or amnesia. If he had a history of alcoholism, there would be some evidence from his physical examination (or in his blood alcohol level).

[49.2] **B.** Travel far from one's home or family distinguishes dissociative fugue from dissociative amnesia; both are precipitated by trauma and are characterized by retrograde amnesia. In neither dissociative fugue nor dissociative amnesia are multiple identities created, as they are in dissociative identity disorder.

[49.3] **A.** A history of head trauma predisposes one to dissociative fugue.

CLINICAL PEARLS

❖ Dissociative fugue is rare, and several disorders must be considered and ruled out before it is definitively diagnosed.

❖ Interviews conducted under hypnosis or Amytal Sodium (amobarbital sodium) or benzodiazpines can confirm the diagnosis if a corroborative history is lacking.

REFERENCES

Kapur N. Amnesia in relation to fugue states: distinguishing a neurological form from a psychogenic basis. Br J Psychiatry 1991;159:872–873.

Saxe GN, van der Kolk VA, Berkowitz R, et al. Dissociative disorders in psychiatric inpatients. Am J Psychiatry 1993;150:1037–1039.

Chefetz R, ed. Neuroscientific and therapeutic advances in dissociative disorders. Psychiatric Annals 2005;35(8):657–665.

CASE 50

A 16 year-old girl comes to the emergency department at the insistence of her parents with a chief complaint of suicidal ideation. She states that for the past week she has felt that life is no longer worth living and that she has been planning to kill herself by getting drunk and taking her mother's Xanax (alprazolam). She says that her mood is depressed, she has no energy, and she is not interested in doing things she normally enjoys. Prior to 1 week ago, she had none of these symptoms. The patient states that she has been sleeping 12 to 14 hours a day for the past week and eating "everything in sight." She says she has never been diagnosed with major depression or has been seen by a psychiatrist and that she has no medical problems of which she is aware. The patient states that up until 9 days ago she used cocaine on a daily basis for a month and then stopped it when school started.

On a mental status examination, the patient appears alert and oriented to person, place, and time. Her speech is normal, but her mood is "depressed" and her affect is constricted and dysphoric. She denies having hallucinations or delusions but has suicidal ideation with a specific intent and plan. She denies having homicidal ideation.

- **What is the most likely diagnosis for this patient?**

- **What is the next step in the treatment?**

ANSWERS TO CASE 50: Substance-Induced Mood Disorder

Summary: A 16-year-old patient presents to the emergency department with suicidal ideation 9 days after she stopped using cocaine. Since 1 week ago, she has noted a depressed mood, hypersomnia, decreased energy, anhedonia, and an increased appetite. She has no medical problems and has never been diagnosed with major depression. On a mental status examination, her mood is seen to be depressed, and her affect is dysphoric and constricted. She has suicidal ideation with a specific intent and a plan.

Most likely diagnosis: Substance-induced mood disorder (cocaine withdrawal).

Next step: Discontinuing use of the offending drug is usually enough to cause the mood disorder symptoms to abate. An antidepressant is generally not needed initially, however, if the depressive symptoms continue, treatment with an antidepressant can be indicated. This patient certainly needs substance abuse treatment to deal with her substance abuse problems. A more detailed substance abuse history should be taken.

Analysis

Objectives

1. Recognize substance-induced mood disorder (see Table 50–1 for diagnostic criteria).
2. Know the treatment recommendations for a patient with this disorder.

Table 50–1

DIAGNOSTIC CRITERIA FOR SUBSTANCE-INDUCED MOOD DISORDER

1. A persistent, prominent disturbance in mood characterized by either (or both) of the following: (a) a depressed mood or markedly decreased interest or pleasure in activities that are usually enjoyable, or (b) an elevated, expansive, or irritable mood.
2. An indication from the patient's history, a physical examination, or laboratory results that the symptoms developed during or within a month of substance intoxication or withdrawal. The symptoms can also be related to the use of a medication.
3. Sufficient evidence is not present indicating that the mood disorder is not substance-induced. This evidence might include symptoms that started before use of the substance, symptoms that persisted well beyond (more than a month) the period of intoxication or withdrawal, symptoms in excess of what would be expected for the type and amount of substance used, or a history of major depression.
5. Symptoms do not occur only during the course of a delirium.

Considerations

The primary consideration in this case is that the patient did not start having mood symptoms until *after* she stopped taking cocaine. On withdrawing from the drug, the patient noted a severely depressed mood with suicidal ideation. In addition, she noted many of the signs/symptoms of cocaine withdrawal, including fatigue, decreased energy, hypersomnia, and an increased appetite. The patient has no history of major depression.

APPROACH TO SUBSTANCE-INDUCED MOOD DISORDER

Definitions

Anhedonia: Loss of interest or pleasure in normally enjoyable activities
Hyperactivity: Excessive level of activity significantly above that expected for the developmental stage and setting
Hypersomnia: An increase in the amount of sleep (and a subjective feeling of a need for sleep) above what is normal for a particular person
Impulsivity: Taking action without appropriate thought and consideration, which often leads to a dangerous situation

Clinical Approach

Cocaine has been used at least once by 25 million people in the United Sates with 2.7% of the population having had cocaine dependence at one time. (The lifetime prevalence of bipolar disorder is only 1.6%.) Cocaine-induced mood disorder can occur during use, intoxication or withdrawal from the drug. During use and intoxication, cocaine is more likely to produce a manic state; depressed states are more common during withdrawal.

Substances, including medications used to treat nonpsychiatric disorders, neuroactive chemicals, or recreational agents can induce mood changes. Antihypertensive agents especially are commonly causative. Depression, mania with or without psychotic symptoms, or mixed depression and mania can result. Both intoxication with and withdrawal from a substance can lead to a mood disturbance.

Differential Diagnosis

Care must be taken to determine if substance intoxication or substance withdrawal is currently present. Realize that patients will often lie to health care providers regarding their substance use. A toxicology screen and ancillary history from family and friends can be extremely helpful in determining actual substance use patterns. If no substance use is identified, a primary mood disorder or depressive disorder not otherwise specified (NOS) should be considered. Mood disorder caused by a general medical condition is diagnosed if a medical condition is thought to account for the depressive symptoms. Finally, a careful review of the patient's history should indicate whether episodes of mania or depression have occurred, and if so, a diagnosis of bipolar disorder should be considered.

Treatment

The main treatment for a substance-induced mood disorder is cessation of use of the causative substance. This is particularly true of alcohol and opioids. On the other hand, cessation of the use of some substances can initially result in a worsening of mood; for instance, discontinuing cocaine use often leads to a "crash," which quite commonly includes a severely dysphoric mood. However, even in such cases, the vast majority of mood symptoms resolve on their own without psychopharmacologic intervention, usually within several weeks. If the symptoms of a substance-induced mood disorder do not resolve with removal of the offending substance, the use of psychotropic medications can be indicated. For example, a patient with this disorder who remains depressed should be treated like a patient with major depression and given antidepressant medication. A patient whose substance-induced mood disorder takes the form of a manic presentation should be treated like a patient with bipolar disease and given a mood stabilizer.

Referral for substance abuse treatment is always indicated. Many patients need more than 10 attempts at substance abuse treatment in order to finally achieve sobriety.

Comprehension Questions

[50.1] Mood disturbances associated with substances can best be described as which of the following?

A. Euthymic
B. Primarily depressed
C. Primarily manic
D. Fluctuating between depressed and manic
E. Substance-specific

[50.2] Which of the following is true of substances that can cause a substance-induced mood disorder?

A. The substance can be a medication prescribed by a physician.
B. The substance is almost always of an illicit nature.
C. It does not matter whether the symptoms are related to the intoxication state.
D. It does not matter whether the symptoms are related to the withdrawal state.
E. The substance should not produce any pleasurable effects for the user.

[50.3] A 23-year-old male comes in to see you because he thinks he is "going crazy." He states that he feels that things around him are "unreal" and that he is "fading out at times." He denies having hallucinations. On examination, he appears relaxed and has reddened conjunctivae. Which of the following is most likely to clarify that drug use is a problem?

A. Physical exam
B. Mental status exam
C. Urine toxicology screen
D. Serum liver panel
E. Magnetic resonance imaging of brain

Answers

[50.1] **E.** Substances vary in their effect on mood. For example, alcohol is primarily a depressant, whereas cocaine can cause euphoria over the short term, but generally depression as it is eliminated from the body and withdrawal is experienced.

[50.2] **A.** Many medications prescribed by physicians have an effect on mood and might be the cause of mood symptoms or a disorder. The substance need not be illicit and can produce many pleasurable effects during the intoxication state. The disorder should not be diagnosed if the intoxication or withdrawal state is still present.

[50.3] **C.** Urine toxicology screens are extremely important to obtain in the emergency center setting.

CLINICAL PEARLS

❖ The symptoms can occur during the period of time the substance is being used or up to a month after use of the substance has ceased.

❖ In order for the mood symptoms to be accurately assessed, the patient should not be acutely intoxicated or undergoing the withdrawal process.

REFERENCES

Jaffe JH. Cocaine-related disorders. In: Sadock BJ, Sadock VA, eds. Kaplan and Sadock's comprehensive textbook of psychiatry, 7th ed. Philadelphia: Lippincott Williams & Wilkins, 2000:999–1015.

Jaffe JH. Introduction and overview of substance-related disorders. In: Sadock BJ, Sadock VA, eds. Kaplan and Sadock's comprehensive textbook of psychiatry, 7th ed. Philadelphia: Lippincott Williams & Wilkins, 2000:924–952.

CASE 51

A 30-year-old woman comes to a psychiatrist with a chief complaint of "I can't seem to finish my PhD." She claims that she has been working on her thesis for the last 5 years but has procrastinated to the point where it seems as if she will not finish it any time soon. Likewise, it took her 6 years to finish college. She says that she sometimes worries that "I'm all messed up" but can only relate this to her general unhappiness with her progress on her thesis and her lack of a long-term love relationship. She states that she is tired of this and wants to "get to the bottom of why I do this to myself." The patient notes that she is doing fine otherwise. She has no problems with sleep, appetite, concentration, or energy level. Her mood has been fine, and she is interested in numerous hobbies. She has no psychiatric history, and her only medical problem is mild hypertension that is well controlled by a diuretic. She lives alone in an apartment with her cat and supports herself by working for the physiology laboratory where she is working on her thesis. She states that she has a good relationship with her parents, who were divorced when she was 9 years old. The patient denies using drugs and drinks two or three glasses of red wine a week because "I was told it is good for my heart." The results of her mental status examination are entirely within normal limits.

 **What is the most likely diagnosis?**

What treatment should be suggested for this woman?

ANSWERS TO CASE 51: Neurosis

Summary: A 30-year-old woman presents with a chief complaint of being unable to finish her thesis. She had difficulty finishing college in 4 years as well. She is afraid that there is something wrong with her, although she cannot pinpoint exactly what it is. She also lacks a long-term love relationship, although she would like to have one. Otherwise, the patient has no psychiatric signs or symptoms. She has no psychiatric history, and her only medical problem is well-controlled hypertension. Her parents were divorced when she was 9 years old. The patient has no history of drug use and drinks two or three glasses of red wine a week.

 **Most likely diagnosis:** No diagnosis is listed in the *Diagnostic and Statistical Manual of Mental Disorders, text revision (DSM-IV-TR).* (The patient might be considered neurotic.)

◆ **Best treatment:** Insight-oriented psychotherapy or psychoanalysis.

Analysis

Objectives

1. Recognize neurotic symptoms in a patient when there is no *DSM-IV-TR* diagnosis.
2. Understand the treatment recommended for a patient with neurosis.

Considerations

This patient exhibits the classic Freudian problems of a patient with neurosis—"trouble working and loving." She procrastinates as a matter of course, resulting in her taking longer than usual to finish college and to complete her thesis. She lacks a long-term love relationship, although she would like one. She has insight into the fact that something that she is doing to herself is causing these problems. Otherwise, she has no signs or symptoms of a *DSM-IV-TR* disorder, and the results of her mental status examination are normal.

APPROACH TO NEUROSIS

Definitions

Insight-oriented psychotherapy: A type of therapy derived from psychoanalytic principles, but the frequency of the sessions can be once or twice a week and the length of the treatment can be as short as several weeks. The goal is still "to make the unconscious conscious," but on a more limited scale and in relation to a circumscribed life problem.

Neurosis: A central concept of psychoanalytic theory that describes "problems in living" not currently part of the *DSM-IV-TR*. It is a chronic, nonpsychotic condition characterized by anxiety. The anxiety can be expressed by way of defense mechanisms, becoming symptoms such as sexual inhibitions, phobias, or obsessions. Neurotic symptoms are thought to be caused by an unconscious conflict that generates anxiety; symptoms develop when an individual's defenses cannot adequately cope with this anxiety. The unconscious conflicts can involve forbidden wishes or feelings, which usually have roots in the individual's early development. For example, the woman cited in the case described can have an unconscious conflict about both competing in the professional world and seeking a love relationship; that is, she feels guilty about her wish to succeed in both, as if success in one would result in failure in the other.

Psychoanalysis: Freud created psychoanalysis for the treatment of neurotic symptoms. It is an intensive therapy usually involving an hour of therapy for 4 or 5 days a week over several years. The goal is to "make the unconscious conscious." Ideally, once patients have gained a full understanding of the roots of their unconscious fears and wishes, they are able to live life more fully. Psychoanalysis is used to treat individuals with neurotic or character pathology—but not those with psychoses or severe depression. It is demanding in terms of time and money, and so the patient must be functioning reasonably well in many areas of life.

Clinical Approach

The individual must experience chronic symptoms of anxiety—or anxiety expressed as inhibitions, fears, phobias, or obsessions—that he or she considers distressing and not acceptable. The anxiety or other symptoms must cause mild to moderate impairment in the individual's work and/or interpersonal life. There must be no psychotic disorder or other axis I or II disorder that can account for the anxiety, and no medical condition or substance use that can explain the condition.

Differential Diagnosis

Neurosis is not listed in the *DSM-IV-TR,* and there can be **considerable overlap** between patients who are considered to have a **neurosis** and those with **generalized anxiety disorder (GAD).** In a neurosis, there is usually evidence in the patient's history of an **intrapsychic conflict,** such as discomfort with achieving success in work. In contrast, patients with GAD can describe themselves as always having been anxious, with no particular focus or area of life as a nodal point. Neurotic obsessions or compulsions can mimic those of obsessive-compulsive disorder (OCD), but individuals with OCD do not have premorbid compulsive symptoms. Neurotic obsessions and compulsions are not as severe and are consistent with lifelong character traits.

In general, neurotic patients have no psychiatric history and function reasonably successfully overall; problems occur in a more circumscribed area of the personality. Patients with borderline personality disorder complain of some of the same symptoms but have serious problems identifying and managing their emotions (especially anger), lack a firm sense of self, and have a history of tumultuous relationships with others. They usually have a history of impulsive behavior, including self-destructive gestures or suicide attempts.

Treatment

Psychoanalysis or intensive psychodynamic therapy is the treatment of choice for neurosis. The unconscious meaning of symptoms becomes evident in the course of treatment, allowing the patient freedom to think, feel, and behave in ways more conducive to achieving life goals and ambitions. The process can be long-term in nature and does not follow a predetermined course; rather, the therapist works with the patient through typically 45-minute sessions to discover how the patient thinks and feels about the world. The theory is that this particular mode of thinking and feeling developed as a reaction to childhood events and to the environment in which the child found himself or herself. Although the particular ways of reacting to the world were adaptive in childhood, they have since become rigid and inflexible and are used in every situation in adulthood, thus precipitating neurotic symptoms and other "clashes" with the outside world. For example, a patient tells his therapist about his father and the unpredictable, harsh, and often punitive attitude his father had toward his son. As an adaptive response in childhood, the boy learned to be meek and to see authority figures as dangerous and something to be avoided. Although this worked well in allowing him to survive his childhood, it does not work well in the present, where as a man he is asked to be assertive with his bosses and colleagues, something he finds almost impossible. In psychotherapy, he learns about the coping skills he developed as a child, and after discussing with the therapist his feelings of anxiety about trying something else, he discovers that there are ways to approach authority figures other than the only one he thought was available.

Comprehension Questions

[51.1] A 27-year-old female teacher with no psychiatric history comes in for treatment with the complaint that a recent relationship with a boyfriend has failed; she states that she has had long-standing problems maintaining relationships with men and wishes to find "a solution." Since the breakup 4 weeks previously, she has had difficulty getting to sleep and frequently wakes up at 3 A.M. She has no appetite and has lost 7 lb. She complains that her concentration in the classroom has deteriorated, that she has lost interest in her students, and that she often has crying spells during the day. She has withdrawn from friends and colleagues recently. Which one of the following diagnoses must the clinician consider first?

A. Sleep disorder
B. Major depression
C. Neurosis
D. Eating disorder

[51.2] A 24-year-old male engineering student comes to the counseling center because of "problems with sex." He is heterosexual, is attracted to women, and is able to begin casual relationships. He experiences normal sexual excitement, but when the opportunity for intercourse occurs, he becomes anxious and cannot maintain an erection. He can masturbate without difficulty, and his family physician has told him that he is "completely normal physically." The man states that his father was a military officer who was absent for several years when the patient was in his early school years; the patient was an only child who was very close to his mother. He has no psychiatric history. Which of the following is the most appropriate treatment for this patient?

A. Cognitive behavioral therapy (CBT)
B. Antidepressant medication
C. Psychodynamic psychotherapy
D. Interpersonal therapy

[51.3] Which of the following best describes the difference between a neurotic patient and a patient with a personality disorder?

A. Neurotic patients are less functional than patients with a personality disorder.
B. Neurotic patients believe that their problems stem from inside themselves, whereas patients with personality disorders believe that their problems are the result of interactions with the people around them.
C. Patients with personality disorders are more easily treated with antidepressants than are neurotic patients.
D. Patients with personality disorders tend to be more motivated to seek psychotherapy than are neurotic patients.
E. Psychotherapy tends to be more successful with patients with personality disorders than with neurotic patients.

Answers

[51.1] **B.** Although there can indeed be a neurotic conflict underlying the patient's difficulty with men, she currently has symptoms of major depression that must be treated before intensive dynamic psychotherapy or psychoanalysis can be considered. Her weight loss is not severe and occurs in the context of the depression. Her sleep problems are also part of the depressive picture.

[51.2] **C.** Psychodynamic psychotherapy is indicated for this young man, who has a circumscribed conflict about performing sexually. Although additional history is needed, there is a suggestion that early conflicts about sexuality arose because his father was absent from the home at a time when normal children entertain fantasies about marrying the parent of the opposite sex. The patient is not depressed, and neither CBT nor interpersonal therapy is likely to elicit the unconscious conflict troubling him.

[51.3] **B.** Neurotic patients see their symptoms as ego-dystonic, that is, objectionable behavior coming from within themselves. Patients with personality disorders, in contrast, see their symptoms as ego-syntonic, that is, objectionable behavior coming from others, not themselves.

CLINICAL PEARLS

❖ Neuroses are seen in individuals who are generally doing well in life although they are **distressed** by their symptoms. They can identify and manage their emotions, have generally good interpersonal relationships, and have a stable sense of self.

❖ Psychodynamic psychotherapy is often helpful in treating individuals who are neurotic.

REFERENCES

Gabbard GO, Psychoanalysis. In: Sadock BJ, Sadock VA, eds., Comprehensive textbook of psychiatry, 7th ed., vol 1. Baltimore: Lippincott Williams & Wilkins, 2000:563–566.

Gabbard GO. Psychodynamic psychiatry in clinical practice, 3rd ed. Washington, DC: American Psychiatric Press, 2000:35–173.

❖ CASE 52

Eight hours after a psychiatric admission because of suicidal ideation, a 32-year-old woman begins to complain of feeling jittery and shaky. Six hours later, she tells staff members that she is hearing the voice of a dead relative shouting at her, although on admission she denied ever having heard voices previously. She complains of an upset stomach, irritability, and sweatiness. Her vital signs are blood pressure 150/95 mm Hg, pulse rate 120/min, respirations 20/min, and temperature 100.0°F (37.8°C). The patient reports no significant medical problems and says that she takes no medications.

- **What is the most likely diagnosis?**

- **What is the next step in the treatment of this disorder?**

ANSWERS TO CASE 52: Alcohol Withdrawal

Summary: Eight hours after admission to a hospital, a 32-year-old woman complains of feeling shaky. Six hours later, she is irritable, has gastrointestinal disturbances and hallucinations, and is diaphoretic. She is hypertensive, mildly febrile, and tachycardic. She reports no previous medical problems.

- **Most likely diagnosis:** Alcohol withdrawal.
- **Next step in treatment:** The patient should be treated with a benzodiazepine immediately, starting with high doses and tapering as she recovers.

Analysis

Objectives

1. Recognize the symptoms of alcohol withdrawal in a patient (see Table 52–1 for diagnostic criteria).
2. Be aware of the treatment recommendations that should be instituted immediately in a patient with this disorder.

Considerations

Because of her admission to the hospital, this patient was unable to continue her alcohol intake, and 8 hours after her last drink, she began to experience the signs and symptoms of alcohol withdrawal, which then worsened over the next 6 hours.

Table 52–1

DIAGNOSTIC CRITERIA FOR ALCOHOL WITHDRAWAL

- Cessation of or reduction in heavy, prolonged, alcohol use.
- Two or more of the following develop within hours to days:
  1. Autonomic hyperactivity
  2. Hand tremor
  3. Insomnia
  4. Nausea or vomiting
  5. Transient hallucinations
  6. Agitation
  7. Anxiety
  8. Seizures
- The symptoms cause distress or impairment in functioning.
- The symptoms are not due to a general medical condition or to another mental disorder.

APPROACH TO ALCOHOL WITHDRAWAL

Definitions

Diaphoresis: Excessive sweating.

Sympathomimetic: A substance that mimics at least some adrenalin or catecholamine responses. Examples of sympathomimetic substances include coffee, ephedrine, and amphetamines.

Clinical Approach

Alcohol functions as a depressant much like benzodiazepines and barbiturates. It has an effect on serotonin and gamma-aminobutyric acid type A (GABA-A) receptors, producing tolerance and habituation. Withdrawal symptoms usually, but not always, occur in stages: tremulousness or jitteriness (6 to 8 hours), psychosis and perceptual symptoms (8 to 12 hours), seizures (12 to 24 hours), and delirium tremens (DTs) (24 to 72 hours). Notably, **alcohol withdrawal, particularly DTs can be fatal.**

Differential Diagnosis

Included in the differential diagnosis for alcohol withdrawal are other drug withdrawal states, especially sedative-hypnotic withdrawal. In fact, the criteria for withdrawal from substances such as benzodiazepines (most commonly short-acting, high-potency drugs) and barbiturates are identical to those for alcohol withdrawal. A carefully recorded history, a physical examination, and laboratory results indicative of long-term, heavy, alcohol use (e.g., evidence of cirrhosis or liver failure, macrocytic anemia, elevated liver transaminase levels) will point to the correct diagnosis.

Medical conditions with similar signs and symptoms must be ruled out. Examples of such conditions include thyroid storm (thyrotoxicosis), pheochromocytoma, and inappropriate use of beta-agonist inhalers or sympathomimetics.

Although hallucinations are rare in alcohol withdrawal without delirium, if present they can be confused with those of schizophrenia. Several features distinguish the two conditions: In alcohol withdrawal, the perceptual disturbances are transient, there is not necessarily a history of a psychotic illness, the associated symptoms of schizophrenia are not present, and the patient's reality testing ability remains intact.

Treatment

Severe alcohol withdrawal with autonomic instability (DTs) has a high mortality and requires stabilization in an acute medical facility. The most common treatment for alcohol withdrawal remains **benzodiazepines,** administered either orally or parenterally. If liver function is not impaired, a long-acting benzodiazepine such as chlordiazepoxide or diazepam can be given, although these drugs are absorbed erratically when injected and should be given orally. If there is concern about decreased liver function, a benzodiazepine such as oxazepam or lorazepam can be administered either orally or parenterally, as their metabolism is not dependent on liver function. Whatever the specific drug used, it should be given as frequently as necessary in order to normalize the vital signs and sedate the patient. The medicine should then be gradually tapered over the next several days, and the patient's vital signs monitored. Anticonvulsants such as carbamazepine and valproic acid are also effective in treating alcohol withdrawal, although it is a much less popular option in the United States given familiarity with treatment with benzodiazepines.

Comprehension Questions

[52.1] Which of the following signs is most characteristic of alcohol withdrawal?

A. Decreased blood pressure
B. Hypersomnia
C. Persistent hallucinations
D. Tremor

[52.2] Withdrawal from which of the following substances shares a similar presentation with withdrawal from alcohol?

A. Alprazolam
B. Cocaine
C. Heroin
D. Lysergic acid diethylamide (LSD)

[52.3] Activation of what neurotransmitter system is used most often in treating alcohol withdrawal?

A. Dopaminergic
B. GABA
C. Noradrenergic
D. Serotonergic

[52.4] A 63-year-old man presents to the emergency department with complaints of anxiety. He describes a long history of daily, heavy, alcohol use, and 2 days ago "quit cold turkey." He appears visibly tremulous, flushed, and diaphoretic. His temperature, blood pressure, and pulse rate are elevated. The results of his physical examination are otherwise unremarkable, but his laboratory tests demonstrate low serum albumin and low protein levels, as well as an elevated prothrombin time/partial prothrombin time value. He is admitted to the medical service for alcohol detoxification. Which of the following medications would be most appropriate in treating this patient?

A. Xanax (alprazolam)
B. Chlordiazepoxide
C. Diazepam
D. Lorazepam

Answers

[52.1] **D.** Tremor is the most characteristic sign of alcohol withdrawal. Vital signs are elevated in alcohol withdrawal because of autonomic hyperactivity. Patients generally have insomnia as a result, not hypersomnia. Although hallucinations are rare, if present, they are transient.

[52.2] **A.** Withdrawal from both benzodiazepines and barbiturates shares criteria identical to those for alcohol withdrawal because alcohol and sedative-hypnotics both act on the GABA system.

[52.3] **B.** Alcohol and sedative-hypnotics both increase GABA output in the brain. GABA is the major inhibitory neurotransmitter in the brain. The cross-tolerance of alcohol and sedative-hypnotics (such as benzodiazepines and barbiturates) allows these medications to be used in treating alcohol withdrawal.

[52.4] **D.** Although all these medications are benzodiazepines, only lorazepam is metabolized solely by glucuronidation, which is not dependent on liver functioning. The metabolism of the other benzodiazepines is much more dependent on liver function. In this patient (who has evidence of poor liver function), using high doses of medications that are dependent on liver function for their degradation could result in excessive drug levels in the blood of an overly sedated patient. Another reason for choosing lorazepam over chlordiazepoxide and diazepam is that its parenteral absorption is not as erratic, and a patient with significant withdrawal symptoms is not able to tolerate the administration of oral medications.

CLINICAL PEARLS

- ❖ Alcohol withdrawal can occur within hours to days after heavy use and can include elevated vitals signs, tremor, transient hallucinations, anxiety, and seizures.
- ❖ The criteria (and symptoms) of alcohol withdrawal are identical to those for sedative-hypnotic withdrawal.
- ❖ The treatment of choice for alcohol withdrawal is benzodiazepines. Anticonvulsants can also be used.
- ❖ Benzodiazepines not dependent on liver function, such as lorazepam and oxazepam, are often preferred in the treatment of alcohol withdrawal.

REFERENCES

Ebert M, Loosen P, Nurcombe B, eds. Current diagnosis and treatment in psychiatry. New York: McGraw-Hill, 2000:245–246.

Kaplan H, Sadock B. Synopsis of psychiatry, 9th ed. Baltimore: Lippincott Williams & Wilkins, 2004:777–779.

Myers H, Anton R. Treatment of alcohol withdrawal. Alcohol Health Res World 1998;22(1):38–43.

❖ CASE 53

A 26-year-old chromosomal male dressed as a woman comes to see a psychiatrist as part of the workup required before he is allowed to have the sex change operation that he desires. He tells the psychiatrist that he has always felt he is a girl. He says, "When I was born, there must have been some mistake. I should have had the body of a girl." Then, he notes that as a child he enjoyed playing with dolls and female playmates; he never seemed to fit in with those of his own male gender. He claims that he has adopted all the mannerisms of a woman, including dressing like one, since leaving home at age 16. He states that he always would have dressed this way but was forbidden to do so by his parents, from whom he is now estranged. He admits that he has had no sexual experiences with women. His first sexual encounter with a man occurred when he was 18 years old, and he is currently in a relationship with another man lasting for the past 4 years. He considers himself a "straight woman" and has never seen himself as a gay man.

On his mental status examination, the patient appears alert and oriented to person, place, and time. He is dressed in a blouse, skirt, jacket, nylons, and high heels and purports himself to be a woman. His grooming is good, and he cooperates fully during the examination. No abnormalities were found on his mental status examination.

◆ **What is the most likely diagnosis?**

◆ **What options are open to the patient other than sex reassignment surgery?**

ANSWERS TO CASE 53: Gender Identity Disorder

Summary: A 26-year-old man is referred to a psychiatrist as part of the workup for a sex change operation. He has a strong, persistent desire to be female and has dressed as a woman since age 16. His sexual experiences have been exclusively with men. The results of his mental status examination are normal.

- **Most likely diagnosis:** Gender identity disorder.
- **Options other than sex reassignment surgery:** Patients can take estrogen to create breasts and other feminine contours and undergo electrolysis to remove their male hair.

Analysis

Objectives

1. Recognize gender identity disorder in a patient (see Table 53–1 for diagnostic criteria).
2. Understand treatment options open to patients with this disorder.

Considerations

This patient has had a persistent desire to be female and has always been uncomfortable with his male body. As soon as he could, he adopted female dress and mannerisms, although this resulted in estrangement from his family. He has requested surgery in order to fulfill his desire to be a woman. His sexual preference is for men, although because he sees himself as a woman, he does not consider himself a homosexual.

Table 53–1
DIAGNOSTIC CRITERIA FOR GENDER IDENTITY DISORDER

1. A strong, persistent, cross-gender identification.
2. In children, this desire is manifested by
   a. Repeatedly stating that one is a member of the other sex
   b. Dressing in the attire of the other sex
   c. A preference for cross-sex roles in make-believe play
   d. A strong preference for playmates of the other sex
3. In adults, this desire is manifested by stated wishes to live and be treated as a member of the other sex.
4. A persistent discomfort with the patient's own sex and a sense of inappropriateness in this gender role; in adults, this is often accompanied by a preoccupation with getting rid of the sex characteristics with which one was born.
5. The disturbance is not concurrent with a physical intersex condition.
6. The disturbance is distressing to or impairs the functioning of the individual.

APPROACH TO GENDER IDENTITY DISORDER

Definition

Androgen Insensitivity syndrome: A type of intersex presentation where the patient is chromosomally a male, but does not respond developmentally to androgen, therefore, develops externally female genitalia.

Intersex: Intersex states are conditions where a newborn's sex organs (genitals) appear unusual, making it impossible to identify the sex of the baby from its outward appearance.

Clinical Approach

There are no epidemiologic data on the prevalence of gender identity disorder in children, adolescents, or adults. Males seem to be more affected than females. These individuals often suffer internal and external conflict and ridicule and need to be approached with sensitivity.

The main item in the differential diagnosis for gender identity disorder is simple nonconformity with stereotypic sex role behavior. For example, this includes being a "tomboy" as a girl or a "sissy" as a boy. Gender identity disorder goes far beyond this type of behavior. There is a profound disturbance in the patient's sense of identity in regard to being a male or a female. Transvestic fetishism, that is, cross-dressing in the clothes of the other sex, serves to create sexual excitement. Patients displaying these behaviors generally do not have other symptoms of gender identity disorder such as childhood cross-gender behaviors. In schizophrenia, delusions can occur in which patients believe that they are members of the other sex. However, these individuals actually believe that they *are* members of the other sex. Patients with gender identity disorder usually say that they *feel* as if they are members of the other sex but do not actually believe that they *are*.

Comprehension Questions

[53.1] Gender identity disorder with a sexual attraction to males has been diagnosed in a 15-year-old boy sent to a psychiatrist. His parents are extremely unhappy with the boy's insistence on wearing women's clothes and want the psychiatrist to provide therapy "so that he won't think like this any more." The boy is willing to talk to the psychiatrist but only if he can discuss the problems caused by the social ostracism he endures because of his wish to be a woman. Which of the following actions should the psychiatrist take?

A. Inform the patient that his gender dysphoria will likely remit in time with psychotherapy alone.
B. Inform the patient that psychotherapy has been found to be helpful but that sexual reassignment surgery is also an option once he is an adult.
C. Inform the parents that their child will likely only experiment with homosexual behavior and will turn to heterosexuality once he is an adult.
D. Inform the parents that they should forbid their son to wear women's clothes.
E. Inform the patient's school that mechanisms must be put in place to reduce his social ostracism.

[53.2] Which of the following disorders has been associated with gender identity disorder?

A. Separation anxiety disorder
B. Schizophrenia
C. Panic disorder
D. Tourette disorder
E. Bipolar disorder, mania

[53.3] A 29-year-old man with a diagnosis of gender identity disorder wishes to undergo sex reassignment surgery. Which of the following treatment steps is strongly related to a positive outcome of sex reassignment?

A. Screening the patient for psychopathology
B. Treating the patient with an antidepressant before surgery
C. Treating the patient with hormones
D. Real-life experience in the community
E. Ongoing supportive psychotherapy

Answers

[53.1] **B.** Gender identity disorders can be treated with psychotherapy and sex reassignment rehabilitation. Psychotherapy alone has not been found to be effective in relieving gender dysphoria and does not stop patients from continuing to be preoccupied with altering their sexual characteristics.

[53.2] **A.** Separation anxiety disorder is also present in many boys with gender identity disorder.

[53.3] **D.** According to the minimum standards of the Harry Benjamin International Gender Dysphoria Association, the real-life experience of living in the community in the desired sex role for at least 3 months before hormonal reassignment, and 12 months before surgical reassignment, is recommended. When participation in a real-life experience is successful, there is a much higher probability of a positive outcome for sex reassignment. Following protocols of this type, 85% to 97% of individuals report being satisfied with their rehabilitation.

CLINICAL PEARLS

- Patients with gender identity disorder feel as if they should have been born a member of the other sex.
- In the diagnosis of gender identity disorder, specifiers are used that identify the sexual attraction of the patient to others: sexually attracted to males, females, both, or neither.
- Psychotherapy should address, primarily, the problems these patients have with social ostracism and conflict.
- Patients with gender identity issues should be asked how they prefer to be referred to.
- Sexual reassignment surgery is an option for such patients.

REFERENCES

Ebert M, Loosen P, Nurcombe B, eds. Current diagnosis and treatment in psychiatry. New York: McGraw-Hill, 2000:584–586.

Goldman HH. Review of general psychiatry, 5th ed. New York: McGraw-Hill, 2000:367–371.

CASE 54

A 47-year-old man is referred to a psychiatrist at his employment assistance program because of continuing conflicts on the job. This is the third time the patient has been referred to a psychiatrist under just such circumstances. He lost two previous jobs because of conflicts with coworkers. The patient states that people do not like him and would like to see him fail. He cites as an example one instance in which one of his colleagues was late in sending him some material he needed, resulting in the patient being unable to complete his assignment in a timely fashion. Although the colleague apologized for the mistake, the patient says that he knows that this man is "out to get me fired." He has since broken off all contact with this coworker and refuses to speak with him directly, preferring to use only written communication.

On a mental status examination, the patient appears somewhat angry and suspicious. He glares intently at the interviewer and sits with his back to the wall. He repeatedly requests a clarification of questions, often asking, "What will this material be used for? I bet you are going to use it against me so that I will be fired." When the interviewer's pager goes off, the patient accuses him of trying to shorten the time allotted to him by arranging to have the pager interrupt them. The patient's mood is described as "fine," but his affect is tense and he appears suspicious and ill at ease. The patient's thought processes and thought content are both within normal limits.

- **What is the most likely diagnosis?**

- **What is the best strategy in approaching this patient?**

ANSWERS TO CASE 54: Paranoid Personality Disorder

Summary: A 47-year-old man comes to a psychiatrist because of conflicts with others at work. He appears suspicious of his colleagues and of the interviewing psychiatrist. He reads hidden meanings into benign remarks or actions (such as the pager going off). The results of his mental status examination are normal except for his paranoia, which does not reach delusional proportions.

◆ **Most likely diagnosis:** Paranoid personality disorder.

◆ **Best approach:** Form a working alliance with the patient.

Analysis

Objectives

1. Recognize paranoid personality disorder.
2. Maintain a respectful alliance in working with a patient with paranoid personality disorder.

Considerations

The presentation in the case vignette is probably one of the most common for these patients, who do not normally seek out mental health treatment. Although pervasive paranoia and suspiciousness characterize this patient, the **absence of any true paranoid delusions or hallucinations make an axis I psychotic disorder unlikely.** The psychiatrist should take a low-key approach and not try to overcompensate by making friends with the patient. He or she should provide clear, straightforward answers to all questions and explain everything that he or she is doing or recommending. When challenged with some kind of paranoid ideation (such as the patient's response to the pager going off), the psychiatrist should provide clear, direct reality testing. (For example, "I'm sorry the pager went off. I did not prearrange for it to go off. I will defer answering it until after we are finished talking.")

APPROACH TO PARANOID PERSONALITY DISORDER

Definitions

Delusions: Fixed, false beliefs about the world that cannot be corrected with reasoning, education, or information.

Hallucinations: False sensory perceptions not associated with any real sensory stimulus. Hallucinations can occur in all five senses (gustatory, olfactory, auditory, visual, tactile).

Ideas of reference: A person's false beliefs that people are talking about him or her.

Paranoid ideation: Suspiciousness that is less than delusional in nature.
Working alliance: A therapeutic relationship formed between patients and their physicians that allow them to interact in a constructive manner.

Clinical Approach

Patients with this disorder have a pervasive tendency to interpret the actions of others as being demeaning or deliberately harmful. These patients are often preoccupied with questioning the loyalty or trustworthiness of friends, even when this is unjustified. Patients are unforgiving of mistakes or slights, and they hold grudges. They believe that the motives of others are malevolent, and they are quick to react to defend their character. These counterattacks are almost always angry and hostile. As in all personality disorders, these symptoms cannot occur exclusively during the course of another psychiatric illness such as schizophrenia, or occur secondary to a general medical condition or the use of a substance.

Differential Diagnosis

Patients with paranoid personality disorder can be differentiated from those with schizophrenia because they do not have frankly psychotic symptoms such as delusions, hallucinations, or a formal thought disorder. They can be differentiated from those with a delusional disorder by the absence of fixed delusions, as the paranoia of patients with a personality disorder never reaches delusional proportions. Although one might consider the possibility of borderline personality disorder (BPD) in a patient who displays angry outbursts toward others, patients with paranoid personality disorder typically do not have other features seen in patients with BPD, such as involvement in many short-lived, tumultuous relationships or chronic feelings of emptiness.

Interview Tips

Patients with paranoid personality disorder can become even more suspicious when a physician tries to become too friendly or close because they wonder about the motives behind this behavior. Therefore, be honest and respectful toward the patient, but use a low-key approach. Acknowledge any mistakes made and expect to explain procedures in detail. Use reality testing where necessary. For example, "No, Mr. Jones, I did not arrange to have my pager go off in the middle of our meeting. Someone from the outside simply needed to speak with me, and therefore my secretary paged me."

Comprehension Questions

[54.1] A 36-year-old man comes to a physician's office with a chief complaint that "people are out to hurt me." Despite being reassured by his wife that this is untrue, the patient is convinced that men are observing his behavior and actions at home and at work, using telescopic lenses and taping devices. He has torn apart his office on more than one occasion looking for "bugs." The patient's wife says that this behavior is relatively new, appearing somewhat suddenly after the patient was robbed on the way to his car approximately 6 months previously. Which of the following symptoms best describes what the patient is experiencing?

A. Ideas of reference
B. Paranoid ideations
C. Paranoid delusions
D. Thought disorder
E. Hallucinations

[54.2] A 24-year-old woman with paranoid personality disorder comes to see her primary care physician for a physical examination. During the examination, the physician notes that the patient has a new systolic murmur. He would like to order an ultrasound examination. Which of the following is the best way to tell this to the patient?

A. Tell the patient she needs a heart test and that she should call the laboratory to request it.
B. Tell the patient that you have heard a heart murmur but that she need not worry because it probably is not serious.
C. Tell the patient that although you think she might be upset by the news, she needs a further examination because you have heard a heart murmur.
D. Do not tell the patient the news until a nurse is present in the room.
E. Tell the patient you have heard a heart murmur and that you will need to order a follow-up ultrasound examination, which you will explain.

[54.3] A 42-year-old woman undergoing psychotherapy storms into her therapist's office for her session and angrily accuses the therapist of "trying to undermine her intelligence." After a discussion with the therapist, it becomes clear that it is the patient who is second-guessing herself, thereby "undermining" her own intelligence. Which of the following defense mechanisms is this patient using?

A. Projection
B. Reaction formation
C. Identification with the aggressor
D. Intellectualization
E. Denial

Answers

[54.1] **C.** This patient's problem is more than mere suspiciousness; he has full-blown paranoid delusions, for example, fixed, false beliefs.

[54.2] **E.** The best way to work with a patient with paranoid personality disorder is to use a low-key approach but be honest and respectful.

[54.3] **A.** Projection is a defense mechanism by which individuals deal with conflict by falsely attributing to another their own unacceptable feelings, impulses, or thoughts. Blaming others for their own sentiments and actions directs the focus away from the person doing the accusing. For example, a patient who is angry with his therapist suddenly starts accusing the therapist of being angry with him.

CLINICAL PEARLS

- Patients with paranoid personality disorder show a pervasive distrust and suspiciousness of others, often interpreting others' motives as malevolent.
- This paranoid personality disorder belongs in cluster A, the "mad" cluster.
- Patients with this paranoid disorder need to be dealt with in a low-key, friendly manner without trying to be too close or friendly, which could increase the patient's suspiciousness.
- The difference between a patient with paranoid personality disorder and a patient with delusional disorder is really a matter of degree, the difference between paranoid ideations and paranoid delusions.

REFERENCES

Ebert M, Loosen P, Nurcombe B, eds. Current diagnosis and treatment in psychiatry. New York: McGraw-Hill, 2000:470–471.

Kaplan H, Sadock B. Synopsis of psychiatry, 9th ed. Baltimore: Lippincott Williams & Wilkins, 2004:1424–1426.

❖ CASE 55

A physician is called to see a 42-year-old man who was jailed on a robbery charge 48 hours previously. Twelve hours before the physician arrived, the patient began to complain of feeling anxious. The guards at the jail noted that he was nauseous, diaphoretic, and had muscle tics, so they called the physician. By the time the physician came to see the patient, the patient had a witnessed generalized tonic-clonic seizure, 30 seconds in duration and is now postictal. The results of a subsequent urine toxicology screening are positive for cocaine, opiates, and benzodiazepines.

◆ **What is the most likely etiology of the patient's seizures?**

◆ **What treatment would you recommend for this patient?**

ANSWERS TO CASE 55: Benzodiazepine Withdrawal

Summary: A 42-year-old man whose urine toxicology screening showed positive results for cocaine, opiates, and benzodiazepines had a seizure 48 hours after he was arrested and put in jail. Twelve hours prior to the seizure, he noted feeling anxious and was observed to be nauseous, diaphoretic, and to have muscle tics.

◆ **Most likely diagnosis:** Benzodiazepine withdrawal. Additionally, cocaine/opioid/benzodiazepine abuse versus dependence should be considered.

◆ **Best treatment:** The patient should be transferred to an acute care medical facility and initially treated with a benzodiazepine that should be slowly tapered so that the withdrawal symptoms do not reappear.

Analysis

Objectives

1. Recognize benzodiazepine withdrawal in a patient (see Table 55–1 for diagnostic criteria).
2. Understand the principles of treatment for patients in this state.

Considerations

Forty-eight hours after he was jailed, this patient began displaying signs and symptoms classic for benzodiazepine withdrawal, namely, anxiety, sweating, intolerance of loud noises or lights, muscle twitching, and ultimately seizures. The other drugs in his system are less likely to contribute to the etiology. Opiate withdrawal (see Case 31) is usually characterized by abdominal cramping, rhinorrhea, diarrhea, nausea, and vomiting. Cocaine withdrawal typically causes depressive symptoms, anxiety, irritability, hypersomnolence, and fatigue. In contrast to benzodiazepine withdrawal, opiate withdrawal and cocaine withdrawal are not life-threatening. Because of the danger involved, the patient should be transferred to a hospital where he can be carefully monitored.

Table 55–1

DIAGNOSTIC CRITERIA FOR ANXIOLYTIC WITHDRAWAL

1. Cessation or reduction in the use of an anxiolytic drug.
2. Two or more of the following symptoms occur following cessation of use of the drug: autonomic hyperactivity, hand tremor, insomnia, nausea, hallucinations, agitation, anxiety, and seizures.
3. Symptoms should not be due to a general medical condition.

APPROACH TO ANXIOLYTIC WITHDRAWAL

Definitions

Anxiolytic drugs: Medications used to treat anxiety. Most commonly, they include the class of drugs called benzodiazepines but can also include barbiturates as well as miscellaneous medications such as buspirone and chloral hydrate.

Flumazenil: A benzodiazepine antagonist that is used in the emergency department to treat benzodiazepine overdose. Its principal danger is that it can precipitate severe withdrawal.

Withdrawal: The pattern of symptoms exhibited by a person after repeated use of a drug and the physiologic effect that occurs on its discontinuation. Withdrawal is also called discontinuance syndrome.

Clinical Approach

A large number of Americans use benzodiazepines, either properly prescribed (as an anxiolytic or hypnotic) or recreationally. Like barbiturates, benzodiazepines have their primary effect on the gamma-aminobutyric acid type A (GABA-A) receptor complex, altering chloride ion influx (Figure 55–1). Withdrawal from both barbiturates and benzodiazepines can be life-threatening. Seizures can result from benzodiazepine withdrawal. The severity

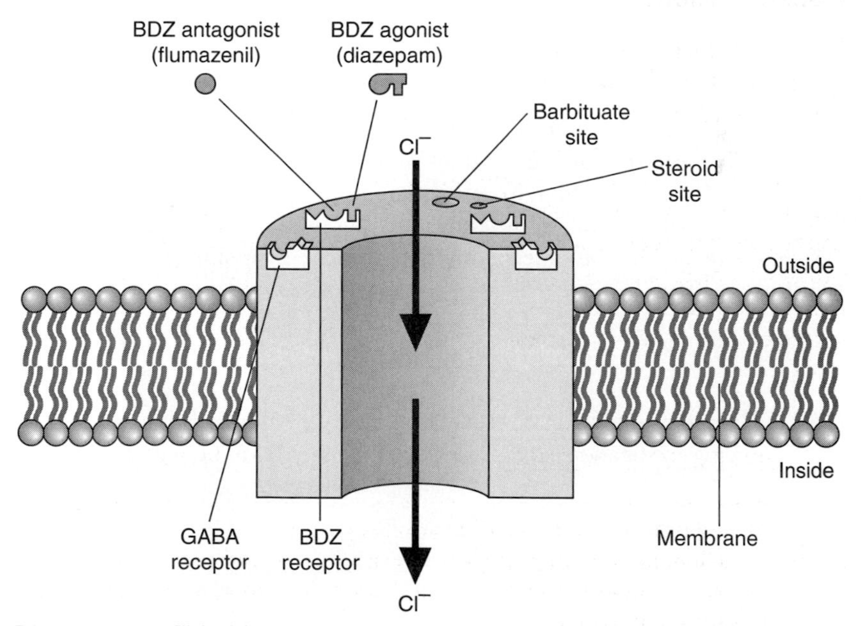

Figure 55–1. Chloride channel showing a benzodiazepine receptor on a cell membrane.

of benzodiazepine withdrawal varies according to duration of use, dose, and the half-life of the agent. Symptoms such as anxiety, photophobia, nausea, diaphoresis, muscle twitching, and seizures can occur.

Differential Diagnosis

Withdrawal from anxiolytics can be confused with withdrawal from other substances, but a carefully recorded history of the symptoms can usually differentiate the two. Opioid withdrawal typically induces abdominal pains, salivation, lacrimation, rhinorrhea, urination, and defecation. Cocaine withdrawal causes a "crash" in which the individual becomes hypersomnic and hyperphagic, in addition to having a strong craving for the drug. Alcohol withdrawal can be manifested by many symptoms similar to those of benzodiazepine withdrawal and can be life-threatening as well, but a history of heavy, sustained use of alcohol is usually present. Panic disorders can cause acute anxiety, diaphoresis, and palpitations, but they typically occur "out of the blue," and a history of a recent cessation of benzodiazepine use is not present. However, since many patients with panic disorder are treated with benzodiazepines, the clinical picture is often confounded.

Treatment

To prevent seizures and other withdrawal symptoms, the clinician should, if possible, **slowly taper the dose of the benzodiazepine** rather than abruptly discontinuing it. Some reports have noted that the addition of carbamazepine can be useful in preventing withdrawal seizures in individuals prone to developing them.

Flumazenil, a benzodiazepine receptor antagonist, reverses the effects of benzodiazepines. Although it may have some future use as an Antabuse (disulfiram)-like medication to help patients addicted to benzodiazepines refrain from using them, it is currently not used in this manner and is **restricted to use in the emergency department in instances of benzodiazepine overdose.**

Comprehension Questions

[55.1] When discontinued after several weeks of treatment, which of the following medications is most likely to cause anxiolytic withdrawal?

A. Propranolol
B. Fluoxetine
C. Clonidine
D. Alprazolam
E. Lithium

[55.2] Which of the following medications is likely to cause the most severe discontinuation syndrome?

A. Clonazepam
B. Alprazolam
C. Temazepam
D. Restoril
E. Librium

[55.3] The patient in the described case vignette is discharged home the next day with appropriate medications to manage his withdrawal. His spouse brings him back to the hospital that evening with the following symptoms: slurred speech, unsteady gait, and nystagmus. Which of the following is the most likely diagnosis for the patient at this time?

A. Withdrawal
B. Discontinuance syndrome
C. Intoxication
D. Dependence
E. Delirium

Answers

[55.1] **D.** Alprazolam is the only anxiolytic listed in the choices. It is the generic name for Xanax and is classified as a benzodiazepine. These medications act on endogenous benzodiazepine receptors, enhancing the effects of GABA.

[55.2] **B.** Medications in the class of drugs called benzodiazepines all have a potential to produce withdrawal syndromes if they are taken long enough and in large enough doses. The ones with the most potential, however, are those with the shortest half-lives and fastest onsets of action. Of the benzodiazepine drugs listed, alprazolam best fits this description. Because seizures are a common occurrence in benzodiazepine withdrawal, Tegretol (carbamazepine) can be useful in its treatment, as well as the administration of a long-acting benzodiazepine, which is then subsequently slowly tapered.

[55.3] **C.** The symptoms and clinical history suggest the acute ingestion and effects of a benzodiazepine drug.

CLINICAL PEARLS

- ❖ Anxiolytic medications include several classes of medication, most commonly benzodiazepines.
- ❖ A withdrawal syndrome is most likely associated with the abuse of benzodiazepines with shorter half-lives and shorter onsets of action.

REFERENCES

Ebert M, Loosen P, Nurcombe B, eds. Current diagnosis and treatment in psychiatry. New York: McGraw-Hill, 2000:234.

Kaplan H, Sadock B. Synopsis of psychiatry, 9th ed. Baltimore: Lippincott Williams & Wilkins, 2004:1333–1334.

❖ CASE 56

An 8-year-old boy is brought to a psychiatrist by his parents because he is having increasing difficulty keeping up academically with his classmates. His parents report that he has always been a slow learner but that they were not really aware of how significant their son's difficulties were until this year, when their other child, a 5-year-old girl, started school. Their daughter is progressing much more quickly and easily than their 8-year-old son did. His teacher says that their son is pleasant but is behind the class in the acquisition of skills in all areas. In preschool, the teacher reported that he had a tendency to hit others, but he does this much less often now. He gets along with other children well, although he seems to enjoy the company of his younger sibling's friends over his same-age peers.

The parents report that their son met all his developmental milestones at the low end of the normally expected range, but their pediatrician told them not to be concerned. He has never had any significant medical illnesses and had an uneventful prenatal period and birth.

◆ **What is the most likely diagnosis?**

◆ **What are the next diagnostic steps?**

 **What is the role of the psychiatrist in the care of this patient?**

ANSWERS TO CASE 56: Mild Mental Retardation

Summary: An 8-year-old boy is brought to a psychiatrist because he is a "slow learner" and has fallen behind his peers in class. He has a history of being aggressive to some degree in preschool, although he seems to have "grown out" of this behavior. His parents do not report any significant current or past medical conditions. He has a younger sister who is doing well and surpasses him in academic and social skills.

- **Most likely diagnosis:** Mental retardation, mild.
- **Diagnostic steps:** Some form of individualized intelligence testing is required in addition to an assessment of the patient's current adaptive functioning. It can be necessary to supplement intelligence testing with other educational testing to assure that the patient does not have learning disabilities that inhibit his performance on the intelligence tests, thus producing a lower intelligence quotient (IQ) score than would otherwise occur.
- **Role of the psychiatrist:** If there are no acute symptoms requiring medication management, a child psychiatrist typically serves in a coordinating or consulting role in cases such as this one. Helping the parents obtain appropriate evaluations and referrals suited to the child's needs is vital. Monitoring for the development of a psychiatric illness in the child is also important.

Analysis

Objectives

1. Understand the diagnostic criteria for mental retardation (Table 56–1).
2. Understand the role of the psychiatrist in the treatment of mental retardation.

Table 56–1
DIAGNOSTIC CRITERIA FOR MENTAL RETARDATION

1. Significantly subaverage intellectual functioning: an intelligence quotient (IQ) of 70 or below on an appropriately administered IQ test (Table 56–2)
2. Concurrent deficits or impairment in adaptive functioning in at least two of the following areas: communication, self-care, home living, social/interpersonal skills, use of community resources, self-direction, functional academic skills, work, leisure, health, and safety
3. Onset occurs before age 18

Considerations

An 8-year-old boy is brought to a psychiatrist because his parents have noticed that he has global deficits in both social and educational skills. They became more aware of their son's deficits after he entered school. The couple now has a younger daughter who surpasses her older brother in skill acquisition and development. When intelligence testing is completed, the child will likely score in the mildly deficient range. On adaptive testing, he will likely score in the deficient range as well.

APPROACH TO MENTAL RETARDATION

Definitions

Adaptive functioning tests: Psychological assessments that measure social, communication, daily living, and community functioning skills. A collateral source who knows the patient well is required to answer questions needed to complete the assessment. Some of these skills can be measured with the Vineland Social Maturity Scale, a test commonly used.

Down syndrome: Trisomy 21, which is associated with hypotonia, language and motor developmental delay, and typical facial features. It is the most common cause of moderate to severe mental retardation in the United States.

Fragile X syndrome: The second most common cause of mental retardation, resulting from a mutation at the *Xq27.3* locus. Males generally have moderate to severe mental retardation, and female carriers are less severely affected.

Intelligence tests: Psychological assessments that measure intellectual capacity. The results of these tests vary based on educational attainment. The most commonly used tests include the Wechsler scales (the Wechsler Preschool and Primary Scale of Intelligence, the Wechsler Intelligence Scale for Children, and the Wechsler Adult Intelligence Scale), and the Stanford-Binet Scale.

Clinical Approach

The prevalence of mental retardation is approximately 1% of the population, with males being more affected than females. There are a multitude of etiologies, including genetics, prenatal infections and toxins, prematurity, and acquired conditions. In one third of individuals, no cause can be identified. Down syndrome, fragile X syndrome, and phenylketonuria (PKU) are common etiologies for moderate to severe mental retardation. Mild mental retardation is often associated with a familial pattern. A diagnosis of this disorder requires a diminished capacity for cognitive functioning measured by an objective intelligence test, as well as a diminished capacity for adaptive functioning in multiple environments (see Table 56–2 for degrees of mental retardation). The causes of mental retardation are numerous, as are the treatments. General causes include genetic prenatal problems such as chromosomal abnormalities or mutations, prenatal causes related to an external source such as toxins or infections, and postnatal causes such as anoxia, infection, or deprivation experienced by an infant after birth.

Differential Diagnosis

Specific communication or learning disorders must be differentiated from mental retardation, which is associated with greater global functional impairment.

Table 56–2
DEGREES OF MENTAL RETARDATION AND FUNCTION

SEVERITY OF RETARDATION	INTELLIGENCE QUOTIENT	CHARACTERISTICS	FUNCTION
Mild	50–55 to about 70	Usually not detected until child attends school; individual usually completes a high level of elementary school	**Can often live and work independently** with social support
Moderate	35–40 to 50–55	Social isolation in elementary school	Can be competent at occupational tasks in supportive setting; **need a high level of supervision**
Severe	20–25 to 35–40	Minimal speech, poor motor development	May accomplish some degree of self-care; needs extensive supervision; **not independent**
Profound	Below 20–25	Absent to minimal speech, poor to absent motor skills	Needs constant supervision; **nursing care needed throughout life**

Patients with pervasive development disorder frequently have uneven areas of deficit, particularly in regard to social interaction skills. Onset must be before the age of 18. If the impairment is noted after the age of 18 years, dementia and its various causes should be considered.

Therapeutic Approach

There are several principles behind the treatment of mental retardation. The first is the concept of **prevention.** Whenever possible, potential causes of mental retardation should be minimized: **Women should abstain from drinking alcohol during pregnancy,** should receive **appropriate immunizations before becoming pregnant and should get proper nutrition including folic acid and other vitamin supplements.** The next specific treatment involves the minimization of causes wherever possible. The best example of this is **diet restrictions for babies born with PKU.** Although the genetic problem cannot be corrected, the environmental exposure that allows this problem to be manifested can be controlled. The next level of treatment involves interventions designed to lessen the impact of mental retardation early in a child's life. These might include early education, speech therapy, occupational therapy, family support, and respite care.

Appropriate medical care should also be provided, as medical problems can complicate the progress of a child with mental retardation. Finally, clinicians should realize that children with mental retardation might also have any one of a number of mental illnesses seen in the nonretarded population. Depression, anxiety, psychosis, and conduct disorders are common in the mentally retarded population but often go undetected. Specific treatments for these disorders in this population do not usually differ from treatments for those in the nonretarded population.

In individuals with moderate to profound retardation, it is important to remember that medical conditions causing pain can result in aggressive or self-destructive behavior in an individual with limited means of communicating. Whenever evaluating a mentally retarded individual for aggressive or self-destructive behavior, a complete physical exam and medical reassessment is indicated rather than immediately proceeding with psychotropic medication.

Comprehension Questions

[56.1] A person with which degree of mental retardation is usually able to hold a job?

A. All levels
B. Mild only
C. Moderate and mild
D. Severe, moderate, and mild

[56.2] Which of the following is the most common cause of mental retardation?

A. Fragile X syndrome
B. Genetic deficits
C. Idiopathic or unknown
D. In utero exposure to toxins
E. Lead intoxication

[56.3] An 18-year-old boy has benefitted from training in social and occupational skills but has been unable to progress beyond the second-grade level in academic subjects. He needs supervision and guidance when under mild social or economic stress. Which level of mental retardation is being described?

A. Mild
B. Moderate
C. Severe
D. Profound

Answers

[56.1] **B.** Although persons with all degrees of mental retardation can require some support to function in the community, those with mild mental retardation are able to hold a job. Individuals with moderate mental retardation are often able to manage small amounts of money and make change. Persons with severe and profound mental retardation have limited abilities to manage themselves and have difficulty learning these skills.

[56.2] **C.** Although each of the conditions listed is associated with mental retardation, the largest percentage continues to be attributed to idiopathic causes.

[56.3] **B.** This description refers to a person with moderate mental retardation.

CLINICAL PEARLS

- Mental retardation is coded on axis II.
- Two pieces of information are needed to make a diagnosis of mental retardation: An intelligence quotient score and evidence of deficits in adaptive functioning are both required.
- **In individuals with moderate to profound retardation, it is important to remember that medical conditions causing pain can result in aggressive or self-destructive behavior in an individual with limited means of communicating.**
- The impairment associated with mental retardation is global and fairly consistent across all areas of functioning.

REFERENCES

King BH, Hodapp RM, Dykens EM. Mental retardation. In: Sadock BJ, Sadock VA, eds. Kaplan and Sadock's comprehensive textbook of psychiatry, 7th ed. Philadelphia: Lippincott Williams & Wilkins, 2000:2587–2613.

❖ CASE 57

A 24-year-old man was admitted to the neurology service with new-onset blindness. The man awoke one morning totally unable to see. A workup by the neurology service revealed no physical reason for this abnormality—the patient was found to be otherwise healthy. A psychiatric consultation was then called.

The patient tells the psychiatrist that he does not know why he is blind. He says that he emigrated from Mexico several years ago, coming to the United States to make some money to support his sick mother. She was ill for several years, but he was not able to send her much money because he became addicted to heroin after arriving in the United States and used all his money to purchase drugs. She died recently, and he became despondent because he would never see her again.

On a mental status examination, the patient is alert and oriented to person, place, and time. His appearance and hygiene are good, and he does not seem to be overly concerned with his blindness. His mood is described as "Okay," and his affect is congruent and full-range. He has normal thought processes and denies having suicidal or homicidal ideation, delusions, or hallucinations.

◆ **What is most likely diagnosis for this patient?**

◆ **What is best therapy for this patient?**

ANSWERS TO CASE 57: Conversion Disorder

Summary: A 24-year-old man presents with new-onset blindness for which there is no physiologic explanation. The patient says that his mother died recently, after he was unable to send her money because he was addicted to drugs. He does not seem to be bothered by his blindness.

- **Most likely diagnosis:** Conversion disorder.
- **Best therapy:** Hypnosis, anxiolytics, or behavioral relaxation exercises may be helpful in treating an acute onset of conversion disorder. Amobarbital or lorazepam administered parenterally may be helpful in obtaining additional information, especially when a patient has recently experienced a traumatic event.

Analysis

Objectives

1. Recognize conversion disorder in a patient (see Table 57–1 for diagnostic criteria).
2. Be familiar with the acute treatment of patients with this disorder.

Considerations

This patient presents with a new onset of blindness following his mother's death, and he realizes that he will never be able to "see" her again. A component of guilt is involved because the patient came to the United States to earn money to help his mother but could not fulfill this obligation because he became addicted to heroin. There is no physiologic explanation for his blindness, and the patient seems to be unconcerned about it, displaying *la belle indifference.*

Table 57–1
DIAGNOSTIC CRITERIA FOR CONVERSION DISORDER

1. One or more sensory or motor deficits suggesting a neurologic or medical illness.
2. Psychological factors are associated because the deficit is preceded by conflicts or stressors.
3. The symptom is not intentionally produced.
4. The deficit cannot be fully explained by a medical condition, a substance of abuse, or a culturally sanctioned response.
5. The deficit causes significant distress and impairment in functioning or warrants medical evaluation.
6. The symptom is not limited to pain or sexual dysfunction and does not occur exclusively during somatization disorder.

APPROACH TO CONVERSION DISORDER

Definition

La belle indifference: Inappropriate lack of concern about one's disability

Clinical Approach

Ruling out an underlying medical or neurologic condition is very important when considering a diagnosis of conversion disorder. It is not unheard of for this disorder to be misdiagnosed in patients who are later found to have multiple sclerosis. However, it is not always a case of either/or. As listed in the criteria, the symptom or deficit cannot be *fully* explained by a general medical condition. In other words, it is quite common for individuals with underlying neurologic diseases to also develop conversion symptoms that do not conform to anatomic or physiologic parameters. For example, a patient with a diagnosed seizure disorder can display additional seizure-like movements without corresponding epileptic discharges appearing on an electroencephalogram. In such cases, conversion symptoms occurring on top of an established illness provide a mode of communication that expresses unconscious conflict.

Also, in the differential diagnosis are other somatoform disorders such as somatization disorder, undifferentiated somatoform disorder, and hypochondriasis, as well as factitious disorders and malingering. Somatization disorder is a chronic disorder that includes many physical symptoms, such as pain in several areas, gastrointestinal complaints, sexual symptoms, and a conversion symptom. In undifferentiated somatoform disorder, one or more physical complaints, such as fatigue, gastrointestinal symptoms, or urinary difficulties, are present that are not neurologic in nature. Hypochondriasis is a chronic fear of having a serious illness as a result of misinterpretation of bodily sensations. Factitious disorders involve the intentional production of physical or psychologic symptoms in order to assume the sick role. **Malingering** involves the intentional production or exaggeration of symptoms motivated by external incentives (avoiding a jail sentence, military duty, or work, or obtaining financial compensation). There is often considerable misunderstanding about the differences among conversion disorder, factitious disorder, and malingering. In the first, there is an *unconscious* production of symptoms because of conflicts or stressors, whereas in the latter two, there is a *conscious* production of symptoms.

Clinical Course and Treatment

In most cases, a conversion symptom resolves on its own, even without treatment. However, it is not at all unusual for the same or similar problems to recur, especially in the presence of a new stressor or conflict. Patients with conversion disorder tend to be highly responsive to suggestion. Reassurance coupled with a comment such as, "Under stress, the body can react in unusual ways; this will likely get better soon on its own," can often result in resolution of the symptoms over several days. It is important not to imply that patients are exaggerating, faking, or consciously producing their symptoms or that their problems are "all in their heads." This approach only tends to alienate the patient, create more stress, and possibly worsen the deficit. Hypnosis or Amytal Sodium (amobarbital sodium) interviews can be helpful in probing deeper into the nature of the unconscious conflict. Hospitalization for conversion disorder is rarely necessary, except in cases where the disability is so severe as to preclude the activities of daily living. In such cases, the patient is usually discharged within several days, after symptoms have resolved.

Comprehension Questions

[57.1] Which of the following characteristics most distinguishes conversion disorder from other somatoform disorders?

A. Symptoms are not fully explained by a medical cause.
B. Symptoms are not intentionally produced.
C. Symptoms involve only motor or sensory neurologic deficits.
D. Psychological factors are related to symptom production.

[57.2] Which of the following is most characteristic of individuals with conversion disorder?

A. Male predominance
B. Higher socioeconomic status
C. Less education
D. Greater psychological insight

[57.3] Which of the following personality disorders is most commonly associated with conversion disorder?

A. Avoidant
B. Histrionic
C. Narcissistic
D. Schizotypal

[57.4] Which of the following is the most effective approach to patients with conversion disorder?

A. Confrontation about intentionally producing symptoms
B. Explaining that their symptoms are not real
C. Reassurance that a neurologic cause will be found
D. Suggestion that symptoms will improve with time

Answers

[57.1] **C.** In all somatoform disorders, the symptoms, pain, deficits, or preoccupation with a serious illness are not fully explained by a medical condition or are out of proportion. None of these symptoms are intentionally produced, as in factitious disorder or malingering. Psychological factors (conflicts or stress) are associated with the creation, exacerbation, and/or maintenance of the symptoms in all these disorders. Although somatization disorder involves a pseudoneurologic symptom, additional symptoms are also required. Conversion disorder is distinguished by having *only* a motor or sensory deficit.

[57.2] **C.** In general, conversion disorder tends to be more common in individuals with less education, a lower socioeconomic status, and less psychological insight. It has a strong female predominance.

[57.3] **B.** Histrionic personality disorder is most commonly associated with conversion disorder. Patients with both types of disorders tend to display a dramatic presentation and are highly responsive to suggestion as well as to hypnosis. Borderline personality disorder is not uncommonly seen in factitious disorder, and antisocial behavior is often found in those who malinger.

[57.4] **D.** Although the deficits often remit spontaneously, suggesting that they will improve can facilitate the process. These patients do not intentionally produce their symptoms, and explaining that their deficits are not real may aggravate the situation and worsen their problems. Whereas reassurance about their likely *improvement* is appropriate, implying that their symptoms are caused by a neurologic illness (assuming that this has been ruled out) may serve only to reinforce their defensive use of a physical illness to express their psychological problems.

CLINICAL PEARLS

- Conversion disorder involves one or more sensory or motor deficits.
- Conversion disorder symptoms are not intentionally produced but rather are the result of an unconscious conflict.
- It is important to rule out an underlying medical or neurologic illness because a significant proportion of individuals initially presenting with conversion symptoms eventually develop an established illness.
- A suggestion by the treating physician that deficits will improve results in the remission of symptoms in most cases.

REFERENCES

Ebert M, Loosen P, Nurcombe B, eds. Current diagnosis and treatment in psychiatry. New York: McGraw-Hill, 2000:366–369.

Kaplan H, Sadock B. Synopsis of psychiatry, 8th ed. Baltimore: Lippincott Williams & Wilkins, 1998:634–637.

❖ CASE 58

A 32-year-old man and his 28-year-old wife come to a psychiatrist because of problems in their relationship. The wife states that the two have been married for 6 months and that they had dated for 2 months prior to that. During all their sexual encounters, the husband insists that the wife wear very high-heeled shoes at all times. Although the wife initially thought that this behavior was sexy, she now worries that it is the shoes that the husband finds attractive and not her. She thinks the behavior is "freaky" and has asked the husband to stop, which he has refused to do. The husband states that he is unable to achieve an erection or orgasm without the presence of the shoes. He notes that for as long as he can remember, he has needed high-heeled shoes as part of his sexual play. He feels no shame or guilt about this behavior, although he is worried that it is causing problems between him and his wife.

◆ **What is the most likely diagnosis for the husband?**

◆ **What is the course of and prognosis for this disorder?**

ANSWERS TO CASE 58: Fetishism

Summary: A 32-year-old man insists that his wife wear very high-heeled shoes during all sexual encounters. This behavior causes problems in their marriage, and the patient has refused to stop because he is unable to achieve an erection or an orgasm without the presence of the shoes. This association with sexual arousal and orgasm has been a long-standing one for the patient. Although he feels no shame or guilt about it, he is concerned about its impact on his marriage.

- **Most likely diagnosis:** Fetishism.
- **Course of and prognosis for this disorder:** The course of this disorder is chronic, and it has a poor prognosis.

Analysis

Objectives

1. Recognize the diagnostic criteria of fetishism in a patient (Table 58–1).
2. Understand the course, prognosis, and mitigating factors of this disorder.

Considerations

The patient has a long history of using high-heeled shoes to achieve erection and orgasm during intercourse. He cannot achieve either without the presence of the shoes. He does not feel guilty about his behavior but is worried that his wife now objects to it and that it is causing friction in his marriage. A poor prognosis is associated with an early age of onset, a high frequency of acts, no guilt or shame about the act, and substance abuse. (The patient has three of these factors.) The course and prognosis are better when the patient has a history of intercourse without paraphilic activity, when the patient has a strong motivation to change, and when the patient is self-referred. (This patient has none of these factors—although he was not referred for treatment by a legal agency, it can be assumed that his wife suggested the visit to the psychiatrist.)

Table 58–1

DIAGNOSTIC CRITERIA FOR FETISHISM

1. An individual has intense, recurring sexual desires or behaviors focused on inanimate objects such as shoes or female underwear; the desires must be present for at least 6 months.
2. The sexual fantasies, desires, or behaviors must be disturbing to the individual or cause a problem with social or occupational functioning (such as marital conflict).
3. The individual does not wear the fetishistic objects (as in transvestic fetishism).

APPROACH TO FETISHISM

Definitions

Erectile dysfunction: Difficulty in obtaining and maintaining an erection can have a psychological or an organic cause. Some studies report that erectile dysfunction has an organic basis in 20% to 50% of men with this disorder. This can include a large number of diseases such as diabetes, malnutrition, cirrhosis, chronic renal failure, atherosclerosis, and a host of others. Medications can also impair male sexual functioning, and many psychiatric drugs (antidepressants, mood stabilizers, and antipsychotics), as well as antihypertensives and other drugs, can be to blame. To differentiate psychological causes from organic ones, a study of nocturnal penile tumescence (erections occurring during sleep) is often made. In patients who **have normal nocturnal erections** but erectile dysfunction during their waking hours, or with a partner, the problem is much more likely to have a **psychological cause.**

Fetishism: A paraphilia in which the individual seeks sexual gratification primarily through contact with an object, such as shoes or underwear, which is closely associated with the body. Fetishists are mostly male, and fetishism usually starts in adolescence. The individual can masturbate with the fetishistic object or incorporate it into sexual intercourse.

Paraphilia: A disorder in which an individual primarily seeks sexual gratification through means considered abnormal by society. Paraphilias include fetishism, voyeurism, exhibitionism, sadism, masochism, transvestism, and pedophilia. What is considered normal sexual behavior varies greatly among different cultures. Many individuals have more than one paraphilia.

Transsexual: A person who feels as if he or she is "trapped in the body of the wrong gender," for example, a man who believes that he is really a woman although genetically and functionally he is male.

Transvestite: A heterosexual male who dresses in female clothing.

Vaginismus: An involuntary muscle constriction of the outer third of the vagina that causes marked distress or interpersonal difficulty and interferes with sexual intercourse. A diagnosis of vaginismus is not made when there is an organic cause for the disorder or when it is better accounted for by another mental disorder such as somatization disorder.

Clinical Approach

Differential Diagnosis

Paraphilias tend to be compound; the presence of one should prompt the clinician to inquire about others. There are few conditions in the differential diagnosis for fetishism; one is transvestism, in which fetishistic clothing is worn to produce sexual excitement.

Treatment

Fetishism, like most paraphilias, is difficult to treat. The presence of only one paraphilia, normal intelligence, an absence of substance dependence, and stable adult relationships are all good prognostic indicators. Fetishists do not usually seek treatment voluntarily. Interventions for fetishism include cognitive behavioral therapy (CBT) and insight-oriented psychotherapy. Cognitive behavioral therapy includes sex education, social skills training, and a reevaluation of the ways in which the individual rationalizes the behavior. Treatment can involve desensitization to the fetish, relaxation techniques, and learning to avoid triggers for the fetishism. Psychodynamic psychotherapy explores the roots of the behavior, the events that caused development of the fetish in childhood or adolescence. This form of therapy also focuses on improving relationships with others.

Comprehension Questions

[58.1] A married pharmacist comes in for treatment at the insistence of his wife, who was disturbed to find that he was wearing some of her undergarments under his clothes. He admitted to her that he often masturbated when wearing her underwear and fantasized about wearing it while having intercourse with her. Which of the following words best define this paraphilia?

A. Exhibitionism
B. Fetishism
C. Transvestism
D. Voyeurism

[58.2] Which of the following is a poor prognostic indicator in the treatment of fetishists?

A. A stable adult relationship
B. Presence of another paraphilia
C. Normal intelligence
D. Self-referral for treatment

[58.3] Which of the following statements can be most accurately applied to fetishism?

A. It is a disorder that tends to last less that 1 year.
B. The object of focus tends to be unrelated to the human body.
C. The disorder occurs predominantly in men.
D. The disorder usually first manifests itself when patients are in their thirties.

[58.4] A 55-year-old man complains of inability to achieve an erection. He has been worried about his health recently and takes antihypertensive medication. Which of the following would most likely differentiate between an organic and psychiatric condition?

A. A lower-extremity myographic examination
B. Magnetic resonance imaging of the lumbosacral spine
C. An erection on awakening in the morning
D. The interpretation of projective tests
E. An electroencephalographic reading

Answers

[58.1] **C.** The patient is a transvestite because he wears the articles of a woman's clothing in order to achieve sexual excitement.

[58.2] **B.** The presence of multiple paraphilias is a poor prognosis indicator.

[58.3] **C.** Fetishism, as do all paraphilias, occurs much more frequently in men.

[58.4] **C.** An erection on awakening is good evidence of a nonorganic etiology.

CLINICAL PEARLS

❖ Fetishists rarely seek treatment and are usually very treatment-resistant.

❖ The presence of one paraphilia should prompt the clinician to inquire about other paraphilias.

❖ Erectile dysfunction is a common disorder in men and has primary, acquired, organic and nonorganic causes. Waking up with an erection is good evidence of a nonorganic etiology.

❖ Vaginismus is an involuntary contraction of vaginal musculature that prevents intercourse; it is best treated with behavioral therapy.

REFERENCES

Feierman JR, Feierman LA. Paraphilias. In: Szuchman LT, Muscarella F, eds. Psychological perspectives on human sexuality. New York: Wiley, 2000:480–484.

Meyer JK. Paraphilias. In: Sadock BJ, Sadock VA, eds. Kaplan and Sadock's comprehensive textbook of psychiatry, 7th ed. Philadelphia: Lippincott Williams & Wilkins, 2000:942–945.

CASE 59

A 26-year-old student is brought to the emergency department after throwing a punch at his best friend in the home they share. The patient states that he must return home to study for his upcoming examinations and quickly becomes angry and belligerent with staff members when they refuse to let him leave. He claims that he has been studying "like a fiend" for the past 3 weeks and has been using some pills given to him by a friend to help him stay awake. The patient's best friend reports that the patient has not slept in days, and he has lost at least 10 lb because he eats only rarely. The patient has no medical or psychiatric problems that the friend is aware of. According to the friend, he was "his normal self until he started taking those pills."

On a physical examination, the patient is found to have a blood pressure of 140/94 mm Hg and a pulse rate of 100/min. His pupils are constricted, he is sweaty, and he has a fine tremor in both hands. The results of the rest of the physical examination are normal, although the patient is uncooperative. On a mental status examination, the patient is seen to be alert and oriented to person, place, and time. He is belligerent and uncooperative, and his speech is rapid and loud. He describes his mood as "just great," but his affect is angry. He denies suicidal or homicidal ideation. He claims to occasionally hear voices tell him about what he is doing and worries that people are staring at him too much.

- **What is most likely diagnosis for this patient?**

- **What is the best diagnostic test?**

ANSWERS TO CASE 59: Amphetamine Intoxication

Summary: A 26-year-old man is brought to the emergency department after becoming physically aggressive with his best friend. He is belligerent, angry, and mildly psychotic. According to the patient and his roommate, he has been taking pills to help him stay alert so that he can study for a series of upcoming examinations. The patient has not been sleeping or eating well, resulting in a weight loss of approximately 10 lb. The patient has no medical or psychiatric history. In the emergency department, he is oriented but belligerent and uncooperative. He states that his mood is fine, although he appears angry. The patient's physical examination shows hypertension and tachycardia, as well as constricted pupils, diaphoresis, and a fine bilateral tremor in his hands.

- **Most likely diagnosis:** Amphetamine intoxication
- **Diagnostic test:** A urine toxicology screening for amphetamines to verify the suspected diagnosis

Analysis

Objectives

1. Recognize amphetamine intoxication in a patient (see diagnostic criteria in Table 59–1).
2. Understand what laboratory tests can be used to confirm this diagnosis.
3. Be aware of the psychological and physical sequelae that can occur as a patient recovers from amphetamine intoxication.

Considerations

This patient has a history of taking pills given to him by a friend to help him stay awake and study. After using these pills consistently for several weeks, he

Table 59–1
DIAGNOSTIC CRITERIA FOR AMPHETAMINE INTOXICATION

1. Recent use of amphetamine or a related substance (e.g., methylphenidate)
2. Clinically significant maladaptive behavioral or psychological changes that developed during or shortly after use of the amphetamine or related substance.
3. Two or more symptoms develop during or shortly after use of the amphetamine or related substance such as a change in heart rate, dilation of pupils, a change in blood pressure, perspiration, chills, nausea or vomiting, weight loss, muscular weakness, respiratory depression, chest pain, arrhythmias, confusion, seizures, dyskinesia, dystonia, or coma.
4. The symptoms are not caused by another medical condition, including another mental disorder.

becomes belligerent and physically violent with a friend. The friend notes that the patient has not been sleeping or eating. His pulse rate and blood pressure are elevated, his pupils are constricted, he is sweaty, and he has a fine tremor in both hands. The patient denies any other psychiatric illnesses and displays psychotic symptoms, making the diagnosis of substance intoxication likely. If the patient stops taking the pills, what will happen? He will probably "crash," with resulting dysphoria, fatigue, psychomotor slowing, an increased appetite, and a need for sleep. But, unlike schizophrenia, his psychosis will likely resolve after discontinuing the amphetamine.

APPROACH TO AMPHETAMINE INTOXICATION

Definitions

Dyskinesias: Abnormal movements

Dystonias: Abnormal contracture of muscle or muscle groups; typically transient but can be life-threatening if the muscles used in breathing are involved

Clinical Approach

Amphetamines were first synthesized to treat medical and mental disorders but have been widely abused. Currently, they are approved for use in attention-deficit/hyperactivity disorder, narcolepsy, and depressive disorders. The classic amphetamines, Dexedrine (dextroamphetamine), Desoxyn (methamphetamine, "crystal meth"), and Ritalin (methylphenidate), affect the dopamine system. Designer amphetamines have both dopaminergic and serotoninergic effects and can cause hallucinations. They include Ecstasy, Eve, and Serenity Tranquility Peace (STP). Amphetamines are quickly absorbed orally, although the illicit varieties are often injected intravenously or smoked. The neurobiochemical response depends on the specific receptor activated; **adrenergic hyperactivity (dilated pupils, elevated blood pressure, weight loss, confusion or seizures) with or without hallucinations** is common. Additionally, they have central acting effects in several areas of the brain, including the orbitofrontal cortex, dorsolateral prefrontal cortex, and amygdala. Tolerance and habituation occur, although to a lesser degree than with cocaine. **Withdrawal symptoms** include **anxiety, tremors, lethargy, fatigue, nightmares, headache, and extreme hunger.**

Differential Diagnosis

Other psychoactive substances can cause behavioral abnormalities; therefore, amphetamine-induced psychotic disorder, cocaine intoxication, hallucinogen intoxication, and phencyclidine intoxication must be ruled out prior to making this diagnosis. Urine toxicology screening can establish the diagnosis if the patient is unable to give a coherent history of which substance has been used. Psychosis related to amphetamine intoxication can be distinguished from schizophrenia best by history, with no premorbid negative symptoms of schizophrenia such as anhedonia, and flat affect.

Treatment

The treatment of amphetamine intoxication is generally supportive, with the elapse of time being the most useful element, because the amphetamine is cleared through the system. The resulting collapse of the patient, with dysphoria, excessive sleepiness, fatigue, and increased appetite, are also time-limited and do not need treatment unless the depressed mood is severe. In this case, an antidepressant can be considered if it does not clear within several weeks. Emergency treatment of amphetamine intoxication can include the use of antipsychotic agents and/or restraints if the psychosis is severe and violent behavior is present. Hospitalization can be necessary if delusions or paranoia are present, and patients are a danger to themselves or others.

Comprehension Questions

[59.1] What factors associated with this case should make the clinician suspicious of amphetamine intoxication?

A. Anorexia, hypotension, pupillary constriction
B. Anorexia, diaphoresis, pupillary dilation
C. Anorexia, hypotension, bradycardia
D. Hyperphagia, hypertension, tachycardia
E. Hyperphagia, hypotension, tachycardia

[59.2] Which of the following tests is required to make a diagnosis of amphetamine intoxication?

A. Blood pressure
B. Electrocardiogram
C. Pulse rate
D. Urine toxicology screening
E. Weighing (for evidence of weight loss)

[59.3] Which of the following is an emergency manifestation of amphetamine intoxication requiring immediate intervention?

A. Sedation
B. Diaphoresis
C. Violence
D. Confabulation
E. Cerebellar ataxia

[59.4] Which centrally acting neurochemical system is most likely implicated in the psychotic symptoms seen with amphetamine intoxication?

A. Dopamine
B. Serotonin
C. Norepinephrine
D. Histamine
E. Cholinergic

Answers

[59.1] **B.** Symptoms of amphetamine intoxication include anorexia, tachycardia, hypertension, pupillary dilation, and diaphoresis.

[59.2] **D.** The best indication that the symptoms are caused by an amphetamine is to document its presence with a urine toxicology screening.

[59.3] **C.** Violence requires immediate attention. Other emergency manifestations can include delusions, paranoia, anxiety, and delirium.

[59.4] **A.** The dopamine system is most often sited as a central focus for psychotic symptoms.

CLINICAL PEARLS

❖ Urine toxicology screening is the definitive test in making a diagnosis of amphetamine intoxication.

❖ The symptoms should resolve once the amphetamine has been eliminated from the body.

REFERENCES

Ebert M, Loosen P, Nurcombe B, eds. Current diagnosis and treatment in psychiatry. New York: McGraw-Hill, 2000:246.

Kaplan H, Sadock B. Synopsis of psychiatry, 9th ed. Baltimore: Lippincott Williams & Wilkins, 2003:407–412.

❖ CASE 60

A 23-year-old woman is admitted to the inpatient psychiatric unit after slashing both wrists when her therapist left for a week's vacation. The cuts were superficial and did not require stitches. The patient says that she is angry with her psychiatrist for "abandoning her." She claims that she is often depressed, although the depressions last "only a couple of hours." When she was first admitted to the hospital, she told the admitting psychiatrist that she heard a voice telling her that "she will never amount to anything," but she subsequently denies having heard the voice. This is the patient's fourth hospital admission, and all of them have been precipitated by someone in her life leaving. After 3 days in the unit, the patient's psychiatry resident gets into an argument with the nursing staff. He says that the patient has been behaving very well, responding to his therapy, and is deserving of a pass. The nurses claim that the patient has not been following unit rules, sleeping through her group meetings, and ignoring the limits set. Both parties go to the unit director complaining about the other.

◆ **What is the most likely diagnosis?**

◆ **What defense mechanism is being employed by the patient?**

◆ **What should the hospital staff do next?**

ANSWERS TO CASE 60: Borderline Personality Disorder

Summary: A 23-year-old woman is admitted to the psychiatric unit after she superficially lacerates her wrists because she feels she was abandoned by her therapist. She was admitted on previous occasions on which she also claimed she was "abandoned." She admits to having a depressed mood that varies by the hour. On admission, she claimed that she heard a voice speaking to her, although she currently denies it. She seems to be at the center of a disagreement between the psychiatric resident and the nursing staff, who have conflicting views of her behavior in the unit.

- **Most likely diagnosis:** Borderline personality disorder (BPD).
- **Defense mechanism used:** Splitting.
- **Next step for hospital staff:** The unit director should mediate a meeting between the psychiatric resident and the staff, at which time he or she should point out that splitting is occurring. The patient should be brought to the meeting, and everyone involved should discuss whether or not she is ready for a pass.

Analysis

Objectives

1. Recognize the defense mechanism of splitting, which is commonly employed by patients with BPD.
2. Understand treatment strategies to contain splitting in an inpatient unit.

Considerations

This young woman displays several classic signs of BPD, including frantic efforts to avoid abandonment, impulsive behavior, suicidal behavior, and transient psychosis. She also uses the defense mechanism of splitting, during which she "sits calmly on the sidelines" while her treatment team splits in half over whether or not she should be allowed to go on a pass. (Each side sees very different patient behavior and reports it, believing that the other side must be misrepresenting the patient's actions because the observations on each side are so completely different.)

APPROACH TO BORDERLINE PERSONALITY DISORDER

Definitions

Countertransference: A set of expectations, beliefs, and emotional responses induced in the physician (often unconsciously) through interactions with a particular patient. For example, a patient comes to a physician and is denigrating and hostile at every interaction. The physician develops a negative countertransference to the patient and finds himself avoiding the patient and forgetting their appointments.

Defense mechanisms: A psychodynamic term which defines various means by which an individual might use to psychologically cope with a difficult situation. These defense mechanisms range from relatively mature ones such as humor to quite immature ones such as often seen with BPD. These might include mechanisms such as devaluation, idealization, projection, projective identification, and splitting.

Dialectical behavioral therapy: A type of cognitive therapy specifically designed to help manage difficult BPD patients. Through individual relationships with a therapist, patients learn skills to confront and manage the volatile emotions and impulses they are feeling.

Clinical Approach

Patients with BPD demonstrate a pervasive instability of mood, interpersonal relationships, and self-image. They are often chronically depressed and are markedly impulsive. Psychosis, including paranoid ideation, can be seen transiently under stress. Patients make frantic efforts to avoid real or perceived abandonment because they have chronic feelings of emptiness. Suicidal behavior, gestures, or threats are common.

Differential Diagnosis

Patients with **BPD can become psychotic,** but these episodes are **generally transient.** There is generally no thought disorder or other signs of schizophrenia, which helps rule out this diagnosis. Patients with paranoid personality disorder **can show paranoid ideation** as well, but these symptoms are generally long-lasting and pervasive. Patients with BPD can appear depressed and have vegetative symptoms—if they do, overlaying their pervasive behavioral patterns, a major depression can be diagnosed. As such, disorders such as impulse control disorders, substance abuse disorders, eating disorders, and sexual/identity disorders can also coexist. These diagnoses must occur as additional signs and symptoms on top of those that fulfill the BPD diagnosis for two (or more) disorders to be diagnosed.

Interviewing Tips

These patients are often extremely difficult to work with, as they have a peculiar ability to "get under the skin" of the clinician (induce countertransference). Give patients clear, nontechnical answers. Do not encourage the patient to idealize you or other members of the treatment team. Strike a balance that is not too close, but not avoidant or punitive. Set limits early and often on what behavior is acceptable.

Comprehension Questions

[60.1] A 24-year-old woman with BPD is admitted to a psychiatric hospital because of suicidal ideation. The physician on call tells the patient about all the rules and regulations in the unit and that "Although it is a great place to get better, it is a lot of work" Which of the following is this physician attempting to do with this patient?

A. Dissuade the patient from signing in voluntarily
B. Discourage the patient from splitting
C. Decrease idealization of the unit and the hospitalization
D. Encourage the patient to seek admission elsewhere
E. Investigate the patient's motivation for desiring admission

[60.2] Which of the following defense mechanisms is commonly associated with BPD?

A. Splitting
B. Sublimation
C. Intellectualization
D. Undoing
E. Altruism

[60.3] A 24-year-old woman is seen in the emergency department after superficially cutting both her wrists. Her explanation is that she was upset because her boyfriend of 3 weeks just broke up with her. When asked about other relationships, she says that she has had numerous sexual partners, both male and female, but none of them lasted more than several weeks. Which type of psychotherapy might she be most likely to respond to?

A. Psychopharmacotherapy
B. Parent assertiveness training
C. Interpersonal psychotherapy
D. Dialectical behavioral therapy
E. Supportive psychotherapy

[60.4] A 22-year-old man with BPD loses his job at a local restaurant, the first job he held for longer than a month. His mother dies suddenly 3 weeks later. One month after his mother's death, the patient tells his therapist, whom he has been seeing once a week, that he has trouble sleeping and wakes up at 3 AM and is unable to go back to sleep. He lost 13 lb in 5 weeks without trying to do so. He reports low energy and a decreased interest in his usual hobbies. He states that he feels depressed but then grins and says, "But I'm always depressed, aren't I?" Based on his history, which of the following should the clinician do next?

A. Start treating the patient with a mood stabilizer such as carbamazepine
B. Hospitalize the patient
C. Begin seeing the patient for daily psychotherapy
D. Start treating the patient with an antidepressant such as paroxetine
E. Ask the patient keep a sleep log

Answers

[60.1] **C.** Decreasing idealization of the unit before admission will help decrease the devaluation that inevitably follows as well.

[60.2] **A.** Individuals with BPD often use the defense mechanism of splitting.

[60.3] **D.** Dialectical behavioral therapy is a form of cognitive therapy shown through controlled studies to be effective in treating BPD.

[60.4] **D.** Comorbidity of major depression with BPD is quite common. When vegetative symptoms or other qualitative changes occur, medication for the major depression is necessary.

CLINICAL PEARLS

❖ Patients with BPD show a pervasive pattern of unstable personal relationships, self-images, and emotions. They can often be markedly impulsive, displaying sexual acting out, suicidal gestures, and substance abuse.

❖ Physicians need to set limits early and often with these patients. They need to be firm but not punitive. They must keep a constant eye on their own countertransference to these patients, as they can be extremely difficult to work with.

❖ Although patients with this disorder can become psychotic, it is transient, and they do not have signs of a thought disorder or other signs of schizophrenia.

❖ These patients can have other coexisting disorders such as eating disorders, major depression, and substance abuse. The specifics of each must be teased out of the multiple signs and symptoms presented by patients with BPD.

❖ Defense mechanisms used by these patients include splitting, projection, projective identification, devaluation, idealization, distortion, and acting out.

REFERENCES

Ebert M, Loosen P, Nurcombe B, eds. Current diagnosis and treatment in psychiatry. New York: McGraw-Hill, 2000:475–477.

Kaplan H, Sadock B. Synopsis of psychiatry, 9th ed. Baltimore: Lippincott Williams & Wilkins, 2003.

Linehan M. Cognitive-behavioral treatment of borderline personality disorder. New York: Guilford Press, 1993:45–49.

SECTION IV

Listing of Cases

LISTING BY CASE NUMBER

LISTING BY DISORDER (ALPHABETICAL)

LISTING BY *DSM-IV* CATEGORIES

GENERAL CATEGORY	CASE DESCRIPTION	CASE NO.	CASE PAGE
	Mood disorder not otherwise specified	39	312
	Bipolar disorder (child)	5	82
	Bipolar disorder, manic (adult)	12	130
	Hypothyroidism with depression	4	74
	Substance-induced mood disorder	50	378
Anxiety disorders	Panic disorder versus thyroid medication overuse	3	64
	Social phobia	8	106
	Obsessive-compulsive disorder (child)	13	138
	Posttraumatic stress disorder	21	192
	Acute stress disorder	30	256
	Generalized anxiety disorder	11	124
	Anxiety disorder caused by asthma	43	336
	neurosis	51	384
Somatoform disorders	Somatization disorder	38	306
	Conversion disorder	57	422
	Pain disorder	32	268
	Hypochondriasis	24	214
Factitious disorders	Factitious disorder	35	286
Dissociative disorder	Dissociative fugue	49	372
Sexual and gender identity disorders	Fetishism	58	428
	Gender identity disorder	53	396
Eating disorders	Anorexia nervosa	44	342
	Bulimia nervosa	29	248
Sleep disorders	Primary insomnia	37	300
	Sleep terror disorder	36	292
Adjustment disorders	Adjustment disorder	34	280
Personality disorders	Paranoid personality disorder	54	402
	Schizoid personality disorder	6	90

GENERAL CATEGORY	CASE DESCRIPTION	CASE NO.	CASE PAGE
	Schizotypal personality disorder	15	152
	Antisocial personality disorder	25	222
	Borderline personality disorder	60	440
	Histrionic personality disorder	33	274
	Narcissistic personality disorder	41	324
	Avoidant personality disorder	47	360
	Dependent personality disorder	10	118
	Obsessive-compulsive personality disorder	20	184
Additional conditions	Malingering	45	348

❖ INDEX

Note: Page numbers followed by *f* or *t* indicate figures or tables, respectively.

B

D